The Nature of
General Family Practice

The Nature of General Family Practice

583 clinical vignettes in family medicine

An alternative approach to syllabus development

Edited by

W. E. Fabb & J. R. Marshall

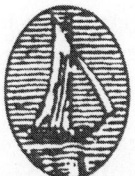

GEORGE A. BOGDEN & SON, INC., PUBLISHERS

45 HUDSON STREET, RIDGEWOOD, NEW JERSEY 07450

Published in USA and Canada by
George A. Bogden & Son, Inc.
45 Hudson Street
Ridgewood,
New Jersey 07450

Published in UK by
MTP Press Limited
Falcon House
Lancaster, England

First published 1983

ISBN-13:978-94-009-6597-3   e-ISBN-13:978-94-009-6595-9
DOI: 10.1007/978-94-009-6595-9

Contents

CONTENTS

Preface

The idea of producing this book of case histories from general family practice was only a twinkle in the editors' eyes until October 1980, when in a room in the Marriott Hotel in New Orleans, the editors met with John Fry, Joseph Levenstein and Bill Jackson to discuss new book projects. The idea was put to the group, which endorsed it enthusiastically. Encouraged by this and by John Fry's advice, the conception of *The Nature of General Family Practice* took place.

It was agreed that to illustrate the universal nature of general family practice it would be useful to collect case histories from all around the world, that for preference they should be brief, and that they should be accompanied by major questions and sub-questions, but no answers. The name 'Vignettes' was applied to these cases and their questions.

Subsequently, well over a hundred family physicians were asked by letter to provide ten vignettes. Sixty doctors from ten countries accepted the invitation and forwarded their contributions during the second half of 1981. Almost all of those who, for a variety of reasons were unable to contribute, said they liked the idea and looked forward to using the final product. Altogether, over 600 vignettes were received, and 583 selected for final inclusion.

In order to preserve the flavour of the cases, the editors have made as few changes as were necessary to comply with the format of presentation. The cases represent each contributor's own words, own expressions and own ways of telling a story. They give a feeling for the doctor and the way he or she thinks and feels.

The gestation of this book has been a long one, but the baby looks to be in good shape. Whether it will be an only child, will depend on how people like the look of this one.

W. E. Fabb,
J. R. Marshall,
Melbourne,
1983

Acknowledgements

The editors wish to place on record their deep appreciation of the efforts of all of those who contributed to this book. Their contributions are acknowledged throughout the book and they are listed in the contributors' pages. Without their support, this book could not have been created. They have given it a truly international flavour. The addresses of the contributors have been provided in the contributors' pages should any reader wish to correspond with them about any of their cases.

We also wish to acknowledge the painstaking way in which Mrs. Judith White and Mrs. Julie Rodman have prepared the manuscript, and the support given by Nadia Gottardo during its final preparation.

To our families, who wondered why the gestation of this book was taking so long and whether it would ever be delivered, we can only say – thank you for your patience.

W. E. Fabb,
J. R. Marshall,
Melbourne,
1983

Contributors

Loren H. Amundson MD Diplomate ABFP Fellow AAFP
Professor of Family Medicine, University of South Dakota School of Medicine, Associate Director, Sioux Falls Family Practice Residency Program
3001 South Holly Avenue, Sioux Falls, SD 57105, USA

Gary Beazley MD CCFP FCFP
Professor and Head, Department of Family Medicine, University of Manitoba
Room E6003, 409 Tache Avenue, Winnipeg, Manitoba, Canada R2H 2A6

Patricia E. Boiko BA Chemistry MD
Third year Resident, Family Medicine Department of Family Practice, Medical University of South Carolina, 171 Ashley Avenue, Charleston, SC 29425, USA

Tommy Bouchier Hayes FRCGP DRCOG
Lieutenant Colonel, British Army
The Hospital, RMA Sandhurst, Camberley, Surrey GU15 4PH, UK

Dennis Gerard Chambers MB ChB (Edin) LRCP LRCS LRFP & S FRACGP
General Practitioner
45 Farrell Flat Road, Clare, South Australia 5453, Australia

Brian H. Connor MB BS FRACGP DCH DObst RCOG DRACOG
General Practitioner
145 Faulkner Street, Armidale, New South Wales 2350, Australia

Zelda Cramer MB ChB
General Practitioner
Department of Family Medicine, Sackler School of Medicine, Tel Aviv University, Israel

Gurna Margaret Dick MB BCh BAO FRACGP
General Practitioner
32 Augusta Road, Lenah Valley, Hobart, Tasmania 7008, Australia

Edward Domovitch MD CCFP
Assistant Professor, Department of Family and Community Medicine, University of Toronto
Wellesley Hospital, Family Practice Unit, 146 Wellesley Street East, Toronto, Ontario, Canada M4Y 1J2

Charles Driscoll MD
Family Physician
Department of Family Practice, The University of Iowa Hospitals and Clinics, The University of Iowa, Iowa City, IA 52242, USA

Earl V. Dunn MD CM
Professor, Department of Family and Community Medicine, University of Toronto
2075 Bayview Avenue, Toronto, Canada M4N 3M5

Wesley E. Fabb MB BS FRACGP FCGPS (Hon) FFGP (SA) (Hon) MCFPC (Hon)
National Director, Family Medicine Programme, Royal Australian College of General Practitioners
70 Jolimont Street, Jolimont, Victoria 3002, Australia

Fred B. Fallis BA MD CCFP FCFP
Director of Continuing Education, Faculty of Medicine, University of Toronto
Fitzgerald Building, Toronto, Canada

Boris Michael (Boz) Fehler MB BCh (Wits.) DCH (RCPS) London MFGP (SA) FRCGP (UK)
President, South African Academy of
Family Practice/Primary Care
P.O. Box 52523, Saxonwold,
2132 Johannesburg, South Africa

Paul Freeling MB BS FRCGP
Head of Sub-Department of
General Practice, St. George's Hospital
Medical School
Cranmer Terrace, Tooting,
London SW17 0RE, UK

John Fry OBE MD FRCS FRCGP
General Practitioner
138 Croydon Road, Beckenham, Kent
BR3 4DG, England, UK

Eric Gambrill MB BS FRCGP DObst RCOG
General Practitioner, Associate Adviser in
General Practice, British Postgraduate
Medical Federation
"Leacroft", Ifield Road, Crawley, Sussex,
England, UK

David A. Game, AO MB BS (Adelaide) FRACGP
General Practitioner
50 Lambert Road, Royston Park,
South Australia 5070, Australia

Peter Leon Gibson, MB ChB (NZ) FRNZCGP
Censor-in-Chief, Royal New Zealand
College of General Practitioners,
Regional Co-ordinator, New Zealand
Family Medicine Training Programme
3 Riverlea Avenue, Pakuranga, Auckland,
New Zealand

Peter Francis Gill MB BS (Melb) MD FRACGP
General Practitioner
67 Hopkins Street, Moonah, Tasmania
7009, Australia

William Francis Glastonbury MB BS FRACGP
General Practitioner
103 Tusmore Avenue, Tusmore,
South Australia 5065, Australia

John Grabinar MB BCh MRCGP
General Practitioner
80 Torridon Road, London SE6 1RB, UK

Peter Grantham BA MD CCFP FCFP
Royal Canadian Legion Professor and
Head, Department of Family Practice,
University of British Columbia
Mather Building, Vancouver,
Canada V6T 1W5

John C. Hasler MB BS DA DCH FRCGP
General Practitioner and Regional
Organiser for General Practice Training,
Oxford Region, UK
Sonning Common Health Centre,
Wood Lane, Sonning Common,
Reading RG4 9SW, England, UK

Michael William Heffernan MB BS FRACGP DObst RCOG MEd
Director of Research, Family Medicine
Programme, Royal Australian College
of General Practitioners
70 Jolimont Street, Jolimont, Victoria 3002,
Australia

Albert Himmelhoch MB BS FRACGP FRCGP
Director of Medical Services,
Hornsby & Ku-ring-gai Hospital
Palmerston Road, Hornsby,
New South Wales 2077, Australia

William D. Jackson MB BS FRACGP
Past President, Royal Australian College
of General Practitioners
Kings Lane, St. Leonards, Tasmania 7250,
Australia

Douglas H. Johnson MD CCFP FCFP
Professor and Head, Department of
Family and Community Medicine,
Sunnybrook, University of Toronto
Sunnybrook Medical Centre, 2075 Bayview
Avenue, Toronto M4N 3M5, Canada

James D. E. Knox MD FRCGP FRCP Ed
Professor of General Practice,
Department of General Practice,
University of Dundee
Westgate Health Centre, Charleston Drive,
Dundee DD2 4AD, Scotland, UK

Campbell Thompson Lamont MD CCFP Dipl ABFP
Professor, Department of Family Medicine,
University of Ottawa
Family Medicine Centre, 175 Bruyere
Street, Ottawa, Ontario, Canada

CONTRIBUTORS

Joseph Henry Levenstein MB ChB MFGP (SA)
Head, Department of General Practice,
University of Cape Town
163 Koeberg Road, Brooklyn,
Cape Town 7405, South Africa

Stanley Levenstein BSc MB ChB MFGP (SA)
General Practitioner
163 Koeberg Road, Brooklyn,
Cape Town 7405, South Africa

Dennis Levet MB ChB (Cape Town) FRACGP
General Practitioner
762 Sandy Bay Road, Sandy Bay, Hobart,
Tasmania 7005, Australia

Mary Deirdre Mahoney MB BS (Qld) FRACGP
State Director, Family Medicine
Programme, Royal Australian College of
General Practitioners
14 Cribb Street, Milton, Brisbane,
Queensland 4064, Australia

Frank Mansfield MA MB B(Chir) MRCP DObst RCOG FRACGP
General Practitioner
Lot 39, Edward Road, Lesmurdie,
Western Australia 6076, Australia

T. Dion Manthorpe MB BS FRACGP MRACGP
General Practitioner
PO Box 692, Port Lincoln, South Australia
5606, Australia

John Robinson Marshall MB BCh FRACGP
Director of Educational Research and
Resource Development, Family Medicine
Programme, Royal Australian College of
General Practitioners
15 Gover Street, North Adelaide,
South Australia 5006, Australia

Roland M. Meyer MB BCh (Wits.) MFGP (SA)
General Practitioner
1206 Lister Buildings, 195 Jeppe Street,
Johannesburg 2001, South Africa

Carl A. Moore BA MD CCFP FCFP
Professor and Chairman,
Department of Family Medicine,
McMaster Faculty of Health Sciences
1200 Main Street West, Hamilton,
Ontario L8N 3Z5, Canada

R. T. Mossop MB ChB FCGP (Zimb)
Senior Lecturer (General Practice),
Department of Community Medicine,
Godfrey Huggins School of Medicine,
University of Zimbabwe
Box A178, Avondale, Zimbabwe

Alistair John Moulds MB ChB MRCGP DObst RCOG
General Practitioner, Trainer
Laindon Health Centre, Basildon, Essex,
England, UK

David S. Muecke MB BS FRACGP
General Practitioner
"Woodlawn", 6 View Road, Walkerville,
South Australia 5081, Australia

John Edward Murtagh BSc BEd MB BS FRACGP DObst RCOG
Senior Lecturer in Community Practice,
Monash University
Community Practice Teaching Unit,
867 Centre Road, East Bentleigh,
Victoria 3165, Australia

E. John H. North MB BS FRACGP
State Director, Family Medicine
Programme, Royal Australian College of
General Practitioners
"Trawalla", 22 Lascelles Avenue, Toorak,
Victoria 3142, Australia

Kenneth C. Nyman MB BS FRACGP MRCS (Eng) LRCP (Lond) DObst RCOG
General Practitioner/part-time
Senior Lecturer
7A The Rise, Drabble Road, City Beach,
Western Australia 6015, Australia

Warren Lambert Ogborne MB BS MRCP (Edin) FRACGP
Medical Educator, Family Medicine
Programme, Royal Australian College of
General Practitioners
"Bagworthy", 31A Carrington Road,
Wahroonga, New South Wales 2076,
Australia

Daryl S. Pedler MB BS DObst RCOG FRACGP
State Director, Family Medicine
Programme, Royal Australian College of
General Practitioners
15 Gover Street, North Adelaide,
South Australia 5006, Australia

Reg. L. Perkin MD CCFP FCFP FRCGP (Hon)
Professor, Department of Family
  and Community Medicine,
  University of Toronto
Family Practice Unit,
751 Dundas Street West,
Toronto, Ontario M6J 1T9, Canada

Max R. Polliack MBChB MPH MRCGP
Professor and Chairman,
  Department of Family Medicine,
  Sackler School of Medicine
Tel Aviv University, Israel

Anthony James Radford MB BS SM FRACP FRCP (Ed) FRACGP FFCM MRCP (Lond) DTM & H
Foundation Professor of Primary Care and
  Community Medicine, The Flinders
  University of South Australia
Flinders Medical Centre, Bedford Park,
South Australia 5042, Australia

A.L.A. (Sandy) Reid MB BS FRACGP
Fellow in Community Medicine, Faculty of
  Medicine, University of Newcastle
Newcastle, New South Wales 2308,
Australia

John Richards MB ChB FRNZCGP FRACGP FRCPE
Associate Professor of General Practice,
  Division of General Practice,
  Department of Community Health
School of Medicine, Private Bag, Auckland,
New Zealand

R. W. (Dick) Roberts MB BS (Melb) FRACGP DCH
Rural General Practitioner
Martin Street, Ravensthorpe,
Western Australia 6346, Australia

Walter W. Rosser MD CCFPC FCFPC
Professor and Chairman Department of
  Family Medicine, University of Ottawa
  School of Medicine
210 Melrose Avenue, Ottawa, Ontario
K1Y 4K7 Canada

J. G. P. Ryan BSc MB BS (Qld) FRACGP
Professor of Community Practice,
  University of Queensland
Medical School, Herston Road, Herston,
Queensland 4006, Australia

John K. Shearman MB CCFP
Associate Professor,
  Department of Family Medicine,
  2V3 McMaster University Medical Center
1200 Main Street West, Hamilton,
Ontario L8N 3Z5, Canada

Denis Shepherd MB BS (Melb) FRACGP FRSH
Senior Lecturer, Department of Community
  Health, University of Melbourne
243 Grattan Street, Carlton, Victoria 3053,
Australia

John Stevens MB BS DObst RCOG FRACGP
General Practitioner
6 Patrick Street, Ulverstone, Tasmania
7315, Australia

Roger Peter Strasser MB BS BMedSc DRACOG
Former Co-State Director, Family Medicine
  Programme, Royal Australian College of
  General Practitioners
2A Boongarry Avenue, Blackburn, Victoria
3130, Australia

A. George Strube MB BChir MRCP (Lond) DObst RCOG
General Practitioner
33 Goffs Park Road, Southgate, Crawley,
Sussex, England, UK

Gillian Strube MB BS DCH
General Practitioner
33 Goffs Park Road, Southgate, Crawley,
Sussex, England, UK

Frank E. H. Tan MB BS (HK) DObst RCOG (Lond) MCGP (Mal)
Examiner, College of General Practitioners
  Malaysia
Kumpulan Medic, 176 Jalan Tunku Abdul
Rahman, Kuala Lumpur, Malaysia

Howard C. Watts MB BS FRACGP DObst RCOG
General Practitioner
8 Canning Road, Kalamunda,
Western Australia 6076, Australia

Karl F. Weyrauch MD
Resident in Family Medicine
Department of Family Medicine,
Medical University of South Carolina,
Charleston, SC 29425, USA

CONTRIBUTORS

Glenys O. Williams MB BCh
Assistant Professor, Department of Family
  Practice, University of Iowa
Iowa City, IA 52240, USA

Natalis C. L. Yuen MB BS DTM & H FICS
Vice-President, Hong Kong College of
  General Practitioners, 1980–1982
22A Junction Road, G/F, Kowloon,
Hong Kong

Introduction

Defining the discipline of family medicine has been a difficult task. Difficult for those within the discipline to describe; even more difficult for those outside the discipline to understand. Many excellent texts are now available from all around the world which describe the concepts of family medicine and the principles and practice of the discipline. By taking an academic approach, they have filled many of the gaps in our understanding of the discipline and how it is practised. There are other ways, however, of describing a discipline. This book exemplifies an alternative approach: describing the discipline through illustrative case histories and the questions they invite.

The Nature of General Family Practice is a collection of almost 600 cases which have presented to general practitioners/family physicians in ten countries around the world. In their own unique way, these cases describe what family medicine is all about. In a sense, they constitute a syllabus for family medicine. Anyone who works through these cases, studying them and answering the numerous accompanying questions, will have gained insight into most of the conditions seen in general family practice. There are some gaps; maybe a second volume will fill them.

The book has been prepared for all who are interested or involved in general family practice, but especially for teachers, vocational trainees and undergraduates. It is believed that the case histories and their questions will provide interesting material for group discussion and personal study. Answering the questions will require the use of a wide range of educational resources, both human and material.

In preparing the material, the editors decided that only the cases and the questions they invite should be published. No answers are supplied, although in some of the sub-questions, the diagnosis or management is hinted at. For some questions, several alternative answers may be appropriate; for some there may be no 'correct answer' at all.

The structure of the book

The book is divided into two sections. The first contains the numbered case histories, followed by several major questions which invite answers. Usually no hint is given in these questions about the nature of the problem and its management; this is for the reader to determine. In the second part of the book, the case number, the patient's identifying initials, age, and where appropriate, occupation, are repeated, together with the major questions, under each of which is listed a series of more detailed sub-questions. In many of these the nature of the problem and its management may be indicated, sometimes directly, sometimes less obviously. The reader will benefit most by tackling these sub-questions *after* answering the major questions. Both types of question have their particular function: the major questions are general and require a broad comprehensive approach; the sub-questions are more detailed and require a more specific approach.

The book has been compiled in 26 chapters, which break the material into manageable groups of cases. In selecting the cases for each chapter, it was recognized that some cases could have been placed in one of several chapters; the editors chose the chapter into which each such case seemed to them to fit most comfortably. Cases have been grouped to show that like presentations may result from very different conditions and that like conditions may present in different ways and require different management.

A comprehensive index is provided to allow access to cases categorized in a number of other ways. By using the index, a series of illustrative cases of a condition, problem or process can be selected with ease. It will be noted that the index pays attention to the *process* of general family practice, as well as the content. Numerous references are made to such processes as the doctor–patient relationship, consulting skills, psychotherapy, counselling, patient education, preventive care, health education, health promotion, and many others. The important *concepts* of family medicine too are indexed for ready reference to illustrative cases: concepts such as 'the child as the presenting symptom of the parent', the ' "While I'm here" syndrome', the 'collusion of anonymity', and so on.

Uses for the book

Teachers will find the cases useful in group discussion. One way of using them would be to distribute a case and its major questions in advance, inviting a response, and then after group discussion of the responses, to introduce the sub-questions for discussion. Alternatively, the material could be introduced for the first time during group discussion. The material will be most useful if used flexibly; teachers are invited to modify the cases, major questions and sub-questions to meet their needs and those of their trainees and students. There is a great variety of cases, some simple and straightforward, and some very complex. It should be possible in most instances to select cases of the appropriate complexity for the group concerned.

Individuals will find it useful to select cases in areas in which they have perceived deficiencies and to answer first the major questions, and then the sub-questions. In the process of doing so, specific deficiencies will be exposed, which can be remedied by reference to educational resources such as colleagues, teachers, books, periodicals, audiovisuals, and the like.

It is hoped that this book will also provide armchair reading with a challenge for the practising family physician and send him to his texts and journals for some of the answers.

The editors hope too that it may be used by our specialist colleagues. It would provide an insight into the discipline of family medicine approaching, but admittedly not equalling, that which would result from practising the discipline. We believe it could lead to a better understanding of the discipline of family medicine and the way its practitioners think, feel and act.

The arrangement of the content

The book begins with a cluster of chapters which exemplify some of the fundamental concepts of family medicine. By beginning with 'Why has the patient really come?', 'Problems of living' and 'Family problems', the focus is placed on the interrelationship between the physical, psychological and social factors in health and illness, and on the influence of the family and the environment – home, work and cultural. These chapters examine the concept that patients often initially present with other than the real reason for their coming; that sometimes it is difficult to tell who the patient is – the one presenting, the parent, the spouse, or the whole family; and that sometimes problems of living – poverty, isolation, marital discord, stress at home, work or school – may present as symptoms apparently unrelated to these family and social problems. The family physician needs to be aware of these presentations, sensitive to the cues which signal them, and skilled in the use of strategies to explore and manage the problems they represent. If the reader does nothing more than learn the concepts illustrated in the first three chapters, the book will have been worthwhile.

The next two chapters form a related cluster. Since so much of the family physician's time is spent in patient education, preventive care and routine examination, chapters are devoted to these activities. Patient education and preventive care are closely linked as so much preventive care relies on effective patient education and the compliance of the patient. The doctor needs to be aware of the numerous opportunities which present for patient education and preventive care and to capitalize on these by employing his or her teaching skills. Apart from those illustrated in these chapters, there are hundreds of other examples of opportunities for patient education and preventive care throughout the book.

The next cluster of chapters constitutes life's crises – emergencies, attempted suicide, and dying and death. These are often crises for the doctor as well as the patient. Learning how to cope with them, especially the crisis of dying and death, is one of the most difficult tasks for the trainee family physician. The cases presented will give insight into the nature of these crises and the strategies the family physician uses for dealing with them, professionally and personally.

The next cluster of chapters on contraception and family planning, sexual problems, and problems of pregnancy in a sense also represent some of life's crises. The request for contraception by under-age adolescents, the unwanted pregnancy, the request for termination of pregnancy, the complications of pregnancy, foetal abnormalities and foetal death in utero, and the problem of sexual dysfunction represent crises for the patient, and often for the doctor too. Each needs understanding and empathic handling.

Thereafter follow more traditional chapters on conditions affecting specific areas or on specific symptoms – headaches, fits, faints and funny turns, eye problems, upper respiratory problems (including ENT), breathing problems, chest pain, abdominal problems, genitourinary problems, skin problems, lumps, musculoskeletal problems, and injuries.

The book concludes with chapters on three common general problems – tiredness, weight loss, and iatrogenic illness. These problems challenge the skills of the family physician, as the underlying cause may be difficult to detect and the condition troublesome to manage.

The book is intended to demonstrate that the discipline of family medicine has a distinctive field of action, an identifiable body of knowledge, some of it unique to the discipline, and a unique area for research. The cases in this book show that the uniqueness of family medicine results from the integration of knowledge and skills from many disciplines, including some outside medicine; from the community orientation of its practitioners; from the family-centred approach that family physicians take; but most of all from the person-centred care which they provide continuously: care which considers simultaneously physical, psychological, social and environmental aspects in the definition of health risks and problems, and which integrates the community's promotive, preventive, curative and rehabilitative health resources in their management.

Taken as a whole, the book is a kaleidoscope of general family practice. It gives insight into its nature and thereby the discipline of family medicine. It demonstrates, as well as is possible with words alone, what actually happens out there in the consulting rooms of family physicians, in the homes and workplaces of their patients, and in the hearts and minds of the practitioners. We hope you enjoy this voyage through family medicine.

W. E. Fabb,
J. R. Marshall,
Melbourne,
1983

In the interest of brevity, throughout the rest of this book the masculine pronoun for family physician has been used.

CHAPTER 1

Why has the Patient Really Come?

Often the family physician is faced with the question, 'Why has the patient really come?' The apparent reason somehow seems not to be the real reason — he senses there is something else that brings the patient along. Sometimes he is not sure who the patient really is. Is it the person who presents as the patient, or is it someone else — one of the parents or the whole family? The cases and questions which follow exemplify these dilemmas, explore why patients often present in this way, give insight into how the family physician senses and defines these situations, and suggest strategies for solving the often complex problems which unfold.

1 **MRS. T. AGED 30 HOUSEWIFE**

Mrs. T. had brought her 6 month old baby to see the general practitioner six times in the past 3 weeks. On each occasion the child had a minor physical symptom such as slight rhinorrhoea, slight regurgitation of food, a mild rash, a few loose stools. She also complained that the baby did not sleep well at nights.

On this occasion the baby had a mild napkin dermatitis. The general practitioner recommended treatment for this. After dressing the baby and sitting down again, Mrs. T. said, 'Before I go, doctor, would you please prescribe something for me to sleep at nights?'.

1. Why had Mrs. T. consulted the general practitioner six times in the past 3 weeks with her baby?
2. What were the reasons for the baby's and the mother's insomnia?
3. How should the general practitioner manage this situation?

S. Levenstein, Cape Town

2 **MRS. E.S. AGED 30 HOUSEWIFE**

Mrs. E.S. was formerly a school teacher and had two young children one aged 2 years and an infant aged 4 months, whom she was still breast feeding. She presented complaining that moles on her back had become itchy and she was concerned about malignancy. She had three innocent pigmented naevi on her back with no clinical features to suggest malignancy.

She seemed troubled and asked 'While I'm here, could I have something to help me sleep?' She had trouble getting off to sleep, was disturbed two or three times to breast feed the baby each night as he was a restless baby, and she felt tired out on awakening in the morning. She started to cry, saying she felt depressed and unable to cope. Her libido was non-existent and intercourse was painful. Her husband did not seem to be able to understand her and she felt they were growing apart.

1. What disorder is she suffering from?
2. What is the prognosis of this condition and what are its risks?
3. How would you manage this condition?
4. Why might she have dyspareunia?
5. Does the baby have a sleep disorder? If so, how would you manage it?

H. C. Watts, Perth, Australia

3 **JOHN McALISTER AGED 9 MONTHS**

For the second day in succession Mary McAlister has brought her son John to see you, complaining that he is always crying, won't sleep and won't eat. She says the medicine (sedative) you prescribed didn't help and that John didn't sleep at all again last night. Again, your examination reveals a well baby.

Mary seems very distraught and comments that she is feeling terrible herself and is not sleeping either. Her husband (Bill), who is a metal worker, spends most evenings at the pub with 'the boys'. Since the baby was born Mary feels Bill has lost interest in her. She has no close friends and her mother lives hundreds of kilometres away.

1. Who is the 'patient' in this case?
2. How would you describe 'the problem(s)' in this case?
3. Outline your management of this case.

R. P. Strasser, Melbourne

MRS. A.B.   AGED 34   HOUSEWIFE

4

A continental European immigrant to Australia presents with her 4 month old, healthy looking daughter and a request for an examination of the child to see if she is developing normally. You have never seen her before.

1. What sort of examination would you undertake?
2. Following a normal examination, what sort of questions would be a reasonable follow up?
3. Who is the patient?
4. Closer observation reveals that mother is very tired and anxious. How might you go about further questioning?
5. The mother had had no sleep for almost 2 weeks, awakening at each movement or cough of the child at night for fear of another sudden infant death syndrome (SIDS) which occurred with her first child 9 years ago. Her marriage is becoming strained. What can you offer?

A. J. Radford, Adelaide

MRS. M.L.   AGED 26   HOUSEWIFE

5

Mrs. M.L., aged 26, presented to the doctor for the first time. She had just moved into the neighbourhood. She complained bitterly of pain in her left shoulder. She had seen numerous doctors but they all had been unsuccessful in treating her. An orthopaedic surgeon had thought she may have had a 'bit of calcification' in her tendon and had injected her with steroids.

This was Mrs. L.'s second marriage, her first husband having died in a motor car accident 4 years previously. She had two children from her first marriage and 'had to get married'. Her first husband had been 'such a good man' – as was her second, she hastened to add.

When asked whether she wanted to talk about her first husband, she responded tearfully. In this and subsequent consultations, she revealed much of her suppressed feelings on the first marriage and towards her late husband.

At the first consultation, she had several of the somatic symptoms of depression including early morning awakening. The doctor, in addition to his counselling, prescribed anti-depressants.

Up till 10 months after her initial visit, she never mentioned her shoulder again.

1. What do you understand by 'organization of disease'?
2. What are the possible organic causes for a painful shoulder?
3. Does depression often present through organic symptoms in family practice?
4. What are the advantages and disadvantages of putting this (a young) patient on anti-depressants?

J. H. Levenstein, Cape Town

6   MRS. K.   AGED 18   SECRETARY

Mrs. K. presented for the first time complaining of painful, lumpy breasts. She had been married for 1 week and was on no contraception because her 'husband did not want her to go onto the pill'. She said her first sexual experience had been on the day of her marriage and she had found sex unsatisfactory. She admitted to a fear of pregnancy. Her sister had had an ante-partum haemorrhage at 30 weeks pregnancy. Examination revealed normal breasts and no other physical abnormalities.

1. What was the patient's actual reason for coming to see the doctor?
2. How should the GP manage this situation?

S. Levenstein, Cape Town

7   MARK B.   AGED 23

'I've come because I've had bad flu for several days'. According to the family records Mark has always been fit. He looks well and apart from some excess mucus in his pharynx there is no clinical abnormality.

1. Why has Mark come to see you?
2. With the story and findings what could be your attitude to this patient?

F. Mansfield, Perth, Australia

8   MRS. G.H.   AGED 26   HOUSEWIFE

Mrs. G.H. who is well known to the doctor presents for an annual contraception check-up. She appears very tense and on questioning confirms that she is quite upset because of the unexpected and unexplained death 4 weeks earlier of a 30 year old married male friend of the family. She will offer no further information and suggests that she does not need help in handling the situation. Physical examination is negative.

1. Is it likely that the need for an annual check-up is the real reason for the visit?
2. What sort of treatment, if any, would you offer?
3. Would you make use of the laboratory in managing this total situation?
4. Is it likely that this patient's distress is related to a normal grief reaction?

G. G. Beazley, Winnipeg

MRS. V.　　AGED 40　*AND*　GLORIA　AGED 18　　　9

As Mrs. V. ushers in her 18 year old daughter into your consulting room, 'It's Gloria's nose again,' she says.

Reference to Gloria's notes is hardly necessary because you well remember the frequent visits this couple have paid you in the recent past, seeking relief for Gloria's persistent complaint of stuffy nose and 'catarrh'. Referral to the local ENT consultant has not resulted in any lasting amelioration of a condition labelled 'chronic nasal catarrh' not associated with significant underlying disease.

1. What significance (if any) may be attached to consultations when more than two people (patient and doctor) are present?
2. What might prompt Gloria and Mrs. V. to consult at this time?
3. What are common causes of nasal complaints such as Gloria's?

J. D. E. Knox, Dundee

MASTER C.M.　　AGED 14　　SCHOOLBOY　　　10

Cecil presented for the first time having had an operation 2 weeks previously for undescended testes.

He was complaining of some tenderness over the scar. When the GP started examining him he asked why they had put 'that thing' in his scrotum. It emerged that only a remnant of the left testis had remained, and the surgeon had inserted a prosthesis in the left side of the scrotum for cosmetic purposes. The right testis had successfully been brought down into the scrotum.

After dressing, Cecil sat on his chair, looking sad. When asked what was troubling him, he shook his head and remained silent. He was asked again and given the assurance that anything he said was permissible and confidential. The boy then said 'Will I ever be able to have children'?

1. What was Cecil's **actual** reason for consulting the GP?
2. How did the GP facilitate the expression of the patient's fantasies?
3. How should the GP have responded when asked 'Will I ever be able to have children'?
4. What lasting psychological effects could the operation be expected to have on Cecil, if any?

S. Levenstein, Cape Town

11   MR. D.C.   AGED 46   BOOKKEEPER

A 46 year old man, who was a bookkeeper in a large firm, presented for a 'check-up'. He was last seen 4 years ago in the practice for back pain.

On questioning him why he had come today, he was evasive and stated that he hadn't seen the doctor 'for a long time'. The doctor asked him whether there was anything in particular he was fearful of and he expressed concern about his heart. He then discussed a pain, which he had had 4 days ago on Sunday afternoon, in his stomach and lasting for an hour – 'Didn't want to bother you, doctor, on a Sunday and, anyway, it was just like indigestion.'

The doctor examined the patient and the significant findings were: pulse 106, sinus arrhythmia, a persistently raised blood pressure of 180/110 and no signs of congestive cardiac failure. There was evidence of a recent inferior myocardial infarction on ECG. The patient also related that things were a bit 'peculiar' at home with 'no' children – his youngest having left for university – and the fact that he may become redundant at work with the introduction of computers. He also felt he was more irritable and snappy of late.

The doctor explained the diagnosis and sent him home to bed with certain medications.

1. Do you agree with the doctor's use of home management for acute myocardial infarction (AMI) in this instance?
2. What type of 'personality' did this patient have?
3. Could anything have been done to prevent this attack?

J. H. Levenstein, Cape Town

12   MS. J.R.   AGED 23   OFFICE SECRETARY

A 23 year old, unmarried woman presented with a history of pain in her lower legs for 3 days and coughing for 6 months. She had been taking the contraceptive birth pill for 6 years. Her fear, she said, was that she had a clot in her lung. Examination revealed tender calves but no varicose veins, and the chest was clear on auscultation and X-ray.

The doctor informed her that he did not believe that she had a clot in her lungs and that she probably had a chest infection. He had no explanation for her calf pain. On asking whether she had any other problems, the woman burst out crying. He reflected and then asked 'Do you feel like talking?' She replied 'It's really nothing. I was fine until I came in, but the way you looked and spoke to me, I just burst out crying.'

The doctor then asked whether she knew why it had happened and what she felt had triggered it off. Also, he felt that something must be bothering her.

She replied, 'Leave me alone!'

The doctor accepted her anger and invited her to come and speak to him anytime she felt she wanted to.

1. What do you feel could be the problem/s in this consultation?
2. Why do you think the patient burst out crying?
3. What do you understand by the 'termination of a consultation'?

J. H. Levenstein, Cape Town

MRS. M.S.   AGED 26   SINGLE MOTHER   13

A deserted wife with two pre-school children wants some sleeping tablets. The three family members frequently present at your office with trivial illness and you have tended to overprescribe medications to satisfy the demands of the mother. The family is poor.

1. What are the aetiological factors in this situation?
2. How would you handle this situation?
3. What social agencies would you use?

R. W. Roberts, Ravensthorpe, Australia

MISS C.   AGED 12   SCHOLAR   14

C. was brought by her mother (Mrs. D.) to the general practitioner early one morning. Mrs. D. requested a 'check' as C. would not go to school because she was feeling sick in the mornings. 'If you say there is nothing wrong, doctor, then I will just make her go to school.'

Despite careful attempts by the general practitioner, C. refused to give any further history, or co-operate in any way.

The parents were very simple people of a low socio-economic status, and had on the surface a happy family unit. They used to go on camping holidays with another family. For a short time, a few months previously, C.'s father left home to live with the other couple because 'they understood him better'. It appears he lived in the house as a second husband, but became disenchanted when he found there were others also filling this role. He subsequently returned to the family fold, and certainly superficially all appeared quite stable.

1. What are the likely causes of C.'s refusal to attend school?
2. What would be your approach to elucidating this problem?

3. What would be your approach to the management of this problem?

D. A. Game, Adelaide

15 ROSEMARY C.   AGED 8   SCHOOLGIRL

Rosemary had a normal birth: she walked, talked and was dry at night at quite an early age. She is the youngest of three children and attends the Catholic primary school where, after a bright enough start, she is now labelled as stupid and lazy and is ridiculed by her teacher. Mr. C. has had a variety of jobs and is only a moderate provider. Mrs. C. smokes and drinks excessively but is kind and supportive. She brings Rosemary to see you because she has been wetting the bed for many months.

1. What are the causes of bedwetting in an 8 year old girl?
2. Why should a bright and intelligent child like Rosemary be labelled as dull and stupid?
3. What is Rosemary's real problem and how may it best be helped?

A. L. A. Reid, Newcastle, Australia

16 MASTER M.P.   AGED 2 YEARS

Mr. K.P. consulted you about his own health. As he was about to leave, he asked if you thought there might be anything wrong with his son Mark who at 2 years has made no attempt to speak. He appears to hear normally and obeys verbal commands from his parents.

1. Is Mark retarded?
2. What is the single most important method of reaching a diagnosis?
3. What is the treatment of the condition?

W. F. Glastonbury, Adelaide

17 MRS. A.B.   AGED 71   PENSIONER

Mrs. A.B., aged 71 years, presented with a history of chronic asthma. She and her husband had just moved into the neighbourhood, and this was her first consultation.

She stated, 'I've heard you're a wonderful doctor; no one can do anything for my asthma. I've been to two university clinics, but they do nothing.'

Mrs. B. was on salbutamol inhaler, two puffs every 6 hours, a long-acting xanthine derivative twice a day, and prednisone, 7.5 mg daily. She was a late onset 'asthmatic', her first attack being at the age of 64 years. She had smoked 20 cigarettes a day for 35 years from the age of 20. She had married Mr. B. 9 years ago, and this was her second marriage. Her first husband had died of a heart attack.

At this first consultation, the doctor performed a physical examination and assessed lung function. He also explored possible reasons as to why the bronchospasm started at this age.

At the next consultation, Mrs. B. complained again about 'her chest.' The doctor reassessed her and found her lung function to be of the same order as at the previous consultation. He then asked her again what she felt could make her so short of breath. She pointed out that this had all started after her second marriage.

'I'm embarrassed to tell you, Doctor,' she stated, 'but my husband is not interested in sex! The doctors at the clinic have told me this happens when you get older, but I can't help it – I still feel the need for sex.'

1. What evidence is there for asthma being a psychosomatic disease?
2. What assessment tools are available to measure lung function in primary care?
3. What would be your assessment of Mrs. B.'s sexual status?
4. How do you feel the doctor should have responded to the fact that he was reputed to be 'wonderful'?

J. H. Levenstein, Cape Town

MISS L.T.   AGED 22   BALLET STUDENT   18

Miss L.T. who had come to the doctor for follow up of pneumonia seemed quite anxious. In the ensuing discussion she admits to eating excessively and compulsively to the point of severe abdominal pain which is relieved only by self-induced vomiting. This has occurred since early adolescence and happens several times a week. She has not told anyone. She lives alone. She had an unhappy childhood. Her mother lives in another city. She was raped at ages 13 and 17. She has never seen a psychiatrist. She is attractive, slightly underweight and denies any recent weight loss. She denies hallucinations, delusions and suicidal ideation. She admits to variable anxiety and depression.

1. Is a consultation indicated?
2. What are the therapeutic goals?
3. When a family physician undertakes extensive psychotherapy with a patient, how does it affect the doctor patient relationship?

E. Domovitch, Toronto

HILDA M.   AGED 58   HOUSEWIFE   19

Mrs. M. is a frequent attender. She has low back pain due to chronic degenerative changes in her lumbar spine, and periods of light-headedness which have been ascribed to vertebrobasilar insufficiency. Recently she had a cholecystectomy. At frequent intervals she has attacks of frequency and dysuria. Micro and culture of her urine are nearly always clear. She has been married for 10 years to a man of her own age, who is most attentive to her. For many years Mrs. M. looked after her very demanding mother. There are no children. Although she has unquestioned organic problems Mrs. M. gives the impression that she is a rather troubled person who is less happy than she should be. She denies that there are any underlying problems in her life and a discreet suggestion to her husband that some of her troubles may be functional is met with indignant rejection.

1. What explanation can be made of the processes going on in this relationship?
2. How far should the general practitioner proceed in trying to unravel the possible psychological disturbances underlying the situation.
3. What are the possible causes of dysuria and frequency in a patient of this age?

J. G. P. Ryan, Brisbane

20 GRAHAM B.   AGED 50   BANK MANAGER

Graham B. recently arrived from a neighbouring town. He is still attending a doctor there for long standing dyspepsia for which a recent endoscopy has confirmed duodenal ulceration. Your colleague, in introducing him, describes him as introspective and has at times given him doxepin and oxazepam. He has also seen a local psychiatrist. His problem today is pruritus ani of such severity as to curtail his weekly golf.

The condition persists despite your several applications and repeated advice and the further ministration of a dermatologist to whom he referred himself. The dermatologist's letter suggests among other things a referral to a psychiatrist and arrives simultaneously with one from the psychiatrist advising a dermatological opinion.

You invite him to come to discuss the problem. He can only come at a given time and cannot be kept waiting. He breaks two appointments and eventually turns up unheralded and by the time he is seen is too far behind his schedule for anything but a brief and unsatisfactory interview. He does not return.

1. How do you establish a therapeutic relationship with such a personality?
2. What are the likely psychodynamics?
3. What is the best approach to managing the total situation?

J. A. Stevens, Ulverstone, Australia

GWENDOLINE W.   AGED 69   HOUSEWIFE   **21**

Gwendoline W. is a neat, shy little woman married to a kind but overbearing husband. 7 years ago she had a hysterectomy for fibroids complicated by a vagino-ureteric fistula eventually requiring ureteric re-implantation. Follow up raised doubts about impaired renal function but eventually both gynaecologist and urologist pronounced her fit and dismissed her continued malaise and vague abdominal pains as 'neurotic'. 4 years ago she had herpes ophthalmicus with a third nerve palsy, disciform keratitis and mild uveitis which was slow to recover and left a chronic neuralgia. She was difficult to wean off analgesics and impossible to withdraw from oxazepam.

About every 6 months she appears with fatigue, generalized headaches and occipito-frontal paraesthesiae. Physical examination is negative and Hb (done at her request) and urea, creatinine and microurine (at the doctor's instigation) are all normal. She accepts the news with resignation and disappears for another 6 months. Over the years she has been given various anti-depressants but found the side-effects intolerable and never complied for more than three days at a time.

1. Is she sick?
2. What is the diagnosis?
3. How can you help?

J. A. Stevens, Ulverstone, Australia

MASTER B.   AGED 8   SCHOOLBOY   **22**

Michael's mother had brought him to see the GP several times with abdominal pain unaccompanied by diarrhoea or vomiting for which no organic cause could be found. The mother had requested anti-helminthic treatment which had been given with no improvement in the symptoms.

Mrs. B. had consulted the GP in the past with tension headaches. She had been having an extra-marital affair a year previously but this had been terminated soon after. The tension headaches had, however, persisted.

1. What was the cause of Michael's abdominal pain?
2. Why did Mrs. B. present with tension headaches?
3. How should the GP manage this situation?

S. Levenstein, Cape Town

KARL Z.   AGED 2   **23**

Karl is brought to you by his mother because he is constipated. She has had difficulty in toilet training him and has tried persuasion, threat and punishment to no avail. He refuses to 'poo in the potty' and prefers to soil his pants. She has tried to relieve his constipation with fruit and bran.

The mother appears to be at her wit's end. The child seems apprehensive and is uncooperative.

1. What is the likely cause of the child's condition?
2. How can the situation be managed?

W. E. Fabb, Melbourne

24 MISS V.   AGED 18   TYPIST

Miss V. presented with pain in her right axilla. Examination revealed cellulitis but no abscess, and antibiotics were prescribed. The patient's mother who was present at the consultation requested a prescription for tranquillizers.

At the next consultation a few days later, the mother was once again present. The mother offered certain suggestions about the condition, such as daughter's use of under-arm deodorants. The daughter was irritated with her mother and snapped back at her repeatedly. Examination now revealed an abscess which was incised and drained. On leaving, the mother told the GP that her nerves had improved since the previous consultation and thanked him for his help.

1. Who was the patient, the 18-year old woman or her mother?
2. What is the diagnosis?
3. How would you manage this situation?

S. Levenstein, Cape Town

25 MRS. J.   AGED 23   *AND*   BABY AGED 20 WEEKS

You delivered Mrs. J. of her first child 20 weeks ago. The pregnancy and delivery were normal and the baby was normal. There were no apparent problems at the 6-week check in history or examination of both. Mrs. J. tells you she has not had one good night's sleep since she got the baby home. She cries as she tells you she can't cope any longer and is frightened she may do harm to the baby. She is breast-feeding and the baby appears to be thriving.

1. What further history or clinical information would you like?
2. What is your response to the tears?
3. What is your management?

F. Mansfield, Perth, Australia

MRS. L. AGED 40 HOUSEWIFE

26

This patient presents the following list: ectopic pregnancy, hysterectomy, nerve troubles, migraine, backache, vulvitis – and there is more. You have learned (with little surprise!) that her marital sexual life is singularly unsatisfactory, that she was assaulted as a young girl, that 'her gynaecologist' has just discovered that she had had an aversion to intercourse throughout her life.

1. How do you begin to manage this problem?
2. Might it be better left alone?
3. What does the final statement suggest to you about
   a. the patient
   b. her gynaecologist?

W. D. Jackson, Launceston, Australia

MRS. ANNA N. AGED 27 RECEPTIONIST

27

Mrs. N. presented with a brief history of epigastric pain similar to a pain she had 12 months previously, which was attributed to oesophageal reflux demonstrated on barium meal. Although not severe, she was worried about why the pain had recurred when she had avoided the precipitating factors which had previously caused pain, such as acid foods, wine and eating late at night.

The only physical abnormality was tenderness over the duodenum and a repeat barium meal revealed oesophageal reflux, but no hiatus hernia or other abnormality. Her pain responded well to antacids.

It was during exploration of her home situation that she revealed a sense of loneliness, at times amounting to despair, following her divorce 18 months previously. Her marriage had been unhappy throughout, due, she said, to 'incompatible personalities', and her husband had finally initiated the divorce. 'I was divorced', she said. When asked what she wanted in the future, she said she would like to re-marry and have children, but as she met few suitable males, she felt her chances were poor. She felt separated from her old circle of friends, who are now all married with children. She works as a receptionist during the day and 'puts on an extroverted front, which comes off at night'.

Her feelings of despondency and depression are at times overwhelming, and she finds herself tearful and desolate. She says she tries to keep her feelings inside, but feels there is 'something dead inside', which she feels she needs to 'get out'. When she expressed these feelings, she began to cry and then chided herself for being a 'blubbering female'. She agreed she needed help and agreed to seeing a counsellor.

1. Why did the doctor seek details of her home life?
2. What are the problems faced by divorced women?

3. What response should the doctor make to self-deprecating remarks?
4. How could one manage this situation in a 10 minute consultation?

W. E. Fabb, Melbourne

28 MRS. FRANCINE S.   AGED 29   HOUSEWIFE

DR. A: 'Good morning Mrs. S. I'm Margaret Ashton. I'm working here in Dr. Binet's surgery. How can I help you?'

MRS. S: 'Well, I've come about this head cold that's been worrying me, doctor'.

DR. A: 'Uhmm'.

MRS. S: 'Actually, I've got these terrible pains up the back of my neck, going up into my head'.

DR. A: 'Yes'
Pause

MRS. S: 'Well, we're actually having a lot of trouble with my husband's mother. She's senile and John wants her to come and live with us'.

DR. A: 'Yes'

MRS. S: 'The real problem is doctor, that John and I are having dread-
(crying) ful trouble over sex. I can't get pregnant . . . it's awful . . .'

1. The consultation appears to have been very effective to the present time. What has made it so?
2. What would you 'do' next?

M. W. Heffernan, Melbourne

29 MRS. M.S.   AGED 71   HOUSEWIFE

Mrs. S., a diabetic for 7 years, has been well controlled on diet and glibenclamide 5 mg b.d. since originally being diagnosed. She presents today because she has been consistently showing 1/10% to 1/4% sugar on at least two urine tests per day for the last month.

1. How do you explain this patient's behaviour?
2. What are the possible causes of her loss of control?
3. Are any further investigations indicated?

W. F. Glastonbury, Adelaide

30 MRS. C.B.   AGED 30   HOUSEWIFE

This patient had a difficult childhood. Her parents divorced and her mother subsequently became alcoholic. The children were taken into care and she lost contact with her brothers and sisters. Her husband's job involves frequent absences from home.

She was married for 10 years and underwent considerable investigation for infertility before becoming pregnant. She did not feel well during the pregnancy and was finally delivered by a difficult forceps manoeuvre.

Since the baby, Josie, a normal female child, was born she has frequently complained that Josie is difficult to feed, suffers from colic and wind, and is restless and irritable, especially in the evenings. She does, however, sleep through the night and appears happy, contented and well cared for. Josie is now 7 months old and takes cow's milk and a good mixed diet. No medicines have been of any help.

1. Who is the patient in this situation?
2. What are the causes of 'wind', 'colic' and irritability in babies under 7 months old?
3. What risks are inherent in this situation?
4. What measures could you take to help this family?

E. C. Gambrill, Crawley, UK

MR. E.S.   AGED 42   TRUCK DRIVER

31

Mr. E.S. presented complaining of a heavy feeling around his chest, dyspnoea, and tiredness for the past 24 hours. The symptoms appeared to be related to effort. Pulse and blood pressure were normal, there were no signs of cardiac failure, and the ECG was within normal limits. The patient who was overweight, reported that he had been previously well but had a history of alcohol abuse. He was single, but was due to get married in a month's time. He was asked to return after 2 days bed-rest.

On returning he was found to have 4 + glycosuria. He was referred to a physician for control of his diabetes. However, he returned to the GP complaining that the physician's pills 'did not agree with him' and he refused to return to him. Subsequent contact with the GP was characterized by difficulty in controlling the diabetes because of poor compliance, and frequent requests for sick certificates. His marriage had been postponed indefinitely.

1. Why did the GP not test for glycosuria at the first consultation?
2. Was a provisional diagnosis of myocardial ischaemia justified at the end of the first consultation?
3. Of what importance was the patient's psycho-social background in the diagnosis and management of the patient's problems?
4. Why was the patient's compliance poor?
5. How would you manage this situation further?

S. Levenstein, Cape Town

32 **MR. A.O.S.   AGED 67   PENSIONER**

Mr. A.O.S. has attended your practice for 2 years. Polio at 15 months left a residual disability in both lower limbs, especially below the knees. He wears calipers and uses a stick.

Listed problems include:
- Pruritis ani for years (addicted to topical steroids)
- Rheumatism in his thumbs, neck, left shoulder (uses enteric coated aspirin and ibuprofen)
- Tendency to seborrheic dermatitis of the face (finds the steroids for pruritis ani help).
- Overweight by 6–7 kg
- Tendency to produce a shopping list.
- A smugness and hearty know-all manner which engenders intense feelings of animosity in his medical adviser.

Presents today with his shopping list and new complaints of a chronic stuffy right nostril (helped by Kenacomb ointment in the past), offensive smelling breath, belching and flatus, watery eyes attributed to blocked tear ducts, and his arm (for a BP check – the BP never having been raised in the past).

1. How does a GP come to terms with an intense feeling of animosity towards his patient?
2. How does a GP distinguish between the wants and needs of his patient?
3. How does a GP effectively apportion his time in this type of situation?

D. Levet, Hobart

33 **BRIAN M.   AGED 55**

Brian M. visited his doctor complaining of feelings of weakness which he had had for many years but which were now more frequent. He described himself as anxious but denied any problems or worries. He had no other specific symptoms.

1. How would you manage Brian in the rest of the consultation?
2. What is the most likely diagnosis?
3. How would you manage Brian in the next few weeks?

J. C. Hasler, Oxford

34 **MRS. P.A.   AGED 44   INVALID PENSIONER**

New to your practice, this lady presents complaining of headache, blocked nose, substernal pain, tightness in the chest, back pain, constipation, flatulence and a heavy feeling in the legs. She is on various medications including diazepam and tricyclic antidepressants. She has been separated from her husband for some years.

Examination reveals a slow moving female with no clinical abnormality detectable.

1. What is the differential diagnosis?
2. What further information would you want?
3. How would you manage this patient?

R. W. Roberts, Ravensthorpe, Australia

CHAPTER 2

Problems of Living

The cases in this chapter are related to those in the previous one. Often patients present with symptoms or problems which are the result of environmental stress — problems of living. Maybe this stress is the result of living with a chronic or terminal illness, or a marital or family problem. Sometimes stress at school, business or work brings the patient along. Sometimes people present because of their inability to cope as age brings illness and disability, or because of social problems such as poverty, housing problems, isolation, loneliness, inability to speak the language of the country, or inability to make friends.

These problems of living may present in many different ways; what they have in common is that the patient presents with symptoms which often initially conceal an underlying problem of living. The cases and questions which follow exemplify these often difficult situations and explore how the family physician senses, defines and manages them.

35 MRS. H. AGED 83 HOUSEWIFE

Mrs. H., aged 83, married and living in comfortable surroundings together with her 85 year old husband (who has had two previous cerebro-vascular accidents) called urgently for a home visit as she was unable to cope with the pain in her leg. She had made several such requests in the past few weeks and had been admitted to hospital for investigation. While the possibility of a lumbar disc had been entertained, X-ray and simple blood tests had been negative. Mrs. H. had last consulted the clinic 5 years prior to this episode of illness and rarely before that.

Mrs. H. appeared agitated and, on inquiry, she volunteered that she was restless, 'humiliated by her illness', 'it was so unfair' and that she found it difficult to relinquish 'control' of her life. She felt 'guilty' that her 'ill' husband, whom she always had to look after now had to manage and he couldn't cook.

She was unable to sleep 'because of the pain', or get around. She felt she would rather be dead than be like this. Re-examination was unremarkable except for pain on movement and a positive straight leg raising test.

1. What do you consider to be the main problem?
2. What would your two priorities be in the management of this patient?
3. What do you understand by 'limit-setting'?
4. How do you think this situation may have been avoided?

J. H. Levenstein, Capetown

36 MRS. D.B. AGED 48 MEDICAL PRACTITIONER'S WIFE

Mrs. D.B. had been married to a general physician for 25 years. They had two children, one married, the other a rebellious daughter attending her first year at university and whom she suspected of smoking 'pot'.

In recent years the marriage had been discordant. While she enjoyed the role of the successful doctor's wife with its accompanying affluence, their relationship had deteriorated to frequent arguments and acts of violence against her. She refused to leave him as it was against her religious principles, although friends, clergy and doctors had advised her to do so. She recounted that recently Dr. A.B.'s popularity was declining. He was becoming completely self-centred, more withdrawn and, at times, appeared disinterested in his work. He had become even more argumentative at home and expressed the view that people are working against him. He was drinking more but she did not feel alcohol was a significant problem.

Wearing dark glasses, she presented with a 'black eye' seeking your help.

1. What other information would you wish to obtain from her?
2. What is the nature of the problem?
3. How would you manage the problem?
4. What problems do doctors and their families have in obtaining medical care?
5. How should doctors reconcile the immediate demands of their work with the needs of their families?

H. C. Watts, Perth, Australia

K.L.   AGED 17   STUDENT   37

K.L., a high school student, complains of fatigue, insomnia and poor school performance for the past several months. He appears sad and admits he has been depressed. He has had episodes of crying almost every day.

1. How high a suicidal risk is this patient?
2. What types of pressure contribute to stress at this age?
3. What other sources are available to assess the situation?
4. How would you proceed to manage his depression?

E. V. Dunn, Toronto.

MALCOLM R.   AGED 16   STUDENT   38

Malcolm R. is the elder son of medical missionaries. Till now his life has been spent on the mission stations in the Pacific islands with his parents. He has always been healthy but, 2 years ago, when the family returned from the mission field, Malcolm became aware of a rift between his parents and began to experience migraines.

12 months ago his parents separated and divorced and Malcolm's migraines worsened. They are especially frequent and severe when he is under stress and, despite a series of specialist consultations and wide range of therapeutic agents, he continues to be severely incapacitated.

1. The increasing pressure of senior school examinations during the past 6 months has seen Malcolm requiring more and more frequent injections, usually of dihydroergotamine, Maxolon and pethidine. What should be the GP's major concerns for this boy?
2. Malcolm is an intelligent lad and has good insight into the relationship between the emergence of his migraine and the family break up. He has tried all the known drug regimes and is very much aware of the risks he runs if the current situation continues. What therapeutic strategies are available to his family doctor?

W. L. Ogborne, Sydney

39 MR. J.A.C. AGED 18 STUDENT

Mr. J.A.C. has been known to you since early childhood. He suffers from mild ankylosing spondylitis (currently quiescent) which afflicts his father severely. For the past few years he has been healthy except for headaches, probably tension or migraine. His parents separated 4 years ago amid bitter wrangling. He and his siblings live with his mother, now a pensioner. His father has been ordered to pay for his secondary education in view of the advisability of a career based on intellect rather than physique. (Tertiary education is free.) He is due to sit his final exams in 2 months.

He is accompanied by his mother who asks for referral to a psychiatrist (initiated by her friend, the wife of a physician) because he is 'depressed' and feels that he is a failure, which his father says the whole family is.

1. How might a GP feel when confronted by such a referral request?
2. What are the possible reasons to explain the 'depression'?
3. What aspects of health promotion/preventive medicine apply to this situation?

D. Levet, Hobart

40 JOHN P. AGED 48 SCHOOLMASTER

John P. is married, a senior master, with two sons – one in the police and one still at school. He is moderately obese and mildly hypertensive. Investigation of his left-sided abdominal pain has disclosed minor diverticulosis.

The local police ring to say that he has disappeared in his car with tent, rifle and toilet gear. Is he, you are asked, likely to commit suicide? There are worries – about his financial position and about his health, specifically the possibility of bowel cancer, and about a personality clash with his headmaster.

2 days later the elder son rings to say that father has returned 'blind drunk', the only clues to his whereabouts being a betting slip and a church service sheet for a village 30 miles away.

1. What is your immediate action (a) on receipt of the first call? (b) on receipt of the second call?
2. What is your further plan of management?
3. What prognosis can you give?

J. A. Stevens, Ulverstone, Australia

41 MR. J.L. AGED 55 STORE PROPRIETOR

Mr. J.L. is married with three children, all of whom have left home. He has been well until 3 months ago, when he began to suffer from frontal headaches 'like a tight band around my head' especially in the evenings. He has owned a small grocery store for the past 10 years. Business has decreased markedly since the opening 6 months ago of a modern supermarket nearby. On examination, the only significant physical sign is a recumbent blood pressure reading of 180/105 in both arms. Two previous readings at weekly intervals did not differ significantly from these.

1. What is the cause of this patient's headaches?
2. What is the effect of medical treatment on the natural history of hypertension?
3. How would you plan your management of this patient?
4. What are the possible implications of your treatment for the patient and his family?

M. R. Polliack, Tel-Aviv, Israel

MR. JOHN T.   AGED 43   SMALL BUSINESS PROPRIETOR   42

This pleasant father of three children has become increasingly 'nervous' lately. He has not performed well in the small business he runs with his wife and feels constantly tired. Prior to this consultation, his wife phones and tells you in confidence that he has been drinking heavily for some time. He complains of nervousness and tremor of his hands and head, and feeling tired. He is flushed, has a slurred speech and tremor, and smells of alcohol at 3 p.m. He asks for a prescription for diazepam to help him cope.

1. How common is alcoholism?
2. How would you approach this situation?
3. What agencies exist in the community to help?
4. What tests would you do?
5. During withdrawal what additional therapies can be used?
6. What long term prognosis would you offer?

K. C. Nyman, Perth, Australia.

MRS. D.F.   AGED 57   RETIRED TEACHER   43

Mrs. D.F. retired from teaching 3 years ago with increasing anxiety and inability to cope. She has been married for 20 years to a kindly inadequate alcoholic. Some months after retirement her anxiety increased. She said that although still potent, her husband was 'holding himself back' for someone else. She described in detail the way her husband signals to someone outside (he may turn on the toilet light, or adjust the curtains, but seemingly varies the time he does this so that she shall not be suspicious). She also knows that at night he administers some noxious gas to her so that he can go out; this gas makes her wake feeling nauseated.

This problem has led Mrs. D.F. to leave home on several occasions for her 'safety' and a year ago the marriage appeared to be ended. Later she returned and for 3 months appeared normal. She then suffered a minor stroke. The initial CT scan showed a lesion in the internal capsule lateral to the putamen. She had made a good recovery from the stroke but is under psychiatric care. She knows she is quite normal but does not know how to cope with her husband's strange behaviour: 'You know what alcoholics are'.

1. What may have caused these psychiatric symptoms?
2. What special difficulties arise from living with a passive dependent alcoholic?
3. What approach should one take in talking to someone who can carry out an entirely rational discussion about a system of beliefs which seem totally irrational?
4. What part do psychotropic drugs play in this kind of problem?

A. L. A. Reid, Newcastle, Australia

44 MRS. E.G. AGED 82 AGED PENSIONER

Mrs. E.G. lived with her husband, an 84 year old retired engineer, who was alert and remarkably fit for his age. They owned their own small house but had no close family. She had suffered from pernicious anaemia for 15 years. In the last 5 years, she had become increasingly frail and socially withdrawn so that she had little contact other than coming to the office for her regular B_{12} injections. Her husband did all the shopping and recently, because of her gradual physical deterioration, the cooking and the housework. She had developed increasing forgetfulness and Parkinsonism and was also prone to falls. After one of these falls, during a home visit, you noticed numerous empty brandy bottles outside and two full ones beside her bed. She admitted to taking brandy and milk several times a day 'to get me going'.

1. When do you suspect someone has an alcohol problem?
2. What could you do to help this couple to manage at home?
3. Should doctors play a role in forming community attitudes towards social problems such as alcohol and tobacco? How?
4. What is the value of home visits?

H. C. Watts, Perth, Australia

45 MR. A. AGED 62 CUSTOMS OFFICER

Mr. A. had spent the last 10 years on the wharves working in the excise department. It was his task to ensure that all the imported alcoholic liquors had had the appropriate duty paid. Over recent months his work associates had noted some falling off in his efficiency.

Mr. A. lived alone and Dr. B. visited him at his home which was in a considerable muddle. It was apparent to Dr. B. that not only had Mr. A. been sampling too many of the beverages he supervised but furthermore that he had a tendency to confabulate. Dr. B. had some definite views about management and so that Mr. A. would not forget his instructions he carefully wrote them all down on a piece of paper and handed them to his patient.

5 days later he returned to check on progress. 'Have you followed my directions?' he asked his patient. 'No', came the reply, 'I couldn't remember where I had put the instructions'!

1. What was the syndrome that Mr. A. was suffering from?
2. What principles would you observe in the management of alcoholism?

J. G. Richards, Auckland.

MRS. B.W.   AGED 55

46

For several years she has had recurring vaginal itch – she has come to you for the first time. On examination there is some excoriation of the external surface of the labia majora but no other external or vaginal abnormalities.

Mrs. B.W. runs a small cafe and lives alone, her husband having left her some years previously.

1. What do you think is the importance of the duration of the symptom?
2. Could this lady's social history be of importance?

F. Mansfield, Perth, Australia

MRS. E.I.   AGED 68   WIDOWED PENSIONER

47

You are requested by a neighbour to visit Mrs. E.I., an Italian, who has just moved into a Housing Commission flat in your area. She has a letter for you from her previous doctor. From the letter, your interview and your examination you learn that she is under treatment for mild cardiac failure. You notice she is somewhat forgetful, speaks little English and has problems cooking meals. Her children live across town, and she is a widow of 25 years. She is occasionally visited by a married daughter. She has no other close relatives and few friends in Australia.

1. Under what circumstances should a doctor accept a request from another person to visit a patient?
2. How can you conduct an interview with this patient?
3. What other arrangements will you have to make concerning her welfare?
4. Is her probable 'isolation' likely to cause any problems?

D. U. Shepherd, Melbourne

48 MRS. K.T. AGED 49 HOUSEWIFE

Mrs. K.T. is a recent Latvian immigrant with a serious communication problem in the English language. A relative has brought her along for a 'check-up' and possible referral to a multi-phasic screening centre. She has felt uncharacteristically nervous and irritable over the past few months. She visited a Latvian speaking doctor who was very abrupt with her and prescribed a tranquillizer for an anxiety state.

1. What is the likely diagnosis?
2. How would you manage this problem?
3. What are special problems faced by immigrants?

J. E. Murtagh, Melbourne

49 MRS. MARGARET C. AGED 55 HOUSEWIFE

Margaret C. consults you clutching a book on 'Vitamins and Foods in Health', heavily marked at a page on Vitamin B, which suggests that people feeling depressed and lacking vitality can be cured by taking thiamine. As you explore the story further, she begins to weep openly.

1. How would you cope with this immediate situation?
2. People commonly hold incorrect views about the role of vitamins in health. As doctors should we always dissuade them?
3. Your detailed history reveals Margaret as a recent migrant without relations in this city and living apart from her husband. In addition she is menopausal. Would these facts influence your probable diagnosis and treatment?
4. What avenues of therapy would you consider in this case?

K. C. Nyman, Perth, Australia

50 MRS. K.L. AGED 28 HOUSEWIFE

Mrs. K.L. is an Indian woman married to a Ukranian. She calls you requesting protection. She says her husband has threatened her harm. She has gone to the police and they will do nothing unless she charges him. She tells you her husband has strung her over a beam, has put paper down her boots and into her sleeves and has set fire to the paper as a threat.

1. What is you response to this cry for help?
2. How do you think the husband will respond to you if you intervene in this situation?

J. K. Shearman, Hamilton, Canada

MRS. V.C.   AGED 29   HOUSEWIFE

51

Over the years, Mrs. V.C. has attended various partners in the practice, mostly with symptoms of tension. She appears quiet and behaves as if unable to cope, although her home and family are well cared for. She says she has been off the pill for a year, and has failed to conceive.

Her periods are irregular, the last being a fortnight ago. Her past history reveals an episode of salpingitis 3 years ago, treated at home with antibiotics. A year later, she presented with infertility, and said then that her husband 'didn't understand'. Pregnancy resulted soon afterwards, and she has a 20-month-old baby.

1. How much investigation does the present problem require?
2. What questions does the diagnosis 'salpingitis' raise?
3. What does her history reveal of her personality?

J. Grabinar, Bromley, UK

MRS. C.A.   AGED 28

52

Mrs. C.A. has three children. The second child died (cot death). She still has bouts of anxiety/depression and difficulties coping with children. She requests sterilization.

1. What is your initial response to this request?
2. How would you follow this through?

W. D. Jackson, Launceston, Australia

DAVID J.   AGED 27   COMPANY EXECUTIVE

53

David presents for 'a second opinion'. For the past 6 months he has complained of lethargy and weakness, insomnia, palpitations, vague aches and pains and occasional difficulty in swallowing. He was examined and investigated by another doctor who could find no physical cause for his symptoms and suggested that they were related to the birth of his first child 6 months ago and to his long working hours and associated stress at that time.

In view of the fact that he has always been a fit fellow who plays regular squash and works out in a gymnasium, Mr. J. cannot easily accept the diagnosis of 'nerves'. In his own words: 'There has to be a cause for the way I feel'.

1. What steps should the doctor take to define the cause of David's symptoms?
2. What is the doctor's responsibility to David's previous doctor?
3. Should the doctor consulted for a second opinion learn that David has also sought the help of a hypnotherapist, what influence will this have on the consultation?

W. L. Ogborne, Sydney

54   MRS. E.M.   AGED 43   HOUSEWIFE

Ever since her first pregnancy 22 years ago, which resulted in a premature delivery of twins (who died at birth), this woman has had symptoms of an obsessional nature. She continually complains of the need to check her washing machine, her food preparations, and her hand washing. She has seen several psychiatrists, has been given ECT, monoamine oxidase inhibitors, diazepam, all to no avail. Vague physical diagnoses, like visceroptosis, cancerophobia and lymphadenopathy are scattered in her notes. Despite all this, she has had five further pregnancies, and four children as a result. She comes monthly for a repeat prescription, which consists now of a tricyclic antidepressant only. She remains talkative, but seems to cope with family duties very well.

1. What is the value of psychotherapy in such cases?
2. Why does she come every month?
3. What non-medical help can be offered?

J. Grabinar, Bromley, UK

55   MR. R.P.   AGED 38   MUNICIPAL WORKER/ LAVATORY ATTENDANT

Mr. R.P. is extremely unattractive in appearance and was diagnosed 20 years ago as suffering from schizophrenia. For the past 2 years he has been treated with 50 mg of flupenthixol decanoate in oil (Depixol: Lundbeck), injected every 2 weeks by a community nurse under the supervision of a psychiatrist, who reviews the case every 6 months. Mr. R.P. consults his G.P. at intervals to complain of feeling 'too tired to do my job'. On one of these occasions Mr. R.P. says he is going to leave his job 'because everyone laughs at me behind my back and calls me a homosexual'.

1. What facts about the natural history of schizophrenia are illustrated by this story?
2. What do you understand by 'the collusion of anonymity'?

P. Freeling, London

56   MS. H.S.   AGED 30

This unmarried lady joins your practice when she is 8 months pregnant. She gives a history of a neglected childhood, of being adopted, her parents having been killed in a car accident at an early age, and of being unable to make new friends at school. She is under the care of the Children's Aid because of problems she has had at school and with drugs. She gives birth to a baby girl and is supported by the father of the child morally and financially. She suffers from a birth canal infection and has to stay in hospital longer than usual. She has difficulties as a mother and reports frequently that the child hates her. She eventually threatens to throw the child off a balcony and you and the Children's Aid remove the child from her care.

1. When do you first start to worry about this mother's potential parenting skills?
2. What factors are important in deciding to remove the child from its parents' care?
3. Having removed this child from the parents, what can one do about subsequent children?

J. K. Shearman, Hamilton, Canada

MRS. J.R.　　AGED 48　　HOUSEWIFE

57

Mrs. J.R. initially presents with rectal bleeding. She denies any other problems apart from some backache. Subsequent meetings over several months reveal that she has marital problems and dislikes intercourse with her husband. Both she and he tend to drink to deal with the areas of conflict within the marriage. Both of them are seen together and given medical therapy at various intervals over the subsequent years. Mrs. J.R. has several somatic complaints usually related to menstruation for which she wants an organic diagnosis. She finds a lover and her husband finds a girlfriend. You hear little from them and then hear dramatically that Mr. J.R. has jumped from a high level bridge and is found dead.

1. Mrs. J.R. presents with a somatic complaint for which no obvious pathology is found. Is this a common way for a life stress problem to present?
2. When faced with marital complaints, is it your job as a physician to help them stay together or help them to part?
3. What do you think Mrs. J.R. will feel on learning of her husband's death?

J. K. Shearman, Hamilton, Canada

MRS. I.M.　　AGED 57

58

Mrs. I.M. comes in weeping. She complains of pain in the chest, frequency of micturition and stress incontinence, pain in the back and itching in the vulva. She has been attending four different specialists and usually attends one of the emergency departments in town each night. She has had a vulvectomy for leukoplakia. Her husband was killed in a fight some years ago. Her only son is married and living some 3000 miles away. He calls infrequently.

1. What do you think is the major problem that has to be dealt with in this lady?

2. What do you think is the most efficient way for the health care system to handle the kind of problem this lady has?
3. How would you approach each of the medical problems she presents with?

J. K. Shearman, Hamilton, Canada

59 MRS. G.R.   AGED 47   HOME DUTIES

The patient who has transferred to your area presents with poor sleeping habits present for more than 10 years. She asks for a repeat of diazepam and flunitrazepam tablets although she admits that they have not helped very much. She has been on these tablets for many years and is unable to sleep without them. She does not admit to any problems except the usual stresses of a housewife and mother of three.

1. How may a busy GP properly manage this first interview?
2. What is the predominant cause of insomnia seen in general practice in this age and sex group?
3. What strategies are available in the long term management of this problem?

T. D. Manthorpe, Port Lincoln, Australia

60 MR. D.N.   AGED 49   INVALID, LIVES AT HOME

He was invalided out of the Public Service 6 years ago because of severe anxiety and depression. His wife is 15 years younger than he is and she is well. They are strict Roman Catholics and they have six boys in the family. Two of these children are mildly mentally retarded – one also being an asthmatic. The mental retardation in the eldest child is thought to be associated with his premature birth. Two other children have exhibited behavioural problems. The family are paying off their own small home.

Mr. N. stands up from the table after a meal and suddenly appears to be unable to move the left side of his body. His speech is unaffected. He has never suffered any major physical illnesses in the past and he has a normal blood pressure.

1. What is the cause of his left-sided paralysis?
2. What physical problems could be responsible for the hemiplegia?
3. Who is responsible for this patient's care?
4. How often do family stresses contribute to physical illness?

B. H. Connor, Armidale, Australia

MR. L.M.   AGED 29   BIRD FANCIER

61

Mr. L.M. suffered an illness when 18 months old which left him paralysed down the left side. Since then he has had numerous orthopaedic procedures on his left arm and leg – including an amputation of his forearm just below the elbow. He had recently been in hospital for sciatica from which he has recovered. As a result of his back problems he can now no longer use his artificial arm. Despite his disabilities, he manages to work part-time and he has been informed by the relevant Government agency that he is no longer eligible for an invalid pension.

He claims to have recurrent diarrhoea which has only been noticed occasionally while in hospital. Full investigation for this symptom revealed no abnormality.

His father died 12 months ago.

Every time arrangements are made to help Mr. M. he changes his mind and at these times he has been quite obviously consuming large amounts of alcohol. His hobby is keeping tropical birds.

1. When is an invalid not an invalid?
2. How can the effects of long-term hospitalization be minimised in a young person with a chronic disability?
3. What is alcoholism?

B. H. Connor, Armidale, Australia.

MRS. O.   AGED 53   HOUSEWIFE

62

Mrs. O. reported to the emergency department of a large public hospital, and was referred to the primary care unit of that hospital. She was seen by the intern who, before arranging for her treatment, discussed the problem with his general practitioner supervisor.

Mrs. O. stated that she had 'arthritis throughout her body'. Further questioning revealed that the manifestation of this was pain in her arms and legs, mainly in the muscle masses. This pain was almost constant but worse after work. She had seen a general practitioner (not her regular doctor) near her home and had been given several courses of antiinflammatory drugs. As these were not effective she was referred to an orthopaedic surgeon.

At the primary care unit Mrs. O. announced that she just wanted some physiotherapy, and to support this she had brought with her the X-ray films of her thoracic and lumbar spines. These showed early degenerative changes. She also had a note from the orthopaedic surgeon which simply stated that Mrs. O. was suffering from arthritis and would benefit from physiotherapy.

The intern suggested to the general practitioner supervisor that he should arrange for physiotherapy. However, the supervisor said that he thought this would be just as unsuccessful as the anti-inflammatory drugs, and suggested alternative management.

1. Why did the general practitioner supervisor say that physiotherapy would be as unsuccessful as the anti-inflammatory drugs.
2. What would have been the correct management of Mrs. O's problems?
3. What is your definition of a general practitioner/family physician?

D. A. Game, Adelaide

63 MISS LINDA W.   AGED 26

As a result of birth injuries, Linda is an epileptic of below normal intelligence. She meets a male of similar intellectual impairment at a sheltered workshop. They decide to marry and live on their meagre workshop income plus welfare payments. She wants children, yet is unable to prepare simple meals for herself. They come to you because of family pressure against marriage and pregnancy.

1. What further information do you want?
2. Identify the problems to be managed.
3. Can/should society intervene?

D. H. Johnson, Toronto

64 MRS. P.   AGED 32

Mrs. P. was a new patient who presented requesting a change of the contraceptive pill on the grounds that her husband was worried the present one she was taking did not suit her. She was reluctant to volunteer any further information insisting all she needed was a change of medication. When the doctor refused to meet her request she did, with great reluctance, volunteer the following history.

- She had four children, the youngest a babe of 5 months.
- She had just moved to town and was living in a caravan park.
- Her marriage had just broken up 3 months ago and she was now living with a man who had just resigned from the police force.

They had been living in a small isolated town and both their marriages had broken up at the same time for different reasons. Only after their individual marriage breakups did they become mutually attracted to each other and started living together but this was not tolerated by the local community which included her parents. The policeman had to resign his job and they had to leave town. At present neither her family nor his family will have anything to do with them.

Examination revealed heavy PV loss suggesting a diagnostic curettage would be the best and immediate form of treatment. The patient refused this advice claiming that any hospitalization at this stage would place in jeopardy this new relationship she was trying to foster and which was so necessary to her because few men would accept her and her four children. An arrangement was made for the patient to see a gynaecologist and a social worker at the local public hospital but she failed to keep the appointment. The doctor later learns the pill has been prescribed elsewhere.

1. Is the contraceptive pill prescribed too easily?
2. Should the doctor, despite the patient's objection, try to treat social and medical problems together?
3. How far does a doctor's responsibility go?

P. F. Gill, Hobart

MR. S.   AGED 76   65

Mr. S., a 76 year old man, became known to me during the terminal illness of his wife, who had been ill for about 2 years preceding her death. He lived with his wife's sister in an apartment since his wife's death.

His son was concerned about his welfare, but lived 250 miles away and was able to visit him only on some weekends. The son brought his father to the office because of weight loss, weakness and noticeable mental deterioration over the preceding 3 months. The history revealed a considerable decline in physical activity, starting about 4 to 5 months after his wife's death. Although the patient appeared to be slightly depressed, both he and his son denied a severe grief reaction or overwhelming depression. The only other complaint he had was that of dyspepsia.

Further fuctional enquiry revealed no abnormalities. Although he had become somewhat socially isolated, he still had friends who visited him and he had some social life. Living with his sister-in-law was a mutually acceptable arrangement but basically they lived independently other than for meals.

His physical examination was normal except for the marked physical deterioration since I had seen him previously. Initial laboratory investigations included a blood count, X-ray, urinalysis and ESR.

1. What is the most likely cause of this man's presenting signs and symptoms?
2. What other information about this man's lifestyle would be valuable to know between his first and subsequent visits?
3. Why would this man deny the aetiology of his problem?

W. W. Rosser, Ottawa

MR. H.S.   AGED 82   RETIRED BUSINESS MAN   66

Mr. H.S. an 82 year old pensioner underwent an elective surgical repair for an inguinal hernia. Even after 10 days in hospital, he continued to complain of excessive pain and was reluctant to be discharged home.

Mr. H.S., previous to coming to hospital, had been caring for his wife at home. His wife suffered from organic brain syndrome. During Mr. H.S.'s hospital stay, his wife has been admitted to a nursing home, but is to return home to his care when he is discharged.

On the planned day of discharge, the patient develops a swollen left leg.

1. Why has an 82 year old man undergone an elective hernia repair?
2. What would be the normal expected length of stay for an uncomplicated hernia repair?
3. What is the likely explanation of this sudden appearance of a swollen leg?

C. A. Moore, Hamilton, Canada

67 MR. J.B. AGED 81 RETIRED PHARMACIST

Mr. J.B. is a retired pharmacist who lives with his wife in a house near your practice. He suffers from chronic congestive heart failure resulting from atherosclerosis. He is presently taking a multitude of drugs to bolster his heart output, including frusemide, digoxin and hydralazine. He has had a permanent pacemaker for the past 5 years because of heart block. He requires admission to hospital occasionally when his heart failure becomes worse.

1. How would you manage this man's congestive heart failure on an ambulatory basis?
2. What advice do you give such a patient about his living conditions?
3. What advice would you give this patient in relation to the future?
4. How will you help his wife cope with his illness?

J. K. Shearman, Hamilton, Canada

68 MRS. P. AGED 84 WIDOW

Mrs. P. lives alone in her own comfortably furnished apartment. She is physically well except for advanced degenerative disease of her cervical spine.

She is cheerful but delightfully vague. She has her midday meal delivered 5 days a week (weekdays); otherwise she prepares her own meals. She never has any idea which day of the week it is, and therefore does not know on any particular day if her meals will be delivered or not.

She is visited regularly by the district nurse who keeps an eye on her, but carries out no actual treatment. She is visited also by a domiciliary visitor. She is meant to do her own housework but this is very badly attended to. She attends a day centre one day a week for social contact. She has no idea where it is, what the name of it is, or on which day she attends. The domiciliary visitor calls in the morning and makes sure she is ready to be picked up by the arranged transport. She is visited regularly by her general practitioner.

She has three children, all married. One daughter lives in the same town, visits her occasionally and sometimes arranges to meet her in town to help her do some shopping. This daughter was visiting her mother recently when the district nurse called. The nurse found the daughter shouting and abusing her mother for not remembering where she had put something away.

Another daughter lives in the country. She occasionally telephones her mother, but otherwise has little contact with her or her brother or sister.

The only son lives in another major city 900 miles away. He visited his mother about 12 months previously and 'fixed everything up', but since then has had little contact with her or his sisters.

The nurse reported the incident of the daughter abusing her mother to the general practitioner. He made contact with this daughter and had a very long conversation with her over the phone, attempting to explain to her the significance of her mother's condition. The daughter dogmatically stated that 'she could not do anything more for her mother', and 'she will have to go into a home, and fix it up quickly'.

This daughter obviously contacted her brother and sister because both within a few hours were on the phone to the general practitioner. Both demanded details of their mother's condition as they did not believe the report their sister had given them. All three criticised each other, told the general practitioner not to take any notice of the others as they did not know what they were talking about. All however implied the general practitioner had not been sufficiently attentive otherwise the situation would not have arisen, and more significantly, what was **he** going to do about it.

1. What are the possible medical conditions from which Mrs. P. is suffering?
2. What is meant by family dynamics?
3. What can the general practitioner do? (as demanded by the daughter).

D. A. Game, Adelaide

MRS. S.W.   AGED 82   RETIRED   69

This elderly lady has lived with her daughter and son-in-law since her husband died 10 years ago. She suffers from some osteoarthritis of her hips and knees and a moderate degree of congestive cardiac failure, controlled by digoxin and diuretics. Over the past 2 years she has become increasingly forgetful, with a tendency to leave taps and switches on and to wander around the house at night. You are unable to find any other physical abnormalities.

1. How would you assess her mental state?
2. How would you advise her relatives?

3. What resources do you have in the community to help in the care of this old lady?
4. On what grounds should elderly people be encouraged to give up their independence and enter some form of sheltered accommodation?

E. C. Gambrill, Crawley, UK.

70 MRS. F.F.   AGED 82   WIDOW

Mrs. F.F. has been living with her daughter, son-in-law and two grand-children since her husband died 6 years ago. She has been functioning well. In the past few months she has changed in personality. She is unkept. She walks around the house during the night. She turns on the stove unnecessarily, accuses her family of stealing her belongings and occasionally has been incontinent of bladder and bowel.

1. Is this likely to be an organic or psychological problem?
2. What are the common causes of rapid deterioration of the mental status of an elderly person?
3. What investigations would you do?
4. How would you manage this patient?

E. V. Dunn, Toronto

71 MISS M.B.   AGED 82   RETIRED NURSE

Miss M.B. who lives alone is being managed for congestive heart failure with digoxin and a diuretic. Over the past several months she has become increasingly weak and unsteady on her feet. She has fallen several times and sustained minor injuries. She has been losing weight due to malnutrition. She is hopeless, helpless, and depressed. Her mental status is otherwise normal. She refuses hospitalization because during her previous admission she was subject to 'unnecessary tests and too many examinations by medical students'. She adamantly refuses institutionalization.

1. Should she be persuaded to have more medical care?
2. Is there any indication for the use of anti-depressants?
3. How can family physicians assist patients requiring considerable care to remain at home and out of institutions?

E. Domovitch, Toronto

72 MRS. A.T.   AGED 83   WIDOW

Mrs. A.T., a widow, had inoperable carcinoma of the rectum. The consultant surgeon recommended that her family doctor give chemotherapy.

Maintenance doses of 5-fluorouracil (5FU) would mean weekly visits to the office for intravenous injections; Mrs. T.'s niece would have to take time off work to drive her aunt for treatment. The niece and her husband were also patients of this family doctor. The niece had just recovered from severe depression and thyrotoxicosis.

As Mrs. T.'s disease progressed, she became weak and incontinent of faeces, but wanted to stay at home. The niece helped with laundry and shopping. One day the niece's husband called the doctor, saying that Mrs. A.T. must be admitted to a nursing home because the strain was too much for his wife; even though the strain was not obvious to anybody else. A grand-daughter also called.

1. Was the surgeon's recommendation of chemotherapy reasonable?
2. What do you think the doctor's reaction to the telephone requests would be?
3. Which of his patients, Mrs. A.T., her niece, and the niece's husband, should the doctor consider most when making decisions about admitting Mrs. A.T. to a nursing home?

G. Williams, Iowa City

OLIVE N.   AGED 61   EXECUTIVE   73

Mrs. Olive N. is divorced from her husband. She works as an executive and lives in her own flat. She has close relationships with her three children who live in the area.

A few weeks ago she consulted you because of 'catarrh in her throat' – she is a heavy smoker. However since then the full nature of her disorder has become apparent. She has developed difficulty in speaking and swallowing, weakness in the hands and difficulty in walking.

Her tongue shows 'bag of worms' contractions.

A diagnosis of motor neurone disease has been made after a spell in hospital.

She comes to see you with her daughter – both are tense, anxious and frightened.

1. How do you propose to conduct this consultation?
2. What is the likely course of her disorder?

J. Fry, Beckenham, UK

CHAPTER 3

Family Problems

The cases in this chapter are related to those in the previous two. Often the family physician is faced with a diagnostic dilemma – the patient who has presented seems to be part of a bigger problem, often a family problem. Sometimes the presenting patient has a physical illness; sometimes a psychological problem or disturbance of behaviour. Often the problem unfolds as a marital disturbance. Less commonly, the problem may be presented overtly as a family problem. Whether the presentation is overt or covert, the family physician needs to be able to sense, explore and manage these family problems.

Every patient has a family of origin and is living in some 'family' environment, whether it be his original family, his family by marriage, or his living companions. The family physician recognizes that the problems which patients present need to be assessed against these family backgrounds. This principle is exemplified by hundreds of cases in this book. This chapter, however, is devoted to those problems which have their major impact on, or origin in, the family – family problems. Sometimes the family is dysfunctional because of the presence of physical illness, often chronic or terminal, in one of its members; sometimes because of a tragedy in the family; sometimes because of a behavioural disorder which may be the result of family, school or work stress; sometimes because of social or cultural problems; and occasionally because of mental illness or retardation.

The cases and questions in this chapter exemplify a variety of family problems and illustrate how the family physician senses and assesses these problems and how he manages them, either himself or with the help of professional colleagues.

74   J.H.   AGED 7   SCHOLAR

An anxious mother brings in her 7 year old son, J.H., who has been wetting his bed nightly for 2 weeks. You had recently done his pre-school examination and nothing was amiss. He is the only child of Mr. (aged 39) and Mrs. H. (aged 37).

In the past, they had consulted in 'clusters' – Mrs. H. bringing the child in with upper respiratory tract infections. The child had had 3 or 4 attacks of 'asthma' between the ages of 3 and 5 years and the mother was always scared that this 'may develop'.

Mrs. H. consulted rarely and only on clearly defined problems. On one occasion, she confessed to her anxiety, fear of losing control and being a bad mother. The counselling appeared to help but she was a 'no show' at the follow up appointment.

Mr. H. was a passive man who stood back when his wife spoke, seemingly to take a 'back seat'. The doctor had canvassed his views when he had seen all three of them together but he was reticent and withdrawn. On the odd occasion that he (the doctor) had seen him alone, he appeared more talkative but only allowed discussion on a superficial level.

1. Could you list the possible causes of this boy's enuresis in order of probability?
2. Do you think this is a 'dysfunctional' family and if so, why?
3. What is/are the natural history/ies for asthma in children?
4. What do you understand by a 'mother presenting through the child'?

J. H. Levenstein, Cape Town

75   MRS. C.B.   AGED 35   HOUSEWIFE, PART-TIME JOB IN NURSING HOME

Mrs. C.B. has a past history of severe puerperal depression following LUSCS for protracted labour. Has only one child. Husband previously married. Always a worrier, houseproud to a fault. Husband says she is a 'nagging b_____', and she admits he is right. Frequently irritable and weepy. Says husband is lazy around house 'won't do anything.' Child is a grizzler, constantly provokes her by refusing meals. He irritates her to the point where she is afraid she will strike him and damage him. He is now 3 years old.

1. Who should you treat first – mother, father, child or the whole family unit?
2. Does the fact that you don't often see father and son mean anything?
3. Given the common problem of multiple patients in a family but access limited to one, what might you achieve?

W. D. Jackson, Launceston, Australia

THE A FAMILY

76

It is just after midnight when Mr. A. rings you on your private number at home. You instantly recognize the family as one into which you have put a great deal of effort, mainly to support Mrs. A. in coping with her family problems. Mr. A. has been discharged from the psychiatric hospital as an 'unemployable incurable inadequate psychopath', who failed to co-operate in attempts at group therapy. The second son, Bill, aged 17, has had a court conviction for illegal use of 'soft drugs'. Throughout it all, Mrs. A. has struggled to keep her job as sales assistant, and to keep the family together. 'Elsie's had a break-down, she's smashing the furniture – please come!' But it's not your night on call . . .

1. What functions does the family doctor discharge in the on-going care of families like the A's?
2. What should be done at this time of night?
3. What psychiatric diagnoses might be represented in this family?

J. D. E. Knox, Dundee

MRS. D.H.   AGED 33   HOUSEWIFE

77

Mrs. D.H. whose 41 year old husband was discovered 3 months ago to have metastatic bronchogenic carcinoma, presents indicating that she thinks she might be pregnant. This seems unlikely as she has been oligomenorrheic and infertile for 10 years. At age 17 (out of wedlock) she gave birth to a male child with Down's syndrome. She was married at age 21 and a year later bore a female child with tracheo-oesophageal fistula and small bowel atresia. This child died at age 6 months. Physical examination reveals breast changes suggestive of pregnancy and a pregnant uterus consistent with a gestational age of about 22 weeks. She is quite upset at the confirmation of the pregnancy.

1. What is one definition of the 'family life cycle'?
2. Other than routine, what additional measures might be utilized regarding the investigation and management of this pregnancy?
3. What is meant by the concept of the 'family as the patient'?

G. G. Beazley, Winnipeg

MRS. L.M.   AGED 28   PROFESSIONAL MODEL

78

Mrs. L.M. has consulted her doctor and gynaecologist for several years with dysmenorrhoea, lower abdominal pain, infertility and several symptoms related to an ongoing anxiety state. Routine investigations have yielded normal results. Her husband, who is a super athlete and football personality has refused sperm analysis. They have two adopted children. After being admitted to the local hospital with an overdose of a minor tranquillizer, she revealed that her husband was having an affair and that their marriage had never been consummated because of her husband's clumsy technique.

1. What is the problem list for this patient?
2. Who is the real patient?
3. What has gone wrong with the management of this family?
4. How should the family doctor manage this problem?

J. E. Murtagh, Melbourne

79 MRS. M.   AGED 45   HOUSEWIFE

Mrs. M. is the member of the family most frequently presenting to the general practitioner. Mr. and Mrs. M. are of Italian extraction but educated in Australia. Mr. M. is a foreman for a building company and is able to provide well for his family.

There are four children, and all have been given good educational opportunities. The three younger children were delivered by the general practitioner.

The eldest, a daughter, T., aged 21, an attractive girl, works as a hairdresser. She has always tended to despise her mother for her poor education, and her (in T's opinion) lack of interest in her personal appearance and dress. She is seeking and gaining independence despite parental disapproval.

M. the elder son, aged 19, lacking motivation did not like school and left but more recently has become an apprentice cabinet maker and is quite keen on his work. He tends to have little drive or ambition for which he is criticized by his older sister T. He is overweight and requires ongoing medical supervision for acne vulgaris.

The other two children, D, a boy aged 14, and S, a girl aged 8, are still at school. D. requires very little medical attention but S. is frequently brought to the general practitioner by her mother with mild respiratory infections.

Mrs. M. lacks confidence in herself, always has expressed dislike for her elder daughter, is overweight, and suffers from hypertension. Also she requires continuing medication for a condition which for the last 5 years has given her painful and stiff wrists, less so the fingers, shoulders and knees. There has been no marked deterioration in this condition.

Mr. M., an only son, appears to be placid and accepts the family situation. There are no apparent or expressed sexual problems within the marriage.

Mr. M.'s mother, also a patient of the general practitioner, is a widow. She lives alone but within walking distance. She speaks little English and suffers from ischaemic heart disease, heart block (treated with a pacemaker), and severe peripheral vascular disease. She and her daughter-in-law rarely speak to or visit each other. Mrs. M. Snr. bestows quite generous monetary gifts (gained through hard saving) on her elder grandson M., but not on the other grandchildren.

Mrs. M. Jnr., is frequently consulting the general practitioner for supervision of her medical condition, and for counselling and advice on her family relationships, particularly her relationship with her daughter T.

1. What is the likely disease process producing Mrs. M.'s painful joints?
2. What is meant by total patient care?
3. What is family medicine?

D. A. Game, Adelaide

MRS. P.B.   AGED 23   HOUSEWIFE   80

Mrs. P.B., mother of two children aged 3 years and 18 months, was a frequent attender at the office. The problem was always minor, involved one or both of the children and usually required no medication. She rarely spoke of her own health and when she did it was to say that she sometimes felt tired. She attributed this very reasonably to the fact that she combined looking after the children and the house with working five evenings a week.

One day she arrived without the children but with mother in tow. Mrs. B. said nothing while her mother launched a tirade at the astonished doctor. 'Something's got to be done for my daughter. She's been coming back and forwards to the office for ages and nothing has been done to help her. She's very run down and she needs something to give her some energy.' Spurred on by this attack Mrs. B. herself offered the observation, 'My friend at work says that if I don't get any satisfaction here I should change my doctor.'

When it was possible to deflect the conversation back to Mrs. B. and away from her mother it transpired that she had two problems – one a vaginal discharge and the second an uncommunicative and unhelpful husband. The doctor treated her thrush and suggested that she should talk to her husband and encourage him to attend the office with her for a joint consultation. She went away apparently happy and none of the family has been seen in the practice since.

1. What is the significance of a patient arriving in the office accompanied by a relative or friend?
2. What conditions would you consider when a patient complains of tiredness?
3. What might lead the family practitioner to suspect a disturbance of family dynamics?

T. A. I. Bouchier Hayes, Camberley, UK

SHELLEY   AGED 14 MONTHS   81

Shelley is an only child of over solicitous parents. Since moving into the district 9 months ago she has been seen in the office on 10 occasions.

Until recently she has not seen one member of the practice constantly. The usual situation is that father has come home from work late in the afternoon and has been informed by mother that Shelley has not been well during the day. The immediate decision is made to take her down to the office where she sees whichever doctor is on duty late in the afternoon.

On all occasions she exhibits signs of URTI, sometimes ascribed to teething but on three occasions reference has been made to mild otitis media. Although 1 month premature Shelley had a normal postnatal period after discharge from the incubator and was breast fed for 5 months. There is a family history of hay fever and the mother has been treated for anxiety. On the last 3 occasions Shelley has been in considerable distress with an otitis media and her symptoms have cleared rapidly with antibiotics. This had led the parents to neglect a review consultation. The examining doctor insisted on review after the last attack and Shelley was found to have a collection of fluid behind the left ear drum.

1. Should this child and family be requested to stay with one doctor except in emergencies?
2. Does Shelley have a chronic ENT problem?
3. Does this family have a problem?

P. F. Gill, Hobart

82   MRS. I.C.   AGED 28   HOUSEWIFE

Mrs. I.C. consults you complaining of marked loss of weight. She weighs only 87 lbs (40 kg). She has had incessant diarrhoea for 6 weeks – admits to forced vomiting and the taking of excessive daily laxatives. She would like to return to being a model – her previous occupation. She is very tearful and informs you that her son aged 10 years is a hyperactive child and suffers with a learning disability. Her husband has recently been overlooked in promotion by his company. This has caused added problems for the patient.

1. What advice would you give to the patient?
2. How do you treat this family unit?
3. Is medical treatment required?
4. What further advice may be required?

B. M. Fehler, Johannesburg

83   MRS. T.   AGED 49   CHINESE MEATSTALL OWNER

Mrs. T. presents with shortness of breath on minimal exertion, tightness in the chest, and swelling of the ankles. Examination reveals she has atrial fibrillation and is in congestive heart failure. She is treated and advised to rest at home.

Further conversation reveals that she has four children, the youngest aged 4 and the eldest 14 and all are at school. Her husband is an alcoholic and a gambler who refuses to work. He takes the children to and from school and occasionally helps at the meat stall. Mrs. T. therefore, being the sole supporter of the family, cannot afford time to go to hospital or to rest at home. She promises her doctor that she will rest as much as possible although she would have to continue managing the meat stall.

1. What are the problems?
2. How would you manage the husband as part of the overall problem?
3. How do you manage this situation?

N. C. L. Yuen, Hong Kong

MRS. D.G.   AGED 42   HOUSEWIFE   84

Mrs. D.G. who has been married 12 years and previously childless, gave birth to a daughter with Down's syndrome. She was very upset and initially rejected the child. After considerable counselling by her family doctor, who managed the confinement, she agreed to take the child home. She attended regularly for counselling and expressed concern about her husband's attitude and the state of tension at home. After 4 months, when she had grown very fond of her baby, she phoned in an agitated state with the news that her husband had eloped with an 18 year old girl.

1. What were the inherent deficiencies in the management of this family?
2. What preventive measures could have been adopted to help this family?
3. How would you manage the present situation?

J. E. Murtagh, Melbourne

PETER B.   AGED 18 MONTHS   85

This child, who is brought to the doctor's surgery for the first time, is obviously suffering from Down's syndrome. The parents state that he has a bad 'cold and cough', that the baby is prone to respiratory tract infection and request that the doctor examine the child thoroughly because he is not keeping up with his cousin of the same age. The doctor suddenly becomes aware that the parents do not know that the child has Down's syndrome, in spite of the fact that he was born in a large hospital in a provincial city. Examination reveals a fever of 38.5 °C, inflammation without exudate of the tonsils and pharynx, nasal blockage and some redness of both tympanic membranes.

1. What sequence of events could have led to the diagnosis of Down's syndrome either having been overlooked or not communicated to the parents?
2. How does the doctor deal with the problem presented by this 18 months old child?

J. G. P. Ryan, Brisbane

86 MASTER ROBERT S.   AGED 2

Robert has been followed since birth by a paediatric neurosurgeon for macrocephaly which is described as benign after a normal CT scan. The child is irritable. He cannot say any intelligible words. He grasps but cannot pile blocks or copy drawings. He can sit unsupported but cannot stand. He has no specific neurological signs.

1. What is wrong with the child?
2. What should the parents be told?
3. Who is the patient?

E. Domovitch, Toronto

87 HANNA W.   AGED 6   SCHOOLGIRL

Mrs. W. has brought her younger daughter Hanna to the family doctor. Hanna was toilet trained by the age of 3 years, but since the birth of her brother, 9 months ago, she began to wet her bed. Mrs. W. lifts Hanna at night, and takes her to the toilet. Lately, Hanna also wets her bed after returning from the toilet at night, and adds the complaint of 'disturbed sleep' to the other numerous reasons for her reluctance to go to school.

1. How should toilet training be done?
2. What is the diagnosis for Hanna's problems?
3. What additional investigations could help to clarify the problems?
4. How would you manage Hanna's problems?

Z. Cramer, Tel-Aviv, Israel

88 MR. M.S.   AGED 18   PAINTER AND DECORATOR

The parents of this young man come to see you. He left school 2 years ago with poor educational attainment, but is employed in his father's painting and decorating business. His work is satisfactory but in the evenings he often gets extremely frustrated, rubs his hands continually and bangs his head against the wall. His brother is studying law.

The pregnancy and delivery were uneventful and there was nothing significant about his childhood except for the educational problem.

1. What is the significance of a couple coming together to see the doctor?
2. What is the problem?
3. What is the likely prognosis?
4. What can you do to help this family?

E. C. Gambrill, Crawley, UK

STEVEN H.   AGED 13   SCHOOLBOY   **89**

Steven was brought in by mother complaining of a wart on his thumb. After discussion of possible treatments Mrs. H. asked Steven to go back to the waiting room. She then burst into tears and stated she and her husband were very worried about Steven, who is an adopted child and very jealous of his sister, who is not adopted. His parents love him and treat him like their natural child, but when they try to discipline him, he becomes angry and accuses them of not loving him because he was adopted. He had several times recently threatened to run away from home to try to find his natural mother.

Last week father was shocked when he found Steven in the stable of his pet mare attempting intercourse with the animal. On discovery Steven had actually run away from home but was found by friends and brought home.

1. What help was the mother seeking?
2. What problems can adoption cause?
3. What problems relating to male puberty might present to the doctor?
4. How should children be given sex education?
5. How would you handle the complaint of bestiality?

D. G. Chambers, Clare, Australia

MRS. H.   AGED 35   HOUSEWIFE   **90**

Mrs. H. is the mother of three children. She has labile essential hypertension and has been under your care for the last 2 years. Her marriage has been unhappy as her husband has a violent temper and has battered her and her children on many occasions. She has contemplated divorce but as she is uneducated she will be unable to support her children. It would also be unbearable for her to be separated from any one of her three children.

Today she is at your clinic requesting you refer her for admission to the hospital as she is unable to tolerate his naggings and wants to feign an illness to keep the peace at home.

1. What other clinical entities may be brought on by continuous psychological stress?

2. How would you manage her dilemma?
3. Would you accede to her request for admission to a hospital? Give your reasons.

F. E. H. Tan, Kuala Lumpur

91 MRS. S.   AGED 22   HOUSEWIFE

Mrs. S. is a Caucasian American married to a wealthy Chinese manufacturer. They met when the husband was studying in the United States. They have been married for 4 years and have a daughter of 3 years.

She presents with feelings of tightness in her chest, 'something crushing my chest', and a choking sensation in her throat. She is very afraid that she might not be able to breathe. She also complains that she often has palpitations, dizziness and has difficulty in sleeping.

Physical examination revealed nothing abnormal apart from bruising on her arms and legs. She tells of a robbery that occurred in the apartment during the week, saying she was bruised during the struggle. Further questioning revealed a husband who does not permit her to go out other than to the supermarket, does not allow any friends, even other women friends to visit her, denies her any financial independence and phone contact with her mother in the USA. On a few occasions, she has quarrelled with her husband who has become quite violent, kicking and punching her. Mrs. S. confesses that she has had difficulties establishing friendly relationships locally because of cultural differences and she has no one she can confide in.

She still loves her husband and feels he returns this love, but is very jealous. She does not think it would help to have her husband consult the doctor, or anybody else. In fact she feels that should her husband become aware that this matter has been discussed with her doctor, she would be made to seek medical help elsewhere.

1. What are her problems?
2. How can the problems be solved?

N. C. L. Yuen, Hong Kong

92 MRS. Y.H.   AGED 42   NURSING SISTER

This attractive nursing sister came to discuss a problem. Her first husband had died 12 years previously and she was left with two children, a girl now aged 18 and a boy of 16. She had remarried 2 years ago, and although this was a happy union, she was feeling depressed. She had a deep fear that shortly she would 'go mad', for her mother had suffered from Huntington's chorea for the last 10 years and was now in a mental hospital. She was anxious and depressed about the future, and worried about her children, especially her daughter who had become romantically involved in the last few months. She wondered if the way she was feeling might be the first symptom of the disease in her.

1. What are the main considerations to be discussed?
2. What responsibilities does the doctor have?

G. M. Dick, Hobart

MR. I.   AGED 32   UNEMPLOYED LABOURER   93

Mr. I. has a complex history, detailed to you by a social worker who persuades you to take Mr. I. as a patient. Mr. I. hates doctors, having seen his grandmother and then his mother die, in mental hospitals, from Huntington's chorea. The social worker is deeply worried because he thinks Mr. I. also suffers from the disease. He has recently separated from his second wife (who lives in a different part of the country) after a stormy and violent marriage. He is living in a condemned property in your practice area, and has his 11 year old son, Ian, with him.

1. How might initial contact be made with Mr. I?
2. What diagnostic problems are inherent in this situation?
3. What legal and ethical issues are raised by the problems inherent in this situation?

J. D. E. Knox, Dundee

MR. W.G.   AGED 40   AIRLINE PILOT   94

This divorced, athletic, asymptomatic commercial airline pilot informs you his mother has just been diagnosed as having Huntington's chorea. He requests (1) an examination (2) advice and (3) that you not inform his employer or the government's pilot-licensing body.

1. What is the natural history of Huntington's chorea?
2. Where do your professional responsibilities lie?

P. R. Grantham, Vancouver

CHAPTER 4

Patient Education and
Preventive Care

Two of the most important tasks of the family physician are patient education and preventive care. The two are linked closely. The cases in this chapter exemplify how the family physician can exploit each opportunity to provide information, answer questions and proffer advice, and his strategies for doing so. They also exemplify the numerous opportunities he has for providing preventive care. Some cases address the vexed question of compliance and how the family physician might achieve this. The cases and questions selected for this chapter illustrate vividly the family physician's educational and preventive role, for example in immunization, pre-marital counselling, the control of chronic illness such as hypertension, diabetes and obesity, and the avoidance of drug-induced illness. Throughout the rest of the book, there are hundreds of other examples of opportunities for patient education and preventive care.

95 MR. A.B. AGED 45 MID-LEVEL EXECUTIVE

Mr. A.B., who has been your patient for 10 years, had his first proven anterior myocardial infarction 4 weeks ago. While in hospital he had no complications. He was discharged home 2 weeks ago and has had no symptoms since being at home. He is on no medication. He is happily married with two teenage children. You are about to carry out the first home visit.

1. What is the minimal history and physical examination you would consider appropriate for this visit?
2. What effect is this episode likely to have on his life style?
3. When would you permit this patient to return to full activities?
4. What opportunities present for patient education, health promotion and preventive care?

E. V. Dunn, Toronto

96 MR. E.L. AGED 47 PIPE FITTER

Mr. E.L., who is separated from his wife and has lived alone for 5 years, has been attending the same physician for about 12 years. Annually he has presented demanding a 'complete check-up'. He almost always leaves the physician's office angry because the physician does no more than a historical review and physical examination and then counsels him about his excessive alcohol and food intake, his obesity, his cigarette smoking, his sedentary existence and his non-use of seatbelts. Mr. L. has never followed any of the physician's suggestions.

One month ago Mr. L. suffered an uncomplicated myocardial infarction and is now at the office for his first visit since discharge from hospital. He is angry that he has had a heart attack and is demanding that the physician 'do something' to prevent him from having another one.

1. At what different stages of the development of a disease can prevention be applied?
2. What therapeutic measures might be useful in managing Mr. L.'s disease?
3. What are lifestyle problems?

G. G. Beazley, Winnipeg

97 SUSAN M. AGED 3 MONTHS

Susan is the first child of an intelligent and very socially aware young couple. Both parents have brought her to the office as they wish to discuss the pros and cons of vaccination against whooping cough. They are particularly concerned that one of her cousins developed infantile spasms at about 5–6 months of age and that these had been ascribed to the pertussis component of her first triple injection.

1. What is the significance of the infantile spasms?
2. What facts would you present to help the parents decide whether their baby should be vaccinated or not?
3. What are contraindications to pertussis vaccine and why?
4. Should the childhood immunization programme be made compulsory for all children?

A. J. Moulds, Basildon, UK

MRS. A.B.   AGED 25   SOUTHERN EUROPEAN MOTHER   98

Mrs. A.B. brings her 8 month old daughter, a first child of whom she is very proud. Her child has a minor problem, which can be resolved in one visit. During the interview, you ascertain that the child has not been immunized. When asked, the mother says she doesn't believe in immunization. 'If it was any good, God would have done it.'

1. How would you react?
2. How will you explain the immunization process?
3. Are there any dangers; if so, would you discuss them?
4. Is immunization always effective?

A. Himmelhoch, Sydney

MR. J.R.   AGED 22   UNIVERSITY STUDENT   99

Mr. J.R. consulted because he has decided to take a year off his study to wander around SE Asia (or Africa) with two or three friends, and thought he might take 'something for protection' against illness.

1. For which three groups of disease should immunization be considered for travellers?
2. Can you give cholera and typhoid immunization in the same syringe?
3. What medicine kit would you advise this young man and his companions to take?

A. J. Radford, Adelaide

JILL B.   AGED 20   STUDENT   100

'Doctor, Mum said I should come for a checkup before I get married.'

1. What range of topics should a pre-marital consultation cover? Should you plan for a long consultation to cover them?

2. Let us assume that you are really uncomfortable on finding out that she is both totally sexually ignorant and minimally experienced. How would you proceed?

A. J. Radford, Adelaide

101 MR. J.B.   AGED 30

Mr. B. has been an insulin dependent diabetic since childhood. He has been a rather unreliable patient. His blood sugars are generally above 300 mg% (16.6 mmol/l). He has microaneurysms but not haemorrhages or exudates in his fundi. He has plus one to two proteinuria, but his renal function tests are otherwise normal. He has no evidence suggestive of diabetic complications in his neurological or cardiovascular systems. He finds it difficult to comply with the standard diabetic diet and has never found the time for formal diabetic teaching. He reports for his routine visit.

1. How can the doctor motivate the patient?
2. What can be determined from the fact that the patient continues to visit his regular family physician albeit irregularly?
3. What is the doctor's role in this patient's life?
4. Should family physicians take the position that patients should be given appropriate advice and the extent to which they follow that advice is their own responsibility?

E. Domovitch, Toronto

102 G.H.   AGED 11   STUDENT

G.H. has had moderately severe diabetes for 4 years. She is presently treated with 37 units of insulin daily. Her course has been stormy. Her mother neglects to bring her daughter for adequate follow-up visits and as a result G.H. requires frequent hospital admissions because of lack of control. She is easily controlled in hospital.

1. What home factors might contribute to poor diabetic control?
2. Do you expect the mother to comply with instructions in this case?
3. How can G.H. be taught to help herself?
4. What other people can be engaged to help?
5. What problems is G.H. likely to encounter during her adolescence?

E. V. Dunn, Toronto

103 L.W.   AGED 42   VOLUNTEER WORKER

L.W. is a 42 year old black Cuban female whom you are seeing for non-insulin dependent diabetes mellitus. She has been treated with insulin in the past but just before joining your practice she had been started on oral hypoglycaemic agents, and tended to maintain blood sugars in the 150–190 mg% (8.3–10.6 mmol/l) range. Although she religiously checked her urine, she loved to eat fried potatoes and despite repeated referrals to a nutritionist for diet teaching, she was unable to lose weight. Mrs. L.W. refused to take insulin and disliked taking pills as well, so that when her prescription expired she did not get it refilled, but presented to clinic 2 weeks later, saying she no longer wanted to take her medicine at all. Her blood sugar off medication had been 220–280 mg% (12.2–15.6 mmol/l) in the past.

1. How would you manage the problem of diabetes control in this patient?
2. How do cultural and personality variables influence your management decision?
3. What do you think is a reasonable treatment goal for this patient?

K. F. Weyrauch, Charleston, SC, USA

MRS. RUTH S.   AGED 54   WIDOW

104

Mrs. S. is a lonely widow with maturity onset diabetes. She trimmed off all excessive weight and is quite compliant with your dietary and exercise instructions. Her fasting blood sugars remained about 250–300 mg% (14–17 mmol/l). Because of her reluctance to start insulin, you started oral hypoglycaemics. On maximum effective dosage, her blood sugar remained about 250 mg% (14 mmol/l). You firmly recommend insulin and she vehemently says 'never'!

1. What model of doctor–patient relationship would you pursue?
2. What further information would you wish?

D. H. Johnson, Toronto

MR. P.B.   AGED 68   NAVY - RETIRED

105

Mr. B. is an alcoholic and diabetic who requires Lente insulin, 22 units daily. He smokes 30 cigarettes a day. He has moderately severe claudication from peripheral vascular insufficiency and has recently stopped drinking. He has no interest in any alcohol programmes including AA.

1. What techniques might increase Mr. B.'s compliance with diet and insulin?
2. What degree of claudication would require angiography?
3. Are there any effective techniques to help Mr. B. discontinue smoking?

C. T. Lamont, Ottawa

106 MR. M. AGED 72 RETIRED SCHOOLTEACHER

Mr. M. was a regular attender at the office with chronic bronchitis and mild left ventricular failure. He was an obvious alcoholic and the young general practitioner had often spoken to him about his excessive drinking. His wife who was also a patient, confirmed the diagnosis, and his breath always reeked of alcohol. He often injured her when under the influence, she said.

On one occasion his usual doctor was away on holiday and the older more experienced partner saw the patient. Mr. M. appeared in his usual state, not actually drunk but obviously having imbibed earlier in the day. The general practitioner enquired about his drinking habits and then laid down the law in no uncertain terms 'You're a bloody alcoholic', he said, 'You're killing yourself and probably killing your wife. A year or two more like this and you'll be dead. It's up to you to decide whether you want to live or die. If you want to live you'll have to stop drinking now and never drink again.' And so he went on elaborating the dire consequences of continuing to drink.

A few weeks later the young doctor returned. His patient had taken the message to heart. His general health was much better and he never touched a drop of alcohol again. His wife was jubilant and there were no significant withdrawal problems in the patient.

1. What is the problem?
2. Is confrontation the answer?
3. What can the doctor do?

J. G. Richards, Auckland

107 MISS S.H. AGED 20 CLERK

This fat and plain looking clerk comes complaining of mild fleeting abdominal pains and loose motions for 2 days. She looks well but is obviously much overweight. She has no previous history of sickness and her family are well. She admits to having two 'heavy' older sisters. She is not on any medication and not on oral contraceptives.

She looks rueful when talking of her weight problem, and states that Weight Watchers and dieting are useless. She has tried them.

On examination, her BP is 150/90; she has gross hips, but all else is normal. She weighs 85 kg and is 1.68 m tall.

1. How much preventive medicine can be carried out at this interview?
2. What aetiological factors induce overweight?
3. What is the programme of treatment?

G. M. Dick, Hobart

DAVID J. AGED 29 FARMER

108

David had for the past few months developed dusky red, tender swellings over the superficial veins of his legs, first in one place and then another.

Some time after these episodes he complained of pain in his left little toe. On examination it was gangrenous and required amputation.

A year later he developed severe abdominal pain and signs of obstruction. At operation a large section of small gut was found to be gangrenous and in spite of resection he died.

1. What pathological conditions might lead to this type of story?
2. Is there any way in which such an outcome might be prevented?
3. Where does responsibility lie?

R. T. Mossop, Harare, Zimbabwe

MRS. JESSIE A. AGED 78

109

Mrs. A. is on a number of medications for arteriosclerotic heart disease with angina, multiple extrasystoles and congestive heart failure. She also has medication for Parkinsonism. Her heart failure is getting out of control and you are worried that she is not complying with her complex regimen of medications. Medications include digoxin 0.125 mg daily, chlorthalidone 100 mg daily, isosorbide dinitrate 10 mg q.i.d., quinidine 200 mg t.i.d. and trihexyphenidyl (Artane) 2 mg q.i.d. for Parkinsonism.

1. How would you verify whether she is taking her drugs?
2. What are some of the patient factors involved in non-compliance particularly in the elderly?
3. What can the physician do to increase compliance in elderly patients?

D. H. Johnson, Toronto

TONY H. AGED 2½

110

This Chinese boy was presented to the doctor by his 60 year old grandmother. Tony has had a persistent cough for months which has worsened in the last 2 weeks. He has seen a few doctors but the cough persists. He has also had chest X-rays which have been described as clear.

Further conversation reveals that Tony is a poor eater, 'hardly eating anything at all', consequently is 'so skinny'. Tony is an only child. Both his parents work and the grandmother looks after him. Despite the preparation of expensive dishes e.g. bird's nest soup, red date soup, special rice congee, he has not gained any weight.

On examination it is obvious that Tony is suffering from malnutrition. He is apathetic and grossly underweight and the abdomen is distended. The grandmother does not give Tony very much meat for fear of constipation, and does not allow vegetables as they would make him 'cough all the more'. However, the doctor is asked to prescribe a tonic for him.

1. What are the possible diagnoses?
2. Are there differences in the management of these conditions?
3. How do you explain the resurgence of this condition in an otherwise well-fed and affluent society?

N. C. L. Yuen, Hong Kong

111 MRS. PATRICIA M.   AGED 36   HOUSEWIFE

Patricia had undergone hysterectomy 3 years before for gross menorrhagia associated with fibromyomata.

Divorced 10 years ago she has been remarried for 2 years. She and her new husband have recently become spiritualists and have been told by their guides through a medium that she had undergone spiritual surgery and she was now pregnant.

She walks into the office radiantly happy, with morning sickness, tingling breasts and a request for confirmation.

1. Is there any chance of a wombless woman conceiving?
2. How can the doctor get her to face reality?

R. T. Mossop, Harare, Zimbabwe

112 SIMON L.   AGED 35

Simon L. had had hypertension diagnosed 2 years ago, no cause for his hypertension had been found and he was on hypotensive therapy. One year ago he had developed allergic bronchopulmonary aspergillosis, for which he had been seen by a specialist, who had altered his hypotensive therapy to a different diuretic. It became apparent that the patient had defaulted on his follow up appointments to his general practitioner and was taking no drugs at all.

1. How far should the responsibility for regular follow-up and management of long term disease rest with the patient?
2. What factors should be considered before starting a patient on long term medication?
3. How far is a general practitioner entitled to interfere with a specialist's proposals for therapy?

J. C. Hasler, Oxford

MR. E.W.   AGED 56   MARINE ENGINEER

While summarizing and filleting Mr. E.W.'s records you note that 10 years previously he had been diagnosed as hypertensive (180/130) and started on treatment. There is no record of systematic BP checks or of repeat drug prescriptions after that time and you make a note to check his BP when next you see him.

Unfortunately his next consultation is an emergency one as he has developed a stroke. His BP is now 200/140 and he volunteers the information that he had high blood pressure in the past. He had been admitted to hospital for 2 weeks of tests and as a result lost his job. The treatment he was given had affected his sex life so when his doctor told him that his BP had gone back to normal he had been delighted to stop the drugs.

1. What constitute 'good' GP records?
2. How would you ensure your own records were of a high standard?
3. What is compliance and how can it be improved?

A. J. Moulds, Basildon, UK

CHAPTER 5

Routine Examination

The cases and questions in this chapter are related to those in the previous one. The cases selected address the question of the value of the routine examination, illustrate some illnesses detected on routine examination, address the vexed question of how information derived from routine examination is used in work situations, and show how routine examination can be used as an inappropriate substitute for listening to what the patient is really saying.

114 **D.L.   AGED 13   STUDENT**

D.L., a 13 year old, and one of two siblings in his family, was seen for a routine pre-high school examination. His family physician has looked after D.L. since his birth and other than an inguinal hernia repair at the age of 6, had treated him for no other illnesses. The child's mother expressed some concern about his small stature and delay in puberty. David, at this time, was in the third percentile in height and weight, but had been so from birth and remained in this range. His older brother, who was an adopted child, was above the 50th percentile and had reached puberty at the age of 13. David's mother is 4' 10". David's social and academic development has been normal, and although the family physician believes he is a normal child, he feels the pressure of the parent's concern, and refers David to the Growth and Development Clinic.

1. How does a family physician clinically assess normalcy in a child?
2. What do you think about the family physician's role in this patient's care?
3. What might you expect from the Growth and Development Clinic?

C. A. Moore, Hamilton, Canada

115 **MRS. SARAH J.   AGED 68   WIDOW**

Mrs. J. a widow, presented to the general practitioner to have the appropriate injections prior to her departure on an overseas trip. She was a healthy woman who was seldom seen by the doctor. The doctor took the opportunity to offer her a brief general examination. In answer to a routine question about her bowel habits, the patient admitted to having had some frequency of motions and a little mucus for some weeks. A rectal examination was performed and the doctor was just able to feel a suspiciously hard lesion high in the rectum. This proved to be a carcinoma which was successfully resected. Mrs. J. has since made several overseas trips and remains well.

1. What are the lessons which should be learnt from this case?
2. What are the factors which prompt a patient to seek medical advice for an illness?

J. G. P. Ryan, Brisbane

116 **MR. P.B.   AGED 30   BUSH FLIER**

This bush flier who suffered multiple fractures in a crash 10 months ago is found on a routine pilot's re-licensing physical by the government agency to have 2+ glycosuria. He is sent for assessment to you, his family doctor. The same occurrence last year had revealed an asymptomatic athlete with negative urinalysis and a fasting blood glucose of 120 mg% (6.67 mmol/l). A letter had been written saying he was fit for re-licensing at that time. Functional enquiry now reveals polydipsia, polyuria and weight loss of 20 lb (9 kg). Urinalysis 4 + glucose, no ketones. Fasting blood glucose is 480 mg% (26.67 mmol/l).

1. What are the problems?
2. What about his flying licence?
3. What questions will his wife have when she appears with him at subsequent visits to the family doctor's office?

P. R. Grantham, Vancouver

MR. S.   AGED 60   TRAIN DRIVER   117

10 years ago, Mr. S. suffered a myocardial infarction. Since then he has been on treatment for mild hypertension with a beta-blocker and a diuretic. He works as a train driver and is very proud of his job and the fact that he overcame considerable difficulties including a poor education and a significant language barrier to rise up from a labourer in the railways to a position of some status. He attends every 3 months for a review of his blood pressure and has never exhibited any symptoms. His blood pressure is 150/90.

On this occasion he is very confused and disturbed because the annual medical examination insisted upon by the railways and performed by a different doctor resulted in him being sent to a heart specialist who reported that, because of his cardiovascular problems he should not be allowed to drive a train. He has been temporarily demoted to fireman and faces the prospect of retrenchment on the grounds of ill health.

1. How does the general practitioner manage the identity crisis that this man now faces, not only in his own mind but the image that he now presents to his family and work mates?
2. Is this man a risk as a train driver?
3. Should the doctor advise the patient to accept the findings?

P. F. Gill, Hobart

MRS. Q.R.   AGED 42   OFFICE MANAGER   118

The personnel manager of a large firm for which Mrs. Q.R. works telephones you as the family doctor of Mrs. Q.R. She is being considered for a promotion for which good health is a criterion. You are asked to provide the personnel manager with a report on Mrs. Q.R.'s health. This information will be kept confidential by the company.

1. Are you justified in discussing a patient's health with others without his or her knowledge?

2. If you obtained Mrs. Q.R.'s permission what information would you send to the personnel manager?
3. Can a pre-employment physical examination screen out employees who might later develop industrial diseases?
4. If a patient developed a serious medical problem which he wished kept secret would you notify others?

E. V. Dunn, Toronto

119 WADE D. AGED 4

4 year old Wade D. and his family have just moved to the city from a remote country town. Wade was discovered to have a heart murmur at birth but his parents were reassured that it was not important. As Wade has enjoyed good health and has been a vigorous and active child there seemed no reason to doubt the doctor's reassurance. But last week Wade's mother took him to the casualty of the local hospital to seek attention for a minor injury and the RMO told her that Wade had a heart murmur and that she should seek specialist advice.

1. Physical examination confirms that Wade has a mid-systolic murmur which is best heard over the upper praecordium. What characteristics of the murmur and what associated findings would enable you to assess its significance?
2. What important issue does this incident raise for Wade and his parents?

W. L. Ogborne, Sydney

120 MR. K.J. AGED 37 PLUMBER

Mr. K.J. had been a fit active man who worked long hours in his own plumbing business. He was happily married with 3 children aged 11, 6 and 4 years.

He had an influenzal illness and attended because he wanted to get back to work as soon as possible. Physical examination revealed no serious complications from his acute illness but on routine testing, he had a blood pressure of 160/105.

1. Describe the correct technique of recording blood pressure.
2. What other information would you wish to obtain?
3. What investigations would you perform?
4. How would you manage this case?
5. What are the long term benefits of treating hypertension?
6. Should general practitioners screen all patients for hypertension?

H. C. Watts, Perth, Australia

MRS. J.B.   AGED 49   HOUSEWIFE

121

A year after this patient was found to have uterine fibroids and iron deficiency anaemia, she presents to her family physician for a routine physical examination. In the past she was offered and turned down a hysterectomy. She has taken her iron medication irregularly. She has had regular rather heavy menses. Her physical examination is unchanged from the previous year. Her haemoglobin is 9 g/dl.

1. Should she have a hysterectomy?
2. Is the iron deficiency adequately rationalized by the fibroids and menorrhagia?
3. How should the physician act if the patient says, 'You are my doctor, I will leave it up to you'?

E. Domovitch, Toronto

MRS. JANICE L.   AGED 28   HOUSEWIFE

122

You have not seen Mrs. Janice L. before.

She has come about a head cold of a week's duration. You notice that she is sitting on the edge of her chair, has a tense body posture and generally looks anxious.

At the end of her opening statement, you say: 'Janice, you seem very tense'.

She begins to sob, and after being comforted explains, 'that things are tense between herself and her husband'. She goes on to note that she wasn't sure whether or not she was going to tell you about this, because she came last year about the problem but the doctor didn't seem interested. Rather than trying to overcome his disinterest, she had a routine vaginal examination, Pap. smear and went home.

1. How will you conduct the immediate portion of the consultation?
2. What circumstances create this kind of patient story?
3. What is the implication of her story for the practice you are working in?

M. W. Heffernan, Melbourne

CHAPTER 6

Emergencies

This chapter comprises a selection of emergencies which the family physician may be called upon to manage, including head and spinal injuries, respiratory obstruction, cardiac crises, severe infections, poisoning, psychiatric crises and other serious illness. It also addresses the question: 'What is an emergency?'.

This chapter, and the two following, which deal with attempted suicide and dying and death, illustrate the major life crises in which the family physician is involved.

123   **MRS. LOUISE A.**   **AGED 47**   **SOCIAL WORKER**

Mrs. A. is brought into your local hospital following a head-on motor accident, in which she was a front seat passenger. She is deeply unconscious and not responding to painful stimuli. She has a 5 cm laceration in the frontal region, which is bleeding steadily.

She is pale and sweating, her BP 60/40, her pulse 135, and her respiration is 24. There is no obvious injury elsewhere.

1. What is your immediate assessment of her condition?
2. What immediate action would you take?

W. E. Fabb, Melbourne

124   **MRS. JANICE B.**   **AGED 70**   **HOUSEWIFE**

You are called to see Mrs. B. who was brought into the casualty department in a country hospital in a shocked condition. She is the mother of a registered staff nurse at that particular hospital. The patient has been injured in a car accident and is bleeding from wounds to the chest. She refuses to have a blood transfusion as she is a Jehovah's Witness.

1. How would you handle this situation?
2. What do you need to do about the refusal of a blood transfusion?
3. What are some other aspects that have to be considered when a Jehovah's Witness patient requires a blood transfusion?

M. D. Mahoney, Brisbane

125   **MR. VICTOR R.**   **AGED 28**   **COUNCIL WORKER**

Mr. R. is brought into the local hospital following a side-on motor accident in which a truck slammed into the driver's side door of his sedan. He has severe pain in his neck, which he holds stiffly, aided by sandbags either side of his head. He was never unconscious.

He is conscious and alert, but in severe pain. His neck is very tender over the whole cervical spine and his paracervical muscles, which are in spasm. He has no other obvious external injury.

1. What injuries would you suspect?
2. What would you do for this man?

W. E. Fabb, Melbourne

126   **MR. R.C.**   **AGED 24**   **DRAFTSMAN**

Mr. R.C. was first seen entrapped in an overturned motor vehicle on a main highway 30 kilometres from the nearest small town with a cottage hospital, and 550 kilometres from a metropolitan centre.

An ambulance with two attendants arrived at the same time. The driver-wife has escaped virtually unscathed. The patient was complaining of extreme pain in his neck and was unable to move.

He was very tender over his lower cervical spine, was unable to move either his arms or his legs and had no sensation in his trunk. He was shocked and had a deformity with swelling in his right thigh.

1. What are the diagnoses?
2. What first aid measures would you adopt?
3. How should this man be evacuated and where to?
4. What measures can be taken to reduce accidents such as this?

R. W. Roberts, Ravensthorpe, Australia

T.H.   AGED 3   MALE CHILD   127

You and a colleague are talking in the driveway one Sunday morning having a beer. A 5-year-old girl from next door runs around and tells you that her brother is choking on some popcorn. You both rush in. The child is choking and unable to speak. He is still breathing, but is in obvious distress and is turning bluer. You make attempts to remove the popcorn, but you cannot find out where it is nor remove it. You take the child to the hospital and perform emergency tracheostomy. The child suffers from a pneumothorax but survives and eventually does well.

1. What should your initial management be in a case like this?
2. Was tracheostomy the correct move, or could some other manoeuvre have been performed?

J. K. Shearman, Hamilton, Canada

MR. BILL S.   AGED 50   ENGINEER   128

You are attending a Rotary Club dinner when one of your patients, Mr. Bill S. who is sitting a couple of tables away, suddenly stands up, bends over and appears breathless. There is a reddish fluid issuing from his mouth.

1. What are some of the thoughts that will be going through your head?
2. What should be your next step?
3. You have ascertained that he has been eating some meat and has had some wine. The assumption is that the meat has stuck in his throat.
4. What is the incidence of death in people who have choked on food?

M. D. Mahoney, Brisbane

129   DARYL A.   AGED 4

The anxious parents of this 4 year-old boy ask you to visit the home at 3 a.m. because Daryl has severe croup. The child was 'off-colour' when he went to bed, woke at midnight with a croupy cough, and now appears quite ill. The cough is not as noisy as before.

The child is sitting up, appears distressed by his respiratory efforts, is restless, and is dribbling saliva.

1. What diagnostic hypotheses are in your mind?
2. How would you establish a diagnosis?
3. How would you manage this situation?
4. What complications must be avoided?

W. E. Fabb, Melbourne

130   MR. C.K.   AGED 52   BUILDER

Mr. C.K. who has a known carcinoma of his lung, suddenly complains of chest pain and shortness of breath. On examination, his neck veins are markedly distended, heart sounds are distant, blood pressure has dropped to 88/56 with a pulse rate of 120 per minute and respiratory rate 40 per minute. Marked peripheral oedema is present.

1. What emergency investigation should be performed?
2. What emergency medical treatment would be administered?
3. What is the most likely diagnosis?

B. M. Fehler, Johannesburg

131   MR. F.R.   AGED 45   BUSINESSMAN

Mr. F.R. a 45 year old chainsmoking, overweight businessman complained to his wife that he was feeling unwell and collapsed on the floor. His wife immediately called for an ambulance and the attendants, who arrived in less than 5 minutes, found Mr. M.R. blue and pulseless. They began cardiopulmonary resuscitation at once and transported him to a nearby hospital where, after several attempts, the patient was successfully defibrillated and admitted to the intensive care unit. He was unconscious and required the constant assistance of a respirator.

Mrs. F.R. described her husband as a compulsive worker, who found it impossible to spend more than 2–3 hours away from his work, even on weekends. She has accepted his conviction, that while he has a business partner, the latter was unable to run the business without Mr. M.R. As a result, the family had not had a holiday in several years and the children and mother were very interdependent.

As Mr. F.R. returned to consciousness, his physician was elated to discover that he seemed not to have suffered any permanent brain damage, and he was likely to eventually return to work. It was however difficult to understand his apparent apathy about his business in light of his previous obsession that he was indispensable to the success of the business.

1. What is the likelihood that a patient will survive such an event?
2. What are the risk factors in such a patient?
3. What residual effects seem apparent and what might you expect in this case?

C. A. Moore, Hamilton, Canada

ERNEST C.   AGED 70   132

You are on call. It is 2 a.m. The phone rings. Mrs. C. calls in distress as Mr. C. has awakened with nausea and diarrhoea and is very breathless. They had been to a party that night.

You know that Mr. C. has had a laryngeal cancer treated by radiotherapy and 20 years ago he had radioactive iodine therapy for thyrotoxicosis. He had been fibrillating for 3 years and is on digoxin.

1. What do you say to Mrs. C.?
2. What would you take with you on a home visit to Mrs. C.?
3. You visit at home and he dies within 5 minutes of your arrival. What would you do?

J. Fry, Beckenham, UK

MRS. C.S.   AGED 68   HOUSEWIFE   133

You have been called urgently to see Mrs. C.S. by a neighbour, who informs you that the patient was eating supper when she suddenly became pale and said her heart was racing. She became breathless. Your examination reveals that the heart rhythm is regular but at a rate of 190 beats per minute. She has had several attacks, starting without warning. She is being treated for myxoedema.

1. How do you establish your diagnosis?
2. How do you stop this present attack?
3. What advice do you give the patient?
4. What complications can occur?

B. M. Fehler, Johannesburg

MR. C.   AGED 34   COMPANY EXECUTIVE   134

Mr. C. is very worried as he has been experiencing frequent palpitations recently. His visit has been precipitated by the recent death at work, from a heart attack, of a colleague. During your examination you note that he suddenly develops a tachycardia of 150 per minute. The remainder of your examination is normal.

1. What are the possible causes of the tachycardia?
2. What simple test may help to decide the nature of the rapid rhythm? How would the various possible causes respond to such a manoeuvre?
3. During the test the rate suddenly changes to 100 per minute. What is your presumed diagnosis?
4. What treatment will you prescribe?

J. R. Marshall, Adelaide

135 MISS J.C. AGED 16 STUDENT

For 13 years she has been aware of episodes of palpitations which seemed to be related to exercise and found it necessary to reduce her physical activity because of the attacks. The attacks began suddenly, usually related to exercise and lasted for periods of 10 to 30 minutes, with mild difficulty in getting her breath, but no chest pain. Once the attack had settled she felt perfectly well. No family or past history of heart trouble.

1. What is the most likely diagnosis?
2. What is the most likely cause?
3. What is the appropriate management?

D. S. Muecke, Adelaide

136 MRS. F.S. AGED 79 WIDOW

Mrs. F.S. lives in an expensive block of flats quite a long way from the nearest shopping centre to which she normally drives herself. Her husband who was 10 years older than Mrs. F.S. and was your patient, died suddenly 10 years ago and his death was certified as due to myocardial infarction. Mrs. F.S. has, since then, put herself under the care of your partner. She sends for a doctor on Sunday morning and you are on duty. Whilst Mrs. F.S. was having breakfast she experienced marked pain in her left arm and numbness in her left hand with which she cannot now grip things. She tells you she has had some claudication in both calves for some years and that your partner has been prescribing a peripheral vasodilator, chlorthalidone 100 mg twice a week, and digoxin 0.125 mg daily.

1. What are the likely diagnoses?
2. What are the possible social consequences of each of your differential diagnoses?
3. Do you have any comments on her present medication?

P. Freeling, London

BABY M.H.   AGED 14 DAYS

137

Mrs H. was formerly a school teacher, happily married, who had worked through the first 32 weeks of her uneventful pregnancy and had a normal vaginal delivery at term of an infant son, M.H., who weighed 3500 g at birth.

He was her first child, had no obvious congenital abnormalities, was fully breastfed and thrived, being discharged on the seventh day from hospital.

At 10.30 p.m. the mother rang to say that the baby had a cold with a snuffly nose for the preceding 36 hours but during the evening had seemed less well and was reluctant to feed. She thought he was quite ill.

1. What possible causes for these symptoms should be considered?
2. How do you recognise a seriously ill baby?
3. How do you arrive at a more precise diagnosis in this case?
4. How often do you make a correct diagnosis from information given in a telephone call?

H. C. Watts, Perth, Australia

DONNA L.   AGED 2

138

This 2 year old girl is brought in by her mother in the early evening because she has been unwell during the afternoon, sleeping most of the time and refusing food and fluids. She has had a mild 'cold' for a few days.

The child is very pale, listless and lies quietly in her mother's lap, often dozing off to sleep. Her skin feels very hot.

1. What diagnostic hypotheses would you entertain?
2. How would you establish a diagnosis?
3. How would you manage the situation?

W. E. Fabb, Melbourne

RODNEY O.   AGED 12 MONTHS

139

Worried parents bring their little boy to late night surgery, with a fever and 'collapsing legs'. He had been given a penicillin mixture five days previously by another doctor for an ear infection, and had seemed to be improving. Today he vomited, was very irritable and drowsy and was unable to stand.

Although neck rigidity is not present, he holds his head in retraction and cries on interference. His ears are normal, his chest clear. He has large, non-inflamed tonsils and enlarged soft cervical glands. His respirations are slightly increased and his temperature is 40 °C. All else is normal, except for a fine punctate erythematous rash on his upper abdomen and chest.

1. How would you manage this situation?
2. What other illnesses besides meningitis may cause neck retraction, or meningismus?

G. M. Dick, Hobart

140 TOM AGED 12 SCHOOLBOY

It was a severe 'flu' epidemic and the patients were very miserable. High fever, sore throat, headache and some stiffness of the neck, together with generalised aches and pains were the order of the day.

On his way home, Dr. D. was asked to see a 12 year old boy Tom who had apparently developed the 'flu'. He examined him carefully and found nothing other than the same picture that he had seen in probably eight or nine other people that day. He explained carefully to the mother how 'flu' was due to a virus and how viruses were unresponsive to antibiotics. A palliative mixture was prescribed.

Early the next morning around 5 a.m. the phone rang. 'Tom seems worse doctor and he has some dark blue patches on his skin'. Dr. D. was out of bed and at Tom's place within 15 minutes. The description was accurate. Dr. D. gave an immediate injection and accompanied Tom in the ambulance to the hospital. He improved initially but died within 48 hours.

1. What was the syndrome this boy suffered from?
2. What is the best treatment of meningococcal meningitis?

J. G. Richards, Auckland

141 DEBBIE G. AGED 3

Mrs. G., who is 6 months pregnant, rings in a panic one Saturday afternoon because she has discovered her daughter, Debbie, playing with some bottles of tablets which she discovered on Mrs. G.'s dressing table.

The tablets were ferrous sulphate tablets, some of which she believes Debbie has eaten, paracetamol tablets, and a packet of oral contraceptives.

Debbie has also spilt Mrs. G.'s nail polish remover all over the dressing table. Debbie appears to be quite well.

1. How would you manage this situation?
2. What measures would you institute after the crisis was over to avoid such a situation in the future?

3. What do you do in your practice to avoid accidental poisoning amongst your patients?

W. E. Fabb, Melbourne

MRS. LOUISE A.   AGED 48   HOUSEWIFE/CLERK   **142**

You have been caring for Louise for 15 months at the time of this incident.

She first came along deeply depressed and has made good progress. You are comfortable in the psychotherapeutic role and have not sought specialist help. After overcoming her initial depression, Louise still attends because she is undergoing significant growth, and finds counselling useful during this time.

A week ago, as a consequence of a major family disruption, she became acutely depressed and went to bed. Her husband rang you from work at 7 a.m. to tell you of this, seeking a home visit. After discussion with him, and after talking to Louise (this phone call was a psychotherapy consultation) you agreed to visit.

At that visit, and in the presence of Louise's daughter, you used neuro-linguistic techniques to 'reframe' Louise, commenced her on the anti-depressant which had previously been effective for her and arranged for her husband to update you later in the day.

She recovered quickly and though distressed, was able to attend an important family gathering the next day.

You saw her the next day (on a Saturday afternoon – the first available time for you) and at that consultation you arranged to be kept in touch by phone, and to see her in four days time.

On this occasion, Louise began the consultation by saying:

'What's the real problem with me?'
'It can't just be depression. You've shown so much concern and consideration.'
'I've never had a house call before. I realise it might just be you and the way you work. Do you do this for all your patients? Are you sure I haven't got something else?'
'I mean . . . I'm a mother. I've had sick children . . . lots of doctors. Nobody has treated me like this before or visited me at home.'

1. What are some of the characteristics of this doctor–patient relationship?
2. What are the implications of this statement for:
   – day-to-day general practice?
   – the vocational training of general practitioners?
   – the vocational training of other specialties?

M. W. Heffernan, Melbourne

143 MRS. R. AGED 82

Mrs. Robinson, 82, was found lying on her bedroom floor one winter morning. She had apparently been there for several hours, was drowsy, and could not remember what had happened.

In the hospital emergency room, she was pale, disoriented and slow. Vital signs: P 60, irregular, R 12, BP 85/50, T 30 °C. Her voice was gruff and hoarse, and speech slurred. Her pupils were contracted. She was able to move all four extremities with difficulty. There was rigidity of the neck muscles. All tendon reflexes were sluggish. The contraction and relaxation phase of the ankle jerk were prolonged. There was tenderness in the epigastrium, some distension of the abdomen, rigidity of the abdominal wall and diminished bowel sounds. Moist sounds were present at both lung bases.

1. What are your working diagnoses?
2. What is your first priority in treatment?
3. What essential information should you find out from the neighbours and relatives?

G. Williams, Iowa City

144 MR. C.R. AGED 31 BUSINESSMAN

Mr. C.R. was admitted to hospital after a three week illness that began with a sore throat and included malaise, myalgia, headache and general weakness. Three days prior to admission he developed a fever with chills and low back pain. His temperature was recorded as high as 41 °C. The patient noted that his urine was dark and his eyes were slightly yellow. The only drugs that he had taken during this illness were aspirin with codeine, and he had not been exposed to any other chemicals. His previous health was excellent. His wife and two small children were not ill and the patient had not, to his knowledge, been exposed to infection.

On initial examination he was acutely ill, pale and sweating. His oral temperature was 39 °C. He had mild scleral icterus. His pharynx appeared normal and there was no cervical lymphadenopathy. He was dyspnoeic with slight exertion but not orthopnoeic, and the lungs were clear. Cardiac rate was 84/min and the BP was 120/65. There were no murmurs and no signs of congestive heart failure. The liver was not enlarged but the edge was tender. The spleen was enlarged 4 cm below the left costal margin and was tender to palpation. There was bilateral costovertebral angle tenderness.

The haemoglobin was 5.8 g/dl, the white blood count was 22,000 with 65% lymphocytes, most of which were atypical. Sedimentation rate was 118 mm/h. Serum bilirubin was 3.0 mg total with 0.6 mg/dl direct. The SGOT was 81 units. The Paul Bunnell test was positive with a high titre.

The patient's blood group was established to be A Rh positive and attempts to transfuse him because of his acute anaemia were difficult unless the blood was pre-warmed and kept warm during transfusion. The direct Coombs' test was positive and the acute haemolytic reaction was determined to be due to a cold agglutinin which was shown to be inactive at temperatures above 32 °C.

The patient's condition worsened over the first 2 days in hospital, and 5 units of blood raised his haemoglobin to only 9 g/dl. Once the characteristics of the cold agglutinin had been identified, it was decided to treat the patient by warming his environment, so he was placed in a private room heated to over 32 °C and maintained at that temperature. Within 12 hours there was dramatic improvement in his clinical condition and within 1 week his spleen was no longer palpably enlarged. The haemoglobin had risen to 11 g/dl. After 2 weeks the cold agglutinins of high thermal amplitude were no longer present in the patient's serum and it was possible to gradually cool his room to normal temperatures. This patient's treatment did not include any drug therapy. His clinical improvement continued and he has not had any further problem with this illness.

1. What steps are important in the management of seriously ill patients?
2. What essential data are required to determine the treatment of this patient?
3. What is the role of the family physician after he has called in a consultant?

R. L. Perkin, Toronto

BABY G. AGED 5 MONTHS 145

Despite being told by the receptionist that you have no free appointments until tomorrow and that only urgent cases can be fitted in, Mrs. G. has insisted that her baby must be seen.

Although you appreciate that he is her first child you are rather surprised to find that the problem is only a moderately severe nappy rash.

1. Who should decide which cases need to see the doctor quickly and which can safely wait?
2. Are barriers between patients and GPs necessary?
3. What possible explanations are there for Mrs. G's behaviour?
4. What are the principles of management of nappy rash?

A. J. Moulds, Basildon, UK

MRS. P.J. AGED 29 TEACHER 146

She phoned for an emergency consultation asking to be added to the end of the evening's list. She was noted to be upset on arrival and crying in the waiting room.

'I don't know what you'll think of me – I've been such a fool!' were her opening words.

She had had intercourse with a fellow teacher after school at his home – at the time of ovulation – the condom had burst – she had been trying to 'fall' pregnant by her husband.

1. What are the patient's two main problems?
2. What types of patient problems need doctor orientation solutions and what need patient orientation solutions?

F. Mansfield, Perth, Australia

CHAPTER 7

Attempted Suicide

This chapter illustrates one of the ways in which some people may respond to stress and disaster – attempted suicide. Some of the attempts are genuine, some are gestures. Whatever the background, these cases place the family physician under considerable personal stress. They constitute, with the cases in the previous chapter on emergencies and in the following chapter on dying and death, the major life crises in which the family physician becomes involved, and address the question of how he responds, both professionally and personally, to these crises.

147   MR. H.C.   AGED 60   RETIRED GENERAL MANAGER

Mr. H.C. has been increasingly depressed over huge losses of his savings in the stock market. You have been called by his family at 2 a.m. as he was found attempting to gas himself in the kitchen of his high rise flat.

On arrival you found him in a severely agitated state having to be restrained by members of his family. You tried to calm him without avail. Your offer of medication to help him feel better was refused. He also refused to be admitted to the hospital.

Being burly and agitated he could not be restrained for long. You have noticed that the door to the balcony is open and that he is heading in that direction.

1. What immediate steps would you take in such a situation?
2. How would you manage him after his discharge from hospital?
3. What are some of the problems associated with high rise flats?

F. E. H. Tan, Kuala Lumpur

148   MR. S.T.   AGED 40   OCCUPATION UNKNOWN

You are on duty in the emergency department (casualty ward) at 2 p.m. You are faced with an apparently inebriated man bleeding from deep cuts on both wrists. He looks shocked – pulse 110, BP 84/50. He is lucid and vehemently refuses any treatment except pressure bandages. You consult a surgeon just finishing in the operating room and you both feel that immediate transfusion is necessary.

1. Can you treat a patient against his will?
2. What is informed consent for treatment?

E. V. Dunn, Toronto

149   MR. B.S.   AGED 44   BUSINESSMAN

The doctor is phoned on his evening off-duty by a policeman to say that he has just taken a gun from your patient, Mr. S. who has threatened to kill himself.

On reviewing matters in Mr. S.'s home unit, it transpires that he has finally separated from his second wife. He states that they had sexual problems after the birth of their only child and that he is under a great deal of pressure in a new job as a result of proposed changes in the way the business is to operate. His managing director does not know about Mr. S.'s personal problems. Mr. S. admits to becoming a workaholic as a substitute for losing his wife. She has stated categorically that she does not want to see him again. He is physically well and follows a strict exercise programme. He lives alone and normally consumes very little alcohol. On this occasion, however, he has drunk a bottle of port wine.

1. What responsibilities are involved when a primary care doctor is committed to continuity of patient care?
2. How often does change in life circumstances induce psychiatric illness?
3. What immediate help does this man require?

B. H. Connor, Armidale, Australia

MRS. A.B.   AGED 34   HOUSEWIFE

150

This woman was brought into a country hospital by her husband with a story of having taken somewhere between 25 and 30 of her husband's Serepax 15 mg tablets 45 minutes ago. She smells of alcohol, is fully conscious, belligerent, non co-operative and does not wish to get out of the car or go into the hospital and have treatment. After some discussion she agrees to stay in hospital for observation only if the husband goes back to look after the seven children, aged 18 months to 14 years left in their caravan. The husband leaves after stating they had a row when his wife had got back from the hotel and there was no meal prepared.

1. What would be the basis of your discussion with the woman in the car?
2. What would be your management of the problem once she was admitted to hospital?
3. What long term management would you suggest?

T. D. Manthorpe, Port Lincoln, Australia

MISS A.G.   AGED 30   BUYER

151

Miss A.G. who is single, last visited the office more than 2 years ago. She is attractive and independent, living alone in a flat which she owns and working as a buyer for a large retail organization. She appears cheerful and complains only of a sore throat. Her throat appears normal and she is reassured and leaves the office after a brief chat. The following day she is admitted to hospital after having taken an overdose of paracetamol and alcohol.

1. To what conditions are the single as opposed to the married members of the population more susceptible?
2. What is the differential diagnosis of sore throat?
3. What is the principal danger of paracetamol overdosage?

T. A. I. Bouchier Hayes, Camberley, UK

MR. & MRS. H.   AGED 40

152

A 40 year old, good-looking, socially prominent, successful insurance agent with a history of unilateral orchidectomy at age 30 for seminoma presents complaining that his wife, a seductively-attractive former airline stewardess, is making his life miserable with accusations of infidelity, which he denies. They are contemplating – and indeed proceeding to – divorce. They have three children, two sons 10 and 15 years old at home and a 17 year old daughter institutionalized with spastic cerebral palsy. Mother takes an overdose of alcohol and sleeping pills four weeks before the custody trial which you are asked to attend.

1. Whose side are you on anyway?
2. Is mother mentally ill?
3. Is father a good risk for a second marriage?

P. R. Grantham, Vancouver

153 SUSAN AGED 19 SCHOOL LEAVER

In the morning's mail is a request from a doctor in occupational health, requesting information on Susan's past health and your opinion on her fitness to undergo training to be a nurse. He encloses a slip of paper with Susan's written permission 'for information from my medical records to be given to the doctor'.

Susan, aged 19 years, has suffered from asthma and eczema since birth. She has not allowed this problem to intrude into her life. She has left school with good academic qualifications. The last entry in her notes reminds you that one month previously she went through an adolescent crisis, in which she took an overdose (60, 0.5 g tabs paracetamol and 20 aspirin tablets), but surprised herself by surviving. Somehow she managed to keep the affair to herself, and indeed the matter only came out as a result of your probing at the consultation.

1. In sharing information with colleagues, what considerations need to be taken into account?
2. Overdose with paracetamol, even if not associated with a fatal outcome, may cause structural damage. Which organs may bear the brunt?
3. What is meant by the term 'adolescent crisis'?

J. D. E. Knox, Dundee

CHAPTER 8

Dying and Death

Of all of life's crises, there can be few which equal that of dying and death. The family physician needs to be able to manage, both professionally and personally, these demanding situations. This and the two previous chapters on emergencies and attempted suicide comprise the major life crises the family physician is called upon to manage.

The cases selected for this chapter illustrate the challenge of terminal care in chronic illness, such as cancer in an adult or a child, address the ethical problem of withholding treatment in terminal illness, illustrate the need for good doctor-patient communication and understanding, deal with the problem of sudden and unexpected death, and consider the bereavement process.

154 MRS. B.C. AGED 31 HOUSEMINDER

Mrs. B.C., aged 31, had been a patient for several years but had emigrated to another country. She returned after 2 years for an extended holiday and came back to her old family physician for a 'check up'.

She stated that she had odd aches and pains in her abdomen and she 'was a bit worried about her periods which had become scanty and she'd had the occasional break-through bleed'. She had been on the contraceptive pill for 7 of the last 11 years.

Her husband, aged 33, was a skilled technician and there were two sons aged 6 and 8 years.

The doctor had originally felt that they had left their country partly as a 'geographical' solution to their problems and this was discussed with Mrs. C. prior to her departure.

Examination revealed a normotensive patient and no breast lumps. Her urine contained no protein or sugar. Vaginal examination revealed a soft well defined cystic mass in the right adnexa. A Papanicolaou smear was taken.

The doctor informed the patient of his findings and said he would like to refer her to a gynaecologist. He felt that this was a benign cystic mass.

At operation, with the doctor assisting, third stage carcinoma of the ovary was found.

The doctor visited the patient in hospital and saw her regularly thereafter. She was also attending the 'Combined Cancer Clinic' at the hospital.

On one occasion, she brought in her two children for minor complaints. They both looked depressed. After they were examined, the mother wanted them to leave the room – 'they know nothing' she said. The doctor stated that he wished to talk with them while mother was there – of course with her permission.

At another consultation 6 months later, she stated that her husband wanted to go back to their adoptive country and she felt guilty about holding him back. Her mother was also getting on her nerves and she'd lost interest in sex.

At several of the consultations, she discussed her prognosis, her hospital management, her fears, thoughts of the future and her 'feelings'.

1. What is the incidence of carcinoma of the ovary in family practice?
2. What possible interactions could have occurred between the doctor and Mrs. C. on informing her of her diagnosis?
3. On diagnosis, should the doctor initiate 'care of the dying'?
4. What changes in family dynamics could you expect in this situation?

J. H. Levenstein, Cape Town

MISS J.C.   AGED 80   RETIRED SECRETARY

155

Miss J.C. previously enjoyed good health, except for peripheral vascular disease with mild claudication (despite being a non-smoker). She lived alone in her own small home and, being in full possession of her mental faculties, lived an active life in the local community.

She presented complaining of difficulty in swallowing all solid food with a sense of obstruction at the level of the lower chest. This had come on increasingly over the preceding 6 weeks. She suspected that she had something 'serious' but declared that if she did, she did not want any surgical procedure as she would like to die in peace. She did agree to have a barium swallow which revealed an annular constriction of the lower oesophagus, highly suspicious of carcinoma of the oesophagus.

1. How would you manage her when she returned for the result of the barium swallow?
2. How would you organize her terminal care in your practice?
3. Should patients with malignancy be told their diagnosis and prognosis?

H. C. Watts, Perth, Australia

MR. G.T.   AGED 48   COMPANY DIRECTOR

156

Mr. G.T. was well known to his general practitioner, who had been treating him for many years for a duodenal ulcer and psoriasis. He was a heavy smoker, a director of his own very successful firm, and worked hard and long hours. He had few other interests. He and his wife had had serious sexual difficulties due to her vaginismus. They had achieved full sexual intercourse only once when their son, now 14 years, was conceived.

He presented with central chest pain on exertion which the doctor thought was probably ischaemic. However, it was not quite typical and he was referred to hospital where he was found to have a pericardial effusion associated with carcinoma of the bronchus with extensive mediastinal spread. He was offered no treatment.

When he returned home, he understood that the diagnosis was heart trouble and expected to recover with rest. His wife saw the doctor on her own before he came home and insisted that he should not be told the diagnosis at any stage. She also insisted that her son should not be told that his father had a serious illness. She was determined to care for her husband at home until he died. She accompanied him on every visit to the office and later never left him alone with the doctor when she called to see him at home. He became increasingly depressed at his lack of progress but did not ask the doctor any direct questions. His physical symptoms were well controlled but although he had previously been on very friendly terms with the doctor, he became more distant and hostile and appeared not to trust her. She felt she was letting him down.

1. Do you think patients should be told when they are suffering from cancer?
2. Do you think this particular situation was made more difficult by the fact that the doctor was a woman?
3. How important is peace of mind to the dying patient?
4. How would you have managed this situation?

G. Strube, Crawley, UK

157 R.C.   AGED 6   PRE-SCHOOL

You practice single-handed in an isolated country town with a cottage hospital.

This child, from a family in your area, is discharged from a metropolitan hospital with terminal illness due to a posterior fossa intracranial tumour. The parents have asked you to treat the condition and are anxious to have the patient at home.

1. What are the main problems involved?
2. What assistance can you mobilize?

R. W. Roberts, Ravensthorpe, Australia

158 MR. J.B.   AGED 72   RETIRED LABOURER

Mr. J.B. an active, pleasant 72 year old, presented at his family physician's office with a history of weight loss, anorexia and an ability to tolerate only very small meals. There was no apparent melaena or vomiting of blood.

A barium meal showed a shrunken stomach which appeared to be thick walled and demonstrated very little peristaltic activity.

When the diagnosis was discussed with the patient and his wife they decided, and the doctor concurred, that he should not undergo a definitive surgical procedure. After the couple went through an agonising spectrum of various emotional responses concerning his diagnosis, they decided that Mr. J.B. would remain at home until either his wife was unable to care for him, or pain release could not be adequately provided in the home setting.

His family physician visited him regularly at home and a number of community services were mobilized to assist the patient and his wife. When towards the end, he was hospitalized, the patient, his wife and the family physician were able to convince the other members of the hospital staff that intravenous, gastric tubes and similar strategies which might prolong life, were not to be part of his management. It was also agreed that a no resuscitation order was to be placed on his chart.

1. What is the likely diagnosis?

2. What are the emotional stages you might expect the patient and his wife to undergo?
3. What resources are available to assist in keeping a patient at home?
4. What are the relative merits of a patient being allowed to die at home versus in the hospital?
5. What is the family physician's role at home and in the hospital?

C. A. Moore, Hamilton, Canada

R.T.   AGED 40   SOLICITOR (MARRIED, YOUNG SON)   159

Mr. R.T. has a past history of a condition running a protracted course for years producing at various times iritis, polyarthritis, urethral discharge. Ultimately presented with severe left lower lobe pneumonia which failed to resolve with treatment. Developed an effusion which was tapped and tomograms revealed a mass near the hilum. Options for further treatment were discussed and pneumonectomy subsequently carried out. Immediate response was good but the patient died nine weeks after initial presentation.

1. What determines whether pneumonia is fully investigated?
2. How might carcinoma of the lung be identified when associated with pneumonia?
3. To whom and by whom should treatment options be presented and discussed?
4. What will influence your management of impending, inevitable death in this relatively young man?

W. D. Jackson, Launceston, Australia

MR. F.   AGED 53   SHOP ASSISTANT   160

Mr. F. presented with a history of coughing for 5 days with slight blood-streaking of the sputum. The GP prescribed antibiotics and asked him to report back in a week's time. At this point he referred him for a chest X-ray. The chest X-ray showed a suspicious shadow and bronchoscopy revealed advanced carcinoma of the bronchus which proved to be inoperable. The patient's wife appeared at the GP's rooms to inform him of the outcome of the investigations and angrily told him that he should have sent him for a chest X-ray when he first saw him with blood-stained sputum.

1. Why did the GP not refer the patient for chest X-ray on the first consultation?
2. How should the GP have managed the situation when confronted by the patient's wife?
3. How would you manage this situation further?

S. Levenstein, Cape Town

161 THE E. FAMILY

The E. family have been patients for the last 12 years. They are a close family unit. There are 3 children, 2 boys and a girl, and all in their teens at the time of presentation of this problem.

Mrs. E. aged 46, came to the office in an agitated state saying that 3 days ago whilst on a short holiday she had felt a lump in her right breast. She had returned as quickly as possible to see her own general practitioner.

Two weeks previously in the absence of her own doctor she had had a routine examination and a cervical cytology smear by another member of the same practice. She had been assured quite specifically that there were no lumps in her breast.

Immediate surgical treatment was arranged. Her general practitioner assisted at the operation. Frozen section biopsy confirmed carcinoma, and immediate mastectomy was performed. Clinically there was axillary glandular involvement. (This was subsequently confirmed by histo-pathology.)

At the conclusion of the operation the general practitioner enquired of the young surgeon who had performed technically a very adequate operation, what arrangements he had made to discuss the outcome with Mr. E. or the family. He replied, 'I expect he will contact me if he wants to know anything'.

The general practitioner on returning to his office from the hospital found Mr. E. and the elder son waiting to discuss the outcome of the operation with him. Both, but particularly the son, were naturally very upset and disturbed at the news. They quickly assessed all the implications.

Mrs. E. quite rapidly developed evidence of local recurrences, followed by liver and extensive bone metastases. She died exactly 2 years after her operation.

1. What is meant by 'responsibility' in general medical practice?
2. What is the role of the general practitioner in terminal care?

D. A. Game, Adelaide

162 MRS. MARY M.   AGED 75   PENSIONER

Mrs. M. has been looked after for 10 years by her general practitioner in a nursing home, where she was admitted suffering from mental confusion. For the last 4 years she has been bedfast, has not communicated with anyone, and is doubly incontinent. Her husband no longer comes to see her because he finds it too distressing. Her physical condition is generally good. The doctor has been called to see her because she has developed a fever of 39 °C, a cough, and some increase in respiratory rate. Auscultation of her chest reveals scattered rhonchi and crepitations.

1.   How should she be treated?
2.   Are there any grounds for withholding antibiotic therapy?
3.   What are the main causes of dementia in elderly patients?

J. G. P. Ryan, Brisbane

MRS. ROSE Y.   AGED 61   HOUSEWIFE   163

For the last 5 years Mrs. Y. had been under treatment for a carcinoma of the right breast. Radical mastectomy and radiation had been carried out initially, but 12 months later the patient developed evidence of lung secondaries with a pleural effusion. Response to high dosage of oestrogen was for some time quite dramatic, but eventually this therapy failed and it was decided after specialist consultation to commence treatment with cytotoxic drugs. This was reasonably successful but the patient still had some pain and the cytotoxics caused considerable distress because of the associated nausea, vomiting and diarrhoea. The patient was seen frequently by the general practitioner and one day she stated that she did not wish to continue with the cytotoxic drugs. She died 5 months later.

1.   What should have been the general practitioner's response to the patient's request to be taken off the chemotherapy?
2.   If specific therapy is ceased, what overall treatment plan must be followed by the general practitioner in the ensuing months?

J. G. P. Ryan, Brisbane

MRS. C.   AGED 76   164

Mrs. C. suffered from severe congestive failure controlled initially by appropriate treatment. It became obvious over some months that she was not taking her tablets and she became very ill. She refused admission to hospital saying she had had a good life, and had nothing further to live for. Finally she asked her doctor if he would give her an injection or tablets to end her life. This was discussed at length and another visit arranged for two days time. At the second visit her son had materialized and expressed concern and she agreed to enter hospital. She died the morning following her admission.

1.   How would you cope with this patient's request?
2.   Although sick, her sudden death was unexpected – or was it?
3.   Could this outcome have been changed in any way?

A. L. A. Reid, Newcastle, Australia

165 PENNY AGED 11

A phone call from Penny's aunt, saying she was calling on behalf of Penny's mother. She said the father had died at work the day before and the child had gone to sleep only in the wee hours of the morning after crying for hours. She had been very excitable all day, not letting her mother out of her sight. Would I please send some Valium round to make her sleep tonight?

1. What would you send?
2. Why is considerable criticism levelled at the family physician/ general practitioner in relation to the bereaved?
3. Is grief a natural physiological process?
4. What would you do if the mother reported six months after her husband's death that the child was still sleeping badly and was also having some behaviour problems?

A. J. Radford, Adelaide

166 NICHOLAS P. AGED 16

This boy, starting his O-level year at school, came to the doctor as he was anxious about his school work. He was worried about exams and about his future ability to find a job. This was discussed with his tutor at school who said that Nicholas was above average in ability and he should have no difficulty in obtaining good grades in his exams. Nevertheless this crisis of confidence interfered with his school work and he became depressed. In spite of every encouragement from the staff he was brought home by a teacher because he was crying at school.

When Nicholas was 5 years old, his mother had died from a cerebral tumour. His father remarried very happily and Nicholas formed a very good relationship with his stepmother and her son.

He was referred to the child psychiatrist, who discovered that what was really bothering Nicholas was his deceased mother. The start of his 'depression' coincided with his secret visit to the local crematorium. As he was only 5 when his mother died he knew very little about her and the stepmother felt that as father had remarried, he had not really mentioned his first wife. There followed a long discussion on the importance of giving Nicholas' mother her right place in the family and to organize a remembrance day so that she would always be remembered. This interview completely changed Nicholas and he became a normal happy extrovert teenager and there was no further difficulty with his school work.

1. What is the importance of a normal grief reaction?

A. G. Strube, Crawley, UK

MRS. G.N.   AGED 53   SHOPKEEPER

Mrs. G.N. rings one of the new doctors in a large group practice with the following request – 'Doctor, what is a myocardial infarction? It is on my late husband's death certificate. He died suddenly 9 months ago on the way to hospital in the ambulance. Dr. W. made the house call, Dr. X. was his doctor, and Dr. Y. is my doctor but I have not been able to bring myself to talk to any of them about it. I thought it would be better to speak to an independent doctor.'

1. What is this person trying to say?
2. Has the medical profession failed in the management of this problem?
3. How should Dr. Z. manage this problem?

J. E. Murtagh, Melbourne

MRS. LUCY O.   AGED 24   HOUSEWIFE

You are called urgently by a frantic mother to a farmhouse 5 miles from your office, where she has found her 3 month-old baby dead in its cot. She had put the baby down for its morning sleep only an hour before discovering it lying on its face, blue and mottled, with vomitus around its lips. She had tried mouth to mouth resuscitation, but wasn't sure how to do it. She called the ambulance, which arrived 15 minutes before you, and the ambulance drivers too had tried unsuccessfully to resuscitate the baby.
On your arrival, you confirm that the baby is dead.

1. What immediate reactions might you anticipate from the mother?
2. What would you do immediately?
3. What long term reactions should you anticipate?
4. What follow up would you organize?

W. E. Fabb, Melbourne

MRS. H.K.   AGED 34   HOUSEWIFE

Mrs. H.K. had been married for 12 years when she finally managed to conceive. After an uneventful pregnancy and uncomplicated delivery she produced a delightful baby boy. Almost as soon as she returned home from hospital she became a frequent attender at the office. Every minor alteration in the baby's behaviour precipitated a consultation and at various times she reported feeding difficulties, cough, snuffles, colic and change in bowel habit. The baby was examined at each visit and no significant abnormality was ever found. On two occasions upper respiratory tract symptoms were treated with nose drops. He appeared to the doctor to be a cheerful, thriving child and mother was constantly reassured about his good health and normal development.

At the age of 7 months, 2 days after one of his frequent office visits when again nothing abnormal had been found, the baby was found dead in his cot in the early hours of the morning.

1. What are your criteria for diagnosing primary infertility?
2. What does this mother's behaviour illustrate?
3. Of what syndrome is this baby's death an example?

T. A. I. Bouchier Hayes, Camberley, UK

170 MRS. MARGARET K.   AGED 36   HOUSEWIFE

Margaret is a distraught young mother of two children. Forty-eight hours previously her 6 year old daughter had come into the house and told her that Daddy, who was out gardening, was lying in a flower bed and making funny noises. She had rushed outside to find her husband of 38 years lying face down, blue in the face and making gurgling noises. She had turned him over and then rushed to a neighbour for help. When they returned there was no sound from her husband, and all attempts to revive him failed. An ambulance took him at speed to hospital, but he was dead on arrival. She is tearful and full of guilt.

1. Discuss cardiopulmonary resuscitation.
2. How would you handle Margaret in this situation?
3. Discuss the impact and consequences of sudden death in a family.

K. C. Nyman, Perth, Australia

171 MR. O.M.   AGED 91   PENSIONER

It is the seventh day of a heat wave (each day has been over 38 °C). You are called by this man's stepson who went to visit his stepfather and found him dead on the floor of his bedroom. The old man, who was unknown to you, was previously a patient of one of your partners and had not been seen by the practice for fifteen months.

When you arrive you find the body lying fully clothed and face down on the floor. A small amount of dried blood has come from an abrasion on his cheek. Although rigor mortis and hypostasis are present the body is noticeably hot.

1. What are the possible causes of death?
2. In your examination how do you determine how long a body has been dead?
3. Can you issue a death certificate?

D. S. Pedler, Adelaide

MISS A.   AGED 81   PENSIONER

172

Miss A., aged 81, put up a game fight with two teenage youths when she was mugged 3 weeks ago. She was treated at casualty for undisplaced fractures of the left humerus and the left inferior pubic ramus. While convalescing at the home of her widowed sister, she suddenly becomes confused, incontinent and has developed a right hemiplegia. You are called back to the house 12 hours later, to find her dead.

1. What does the family doctor take into account in 'diagnosing' death?
2. What medico-legal implications are there in Miss A.'s case?
3. What assistance can the family doctor provide for Miss A.'s sister?

J. D. E. Knox, Dundee

CHAPTER 9

Contraception and Family Planning

Contraception and family planning constitute a major part of the family physician's work. The cases and questions in this chapter illustrate the variety of issues which he faces – advising on different contraceptive methods, providing contraception for adolescents including those below the age of consent, dealing with unwanted pregnancy and requests for abortion, responding to requests for sterilization and the problems this may create, and dealing with the problem of infertility. The vexed questions of confidentiality and the rights of parents in teenage pregnancy and contraception are addressed in several cases.

173   MISS M.N.   AGED 18   SHOP ASSISTANT

Miss M.N. presented in a state of great consternation. 'Doctor, I'm scared I'm pregnant. But how can I be? I'm on the pill?'

1. List in rank order the level of efficacy of the usual methods of contraception.
2. Pill failure does occur. List the reasons.
3. List the contraindications (relative and absolute) for giving oral contraceptives. There are over 15 of each!

A. J. Radford, Adelaide

174   MISS I.J.   AGED 20   STORE CLERK

Miss I.J. is a sexually active unmarried woman living with two female friends. She suffers from moderately severe acne and migraine headaches. She had one episode of pelvic inflammatory disease 18 months ago. She presents in your office requesting birth control advice.

1. What are the relatively effective birth control modalities?
2. Does I.J. have absolute contraindications to any of these methods?
3. How can you help I.J. to decide what is best for her?
4. How would you follow-up the patient with each method you might use?

E. V. Dunn, Toronto

175   THREE MISSES

Miss J.P. aged 19 is a beautifully groomed casino croupier. Works until 3 a.m. each morning. She lives in a flat with her boyfriend who is a waiter at the same hotel. She requests sleeping pills, and a repeat of her contraceptive pill.

Miss V.C. is 18 years old, has left home and lives in a flat with her boyfriend. They are both out of work. She is on the pill from the family planning clinic. She requests 'nerve pills' and a repeat of her contraceptive pill.

Miss M.B. an 18 year old, sensible, friendly computer programmer, living at home, has a boy friend and is on the pill. She complains of frequent headaches. On thorough physical examination, she passes as a healthy young adult. She wants headache pills ('aspirin and codeine don't work'), and a repeat of her contraceptive pill.

1. Are all these young women suffering from similar problems?
2. Should any of these patients achieve their initial expectations?
3. What problems has the doctor at these interviews?

G. M. Dick, Hobart

MISS C.M.   AGED 15   SCHOOLGIRL

176

This young girl, rather mature for her age, consults you with a request for oral contraception. She has recently started having intercourse with her boyfriend, aged 17 years. She has a stable background, no history of physical or psychological abnormality and no significant family history.

1. What are the legal and moral implications of advising this girl on contraception?
2. What further questions would you wish to ask her?
3. What examination would you perform and why?
4. If you decide to prescribe an oral contraceptive, which product would you choose?
5. What routine surveillance procedures would be appropriate?

E. C. Gambrill, Crawley, UK

DIANA W.   AGED 15

177

Diana W. came to see her doctor asking if she could be put on an oral contraceptive. Her mother, who was a teacher and known to the doctor personally, had telephoned earlier to say she did not wish her daughter to be given contraception, and asked that her intervention be kept confidential.

1. What are the pros and cons of putting a teenager on an oral contraceptive?
2. How do you supervise patients on oral contraceptives?
3. How would you respond to the mother's request?

J. C. Hasler, Oxford

MISS J.E.   AGED 15   SCHOOLGIRL

178

Although 15, Miss J.E. could pass for a mature 18 year old. The first time you saw her you asked a number of standard information gathering questions, one of which was 'Are you using any form of contraception?' She replied in the negative.

About 2 weeks later her mother came to see you to tell you politely but firmly that her daughter did not need contraception and that she would prefer you not to offer it again. You explained you did not offer but merely asked if it was already being used, and parted amicably.

The next week Miss J.E. returned to ask you to prescribe the pill. She had been 'sleeping with her boyfriend' for 3 months and has used your remark about contraception to see how her parents reacted. The fuss convinced her that she was better not to tell them that she was going to start the pill.

When you try to persuade her to talk the matter over with her parents she is adamant that she will not and wants your assurance that her consultation is confidential.

1. Is confidentiality an outdated concept?
2. Should you prescribe the pill for her?
3. What factors should be considered before starting a young girl on the pill?

A. J. Moulds, Basildon, UK

179 JANET R.   AGED 15   SCHOOLGIRL

Janet R., is the youngest of seven brothers and sisters. Her father works as an unskilled labourer, and her mother as a domestic help. Her parents were born in Morocco. 'Doctor' she says, 'I need a prescription for the pill'.

1. What is the family doctor's professional responsibility to a legal minor?
2. What other factors could affect the doctor's response to her request?
3. What are the special risks of teenage pregnancies?
4. What other problems of adolescents are relevant to the family physician?

Z. Cramer, Tel-Aviv, Israel

180 HIGH SCHOOL STUDENTS

You lecture regularly, at a local high school counsellor's request, to mixed classes of 17-year olds on human sexuality, including contraception. One Sunday at 8.00 a.m. you are phoned at home by what sounds like an adolescent male who 'has a friend whose condom broke last night' wanting to know what to do.

1. Is it appropriate to manage this problem over the phone?
2. How effective are the various methods of contraception?
3. Should doctors give sex education lectures in schools?

P. R. Grantham, Vancouver

181 MRS. R.D.   AGED 22   HOUSEWIFE

Mrs. R.D. has difficulties in coping with her three children who are all under 5 years old. She also has difficulties in coping with contraception. She will not take the pill ('it makes me too fat'); will not use the cap ('don't ask me to put that inside me') and will not even consider the coil or sheath. Sterilization is what she wants and she has been referred for this to the gynaecology department of a teaching hospital.

There, while she is immobilized by a speculum, the doctor has said 'I am just going to see if this fits' and has popped in a coil. Although she does not demand its removal, she has complained bitterly about dysmenorrhoea, dyspareunia and menorrhagia ever since.

1. What is 'consent' and how does it affect our day to day work?
2. What right has the gynaecologist, rather than the patient, to make the final decision about sterilization?
3. How would you proceed to manage the patient's gynaecological symptoms?

A. J. Moulds, Basildon, UK

MR. G.P.　　AGED 33　　ARCHITECT　　　182

A Jewish, married female patient with twin sons aged 2 years, has a nocturnal grand mal seizure and is subsequently found to have a non-resectable astrocytoma of her right frontal lobe that will be treated by radiation only. She makes an appointment for her husband, a 36 year old self-employed architect whom you have not previously met, to discuss vasectomy.

1. What constitute acceptable indications and contraindications for sterilization?
2. How can marital health be assessed?
3. Who should be sterilized here, if anyone?

P. R. Grantham, Vancouver

MRS. S.C.　　AGED 29　　HOUSEWIFE　　　183

Mrs. S.C. is a 29 year old mother of three. The two older children, both boys, are the product of her first marriage which ended in divorce. The third child, a girl, was born 14 months ago and is the product of an apparently happy second marriage. Following delivery of her daughter, Mrs. C. had an immediate post-partum tubal ligation. At 2 months of age the child developed a severe respiratory illness and required immediate hospitalization and tracheostomy. She has been hospitalized ever since with what was ultimately diagnosed as cystic fibrosis. She requires almost daily assisted ventilation via tracheostomy tube and is currently recovering from a severe *Pseudomonas* meningitis.

Mrs. C. presents at this time for her annual check-up, seems in good spirits and has no complaints.

1. Is immediate post-partum tubal ligation generally a good idea?
2. On whom should a sterilization procedure be performed?
3. What might be the explanation for Mrs. C.'s apparently good mood.

G. G. Beazley, Winnipeg

184 MR. ARAN W. AGED 29 BUS DRIVER

Aran W. married, with 2 children (a girl of 8 years and another of 6 years), presents with a request for vasectomy. He has been married for 9 years and you know the family well. 4 years ago there was a period of strain in the marriage, mainly over the question of another pregnancy, but this has settled. The doctor explained briefly the mechanics of vasectomy and then asked if he could see Aran again with his wife for a fuller discussion.

1. Do you agree with the doctor's attitude?
2. Assuming you have a joint consultation, what points would you make?
3. Discuss your attitude to 'reversal procedures' for sterilized patients.

K. C. Nyman, Perth, Australia

185 MRS. G.E. AGED 35 HOUSEWIFE

After the birth of their third child, who seemed to be constantly ill with multiple minor problems necessitating the mother visiting her family physician, a college professor and his wife mutually decided that he would have a vasectomy. When the couple were interviewed by their family physician, they reported that neither one of them could bear the thought of additional children. The physician subsequently performed a vasectomy as he had done on a hundred other patients in his practice.

Six months later, the family physician received a desperate phone call from the couple who were at their summer cottage. Mrs. E. having missed a period, had visited a local physician, who indicated that she was pregnant and had confirmed this with a pregnancy test. On the phone they expressed the desire to see their own family physician as soon as possible, both to confirm the diagnosis and to discuss the pregnancy further. The husband reminded the family physician that his wife was an avid member of the Right to Life Group – an anti-abortion movement.

1. What is the possible explanation of the mother bringing the child for frequent visits to her family physician, for what seemed like minor, inappropriate problems?
2. What are the issues surrounding male/female sterilization?
3. Is the physician performing a failed sterilization, legally culpable?
4. What are the implication of this woman's membership in Right to Life?

C. A. Moore, Hamilton, Canada

MRS. T.G.   AGED 23   RECEPTIONIST   **186**

This lady presents with her husband because they are unable to achieve a pregnancy. She ceased the oral contraceptive pill 15 months earlier and has only had three periods since then. Her periods had been irregular (approximately two monthly) before going on the pill. Intercourse has been frequent and regular. General examination of both partners is normal.

1. What are the possible causes of infertility in this case?
2. What would be the initial investigations of this couple?
3. What other aspects of management should be adopted in this case?

D. S. Pedler, Adelaide

MRS. C.B.   AGED 27   HOUSEWIFE   **187**

Mrs. C.B. has been off the pill for 18 months, but unable to conceive. Physical examination revealed a little yellow cervical discharge but was otherwise normal. Appendectomy was performed some years before.

1. What would you do next?
2. Would you want to see her husband, if so when?
3. If you find no barriers to conception how would you structure future management?

W. D. Jackson, Launceston, Australia

CHAPTER 10

Sexual Problems

Sexual problems present to the family physician in many guises, as is illustrated by dozens of cases elsewhere in this book. This chapter exemplifies a number of common sexual problems, including female orgasmic dysfunction and impotence, and illustrates how some of these may present covertly.

188 SALLY THOMPSON   AGED 23   HOUSEWIFE

This patient presented with headaches that were mainly occipital. They did not keep the patient awake and appeared to be made worse by worry. She was anxious and tearful. She was normotensive and physical examination revealed no abnormality. The mother of three children under 5, Mrs. Thompson had been a perfect patient throughout her pregnancies and confinement. A provisional diagnosis of tension headache was made. Further probing resulted in an admission that there were considerable problems in the marriage and eventually to the doctor's surprise the patient admitted that these were due to sexual difficulties. The husband was obviously considerate enough but ignorant of normal female sexual response, while Mrs. Thompson was anorgasmic, apart from one or two occasions early in her marriage. She was extremely inhibited about sexual matters as a result of a very rigid upbringing. She would not permit any foreplay involving the genital area prior to coitus.

1. Is it appropriate for a general practitioner to attempt to deal with this problem?
2. If he decided to attempt to solve the sexual problems in this marriage, how would the general practitioner go about it?
3. What are some of the factors that might lead to failure of this treatment plan?

J. G. P. Ryan, Brisbane

189 MRS. J.B.   AGED 29   HOUSEWIFE

Mrs. J.B. made an appointment at her husband's request, she says, because she wanted to be checked for vaginal infection. Further questioning reveals that her vaginal discomfort occurs when she has intercourse with her husband, specifically when he attempts penile penetration of her introitus. She blushes easily and admits to being very uncomfortable about the topic of sex since childhood and having had two painful sexual encounters as a young adult and having never really enjoyed sexual relations at all.

Physical pelvic exam is unremarkable except for a small vagina with a mildly tender 1 cm diameter cyst at the posterior fourchette.

1. How common are sexual problems in the general population?
2. How well founded are this patient's fears that her vagina is just 'too small' for her husband?
3. How would you intervene to help this patient?

K. F. Weyrauch, Charleston, SC, USA

190 MR. DOUG M.   AGED 28

This athletic fellow is built like a Greek god. He has had a series of intimate girl friends and enjoys 'living it up'. Recently he has been thinking of proposing marriage to his girlfriend of 2 years' duration, but feels the relationship might deteriorate because he has now become impotent.

1. What is the normal physiology of penile erection?
2. What examination would you do?
3. What treatment plan would you offer?

D. H. Johnson, Toronto

MR. O.P.   AGED 32   LAWYER

191

Mr. O.P. is a hard-driving, achievement oriented lawyer. He is concerned that, after a long evening party, he was impotent with a recent female companion. Two days later a similar occurrence took place.

1. Is this a normal sexual response for a man of this age?
2. What are the common male sexual psychological changes with age?
3. What is the most probable cause for the second episode of impotence?
4. Does Mr. O.P. require chemotherapy, long term sexual counselling or reassurance?

E. V. Dunn, Toronto

MR. W.T.   AGED 48

192

Mr. W.T. complains to his doctor of failing sex drive. He and his wife have intercourse less and less often and, if foreplay is prolonged, he loses his erection without orgasm and cannot regain it. He is physically fit and has no other symptoms. He has been married for 18 years and has children aged 12 and 10. His mother died a year ago following a stroke.

1. What is the likely cause of this man's reduced libido?
2. Why does he come to a doctor about it?
3. Should doctors expect to be able to deal with this sort of problem?

G. Strube, Crawley, UK

MR. ROBERT R.   AGED 51

193

Robert presents with a sore throat, but as the consultation is about to end he says that lately his sexual drive has failed. He has been married for 27 years and has three children. He is still very fond of his wife. After a recent tiff in the marriage he slept on his own for 3 weeks. On returning to the marital bed he found that he could not achieve erection. Normally they have had intercourse 2–3 times weekly. He confesses to being under considerable pressure in his business and feeling very tired of late.

1. Is this a common problem of the male in his 50s?
2. Is the condition reversible?
3. Would you arrange to see this patient's wife?
4. What advice would you offer to the patient?

K. C. Nyman, Perth, Australia

194 J.G.   AGED 55   CLERK

You have known J.G. for over 30 years. You knew him as a young clerk who suddenly came into a fortune 20 years ago when he scooped a football pool.

Over the years he has come with multiple minor problems 2–3 times a year. He has three daughters, a nice wife who has otosclerosis but who is busy with many community affairs outside the house. As far as you know it has been a very happy marriage.

He is embarrassed when he complains of frequency of micturition, aching in his testicles and impotence – all over the past 3 months.

1. Give your assessment of J.G. and the likely pathologies.
2. How do you manage the situation?
3. He comes back to see you for the results of the investigations saying that his frequency and aching have cleared but he is still impotent. Why is he impotent and what do you do about it?

J. Fry, Beckenham, UK

195 MR. JOHN P.   AGED 52   ELECTRICIAN

The main complaint of Mr. P. was secondary impotence. For the last three months he was unable to sustain an erection during intercourse. There was no previous impotence and he was very happily married to a woman of the same age. He considered sexual relations with his wife previously satisfactory. Questioning revealed extremely limited knowledge of sexuality; it was apparent that his wife had never achieved orgasm; she was increasingly frustrated. She was under treatment from another doctor for chronic pelvic pain to date undiagnosed. Mr. P. still experienced morning erections and masturbated to relieve tension, causing guilt; no extramarital sex was involved.

1. What are the causes of secondary impotence?
2. What are the factors involved in female orgasmic dysfunction?
3. How should this couple's sexual dysfunction be treated?

D. G. Chambers, Clare, Australia

MR. J.S.   AGED 57   UNEMPLOYED/WIDOWER

196

Three and a half years ago Mr. J.S. presented requiring a check-up because of impotence of 6 months' duration. Complete physical examination was normal except for a solitary prostatic nodule. Subsequent investigation revealed prostatic cancer with extension to local nodes (stage D). He was treated with radiotherapy. For the next 3 years he was relatively symptom free. During the past 6 months bony metastases have been discovered. He underwent bilateral orchidectomy 1 month ago.

He presents indicating that the urologist did not seem willing to answer many of his questions.

1. What concerns or questions might this man wish to voice?
2. What is the prognosis in this case in terms of life expectancy?
3. Could this disease have been cured if discovered earlier?

G. G. Beazley, Winnipeg

MR. H.H.   AGED 46

197

Mr. H.H. has been a patient of the practice for 1 year. He has had multiple sclerosis for 12 years and at this point in time has no use of his legs. He has difficulty with voiding but is able to use a urinal if he gets it in place in time. He lives at home where his mother feeds him and he is pretty mobile in his wheel chair. He is attending a local university working at a degree course. He has been doing this for some time. He presents to the office one day complaining that he had been crossing one leg over the other and had heard a snap. Examination shows some swelling two-thirds of the way down the femur and X-ray shows an oblique fracture. He is admitted for plating of this fracture. While he is in the hospital, a hardworking family medicine resident ascertains that he has a lot of problems about his own sexuality. He has never felt very sure of his own sexuality even before having MS. He would like to talk about it and work out where he should go with this problem.

1. How can society best help the patient with multiple sclerosis?
2. Why do you think this man's leg fractured with such apparent ease? (prior to this major fracture, he sustained a tibial plateau fracture in the same leg by bringing his leg down too hard and after this hospital admission, he sustained an above knee femoral fracture while receiving physiotherapy).
3. How can we help this man with his sexuality?

J. K. Shearman, Hamilton, Canada

MR. C.S.Y.   AGED 26   BARTENDER

198

A not unattractive 'lady' with long hair, high heeled shoes and dressed in a skirt and blouse enters your consulting room. 'She' is having an asthmatic wheeze. You check your medical record card to ensure you have the correct patient.

He tells you that he is in fact a male. His asthma is of recent onset, only coming on in the last 6 months. He tells you that he feels like a woman being trapped in a man's body and besides wanting you to treat him for his asthma, also needs your advice on whether he should have a sex change operation. He has a male homosexual partner waiting outside your consulting room. They have been living together for the last 6 months.

1. Identify the problems presented by this patient.
2. What further history would you like to obtain from this patient?
3. What would you look for in particular at physical examination?
4. How do you propose to manage this patient?

F. E. H. Tan, Kuala Lumpur

CHAPTER 11

Problems of Pregnancy

This chapter illustrates many of the problems of pregnancy which the family physician needs to be able to manage. It deals with the diagnosis of pregnancy, pregnancy in the unmarried woman, unwanted pregnancy and abortion, pregnancy in the mentally retarded, determination of paternity, rubella in pregnancy, the effects of radiation on the foetus, foetal abnormalities, complications of pregnancy and neonatal problems. It concludes by addressing the contemporary issue of surrogate mothers and test-tube babies.

Diagnosis of pregnancy
---

99 **DORIS J.**   **AGED 18**   **CIRCUS HAND**

Doris presents to you for the first time with a 10 day history of nausea and vomiting. For the last few days she has had difficulty keeping any food down at all. The circus arrived in town yesterday and has set up in the field behind your office. No one else in the circus has been ill. With systematic questioning you discover she has not had a menstrual period for nearly 6 weeks.

The circus is Doris' home. She ran away from her parents 3 years ago and has travelled with the circus ever since. They move on in a week's time.

1. What other history would support your suspected diagnosis?
2. How would you confirm the diagnosis?
3. What factors affect the management of this patient?
4. What preventive measures are relevant to this patient?

R. P. Strasser, Melbourne

200 **MRS. E.R.**   **AGED 36**   **HOUSEWIFE**

Mrs. E.R. was a migrant wife, joining her husband in Australia 2 months previously, after 2 years' separation. He had come to a remote country town, some 360 miles from a metropolitan centre, to work as a mechanic.

She stated that she was nauseated and had 9 weeks amenorrhoea. No previous pregnancies. Examination reveals a 16 week uterus, smooth and non tender. Foetal parts were not palpable.

1. What are the possible diagnoses?
2. What investigations would you order?
3. What are the possible risk factors in this patient?

R. W. Roberts, Ravensthorpe, Australia

Unwanted pregnancy

MS. E.F.   AGED 17   STUDENT

201

Ms. E.F., a 17 year old patient presents with a story of 7 weeks amenorrhoea. You have been looking after her and her family for 11 years. She is about to go into first year medicine and has just finished her final year of school with spectacular academic results.

She exclaims, 'Doctor, you've got to help me, otherwise I'll kill myself!'

While she is passing urine and then getting undressed, you look through the family notes and notice that your partner has recently given her mother, a low user, some tranquillizers. Her father is a commercial traveller and is often away for long periods. She has an older sister and a sister younger than herself. You last saw her 2 years ago for a chest infection.

1.   What are the abortion laws in your country?
2.   Is unwanted pregnancy an accident or illness?
3.   Are there any risks to putting a young girl on oral contraceptives?

J. H. Levenstein, Cape Town

MISS N.   AGED 15   SCHOOLGIRL

202

Miss N. presented to the office with a history of 3 weeks' amenorrhoea. She was very upset. I had seen her on two previous occasions for minor complaints. Her father was well known to me. He had been a physical education instructor and was recently promoted to the principalship of a Catholic school. He was well known in the athletic community, and participated actively in the lung association and planned parenthood anti-abortion groups. Her mother was not well known to me as she had been seen on only two occasions for minor complaints by other physicians in our office. On further questioning the patient, she had had intercourse on three occasions and subsequently her pregnancy test was found to be positive. We tried to discuss the options that were open to her on this first visit but this was not productive because she was very upset. I advised her to discuss this with her parents as soon as possible, and suggested that I would be willing to do this with her if that would be helpful.

She subsequently first spoke to her father. After giving the news to her mother, her mother stopped speaking to her and did not speak to her again throughout the entire pregnancy. Subsequently, we had three sessions with both parents and the patient to discuss how to manage the problem. Miss N. was strongly in favour of having an abortion, but her father said that was not possible because she was 15½ and would not turn 16 for another 5 months. Any further procedures until the age of majority (16) would require parental consent.

1. How would you advise this girl in the management of her pregnancy?
2. If her father refused to allow her to abort the pregnancy, what would be your main objective in subsequent management?
3. What are the risks of an unwanted pregnancy in a 15 year old?

W. W. Rosser, Ottawa

203 R.D. AGED 18 WAITRESS

R.D. is an 18 year old black female whom you have seen in your office on several previous occasions. You have treated her for a urinary tract infection and given dietary counselling in response to her request for help in weight reduction. At each of these encounters, you have inquired about her need for birth control, have given her several pamphlets describing various birth control options and have even offered her free birth control pills. Her response has always been to shyly deny that she was in need of birth control at that time. One day you are surprised to find that she has scheduled herself for a 30 minute appointment. She arrives flushed and reports that she has been having unprotected intercourse and her menstrual period is 5 weeks overdue. She seems excited at the prospect of pregnancy and although she is unmarried and living at home with her parents, she flatly refuses to inform her parents of her plans to keep the baby. Her mother is scheduled to see you in 45 minutes.

1. As a family physician, how do you approach the topic of adolescent sexuality?
2. What is your responsibility towards the patient, her mother, the unborn child?
3. How will you manage the present visit and her mother's concerned inquiries?

K. F. Weyrauch, Charleston, SC, USA

204 MAUREEN T. AGED 19 STUDENT TEACHER

Maureen, a second year student teacher living at home, presents with amenorrhoea, nausea and frequency of micturition. On examination she is 10 weeks pregnant, a possibility she doesn't deny. She is of the Catholic faith and her immediate reaction is that she will go on with the pregnancy, as her boy friend aged 20 years, also a student teacher, is anxious to marry her. She leaves to discuss this with him. Soon after, her mother telephones you and says that Maureen's pregnancy must be terminated at all costs or her life would be ruined.

1. What comments would you make to Maureen's mother?
2. Should you arrange a full discussion with Maureen and her boy friend?
3. How would you react to a request for termination?
4. Should you arrange other opinions for Maureen if you feel that you are basically prejudiced in her case?

K. C. Nyman, Perth, Australia

MISS G.G.   AGED 24   MENTALLY RETARDED   205

Miss G.G. was recognized to be mentally retarded at 3 years of age and was institutionalized until about 6 years ago. She is currently living in a supervised community residence with seven other mentally retarded individuals. She is judged to have a mental age of about 8 years. For the past year she has asked questions about oral contraceptives and 3 months ago the physician started her on them as he was concerned about the possibility of her becoming pregnant. She presents with a vague history of amenorrhoea and on examination is found to be approximately 10 weeks pregnant.

1. What options are there for the management of this pregnancy?
2. What contraceptive measures might be adopted in the future?
3. Is it generally accepted that all babies born to mentally retarded mothers should be apprehended?

G. G. Beazley, Winnipeg

MRS. K.L.N.   AGED 25   HOUSEWIFE   206

The patient is a gravida 2 para 1. Her first child is a girl aged 3 years. Her last menstrual period was on 3rd March. Her pregnancy was progressing well. At 16 weeks maturity, she looked distressed and burst into tears. She said she was unsure who the father of her second child was.

Her last 3 years of marriage were unhappy ones. She and her husband had frequent quarrels. She had an affair with a married man and they had sexual intercourse only once in March. Thereafter he avoided her completely, refusing even to answer her phone calls and letters. She wants you to tell her whose child she is carrying.

1. How would you answer her?
2. Should she request termination of pregnancy, how would you advise her?
3. What medico-legal problems may arise after the delivery?

F. E. H. Tan, Kuala Lumpur.

207 MRS. K.W. AGED 28 HOUSEWIFE

Mrs. K.W. has had some difficulty conceiving and in the past 10 years has had three pregnancies. The first pregnancy 10 years previously ended by Caesarean section for cephalo-pelvic disproportion when a healthy boy was delivered. The next pregnancy 7 years later resulted in the normal delivery of a very premature baby who died. A baby girl was delivered by Caesarean section for foetal distress 15 months ago. This baby appears to be mentally retarded and extensive investigations have not revealed any specific reason for this.

Mrs. W. is now pregnant again for the fourth time. She states emphatically that she cannot face another pregnancy – especially with the prospect of requiring to spend extra time with her retarded daughter. A local consultant obstetrician feels that this is a legitimate reason for termination of the pregnancy. There is industrial action involving the nursing staff at the local hospital and no surgery can be performed without the prior approval of the acting medical superintendent who is a strict Roman Catholic.

Mr. W. is a labourer and the family income is limited. They cannot afford the cost of any alternative care which would only be available in a centre several hundred kilometres away.

1. Who decides how a patient should be treated?
2. How does a retarded child affect a family?
3. How does a history of infertility affect the management of subsequent pregnancies?

B. H. Connor, Armidale, Australia

208 MRS. D.C. AGED 32 HOUSEWIFE

Mrs. D.C. was a rather shy 32 year old whose religious convictions prevented her from using any contraception other than the rhythm method. She had married at the age of 27 and in her comparatively short reproductive career had already produced 5 children – first a son, then a daughter closely followed by triplets. Mrs. C. was a highly conscientious housewife and mother and all the children were beautifully turned out and well behaved. From time to time Mrs. C. displayed features of anxiety, but she was determined to cope without recourse to tranquillizers and had even managed to give up smoking with the help of nicotine chewing gum. One day she arrived in an uncharacteristically agitated and tearful state and blurted out almost immediately that her period was five days late and she thought she might be pregnant. As she told her story she wrung her hands and rose constantly to her feet and made to pace around the surgery. She could not, she said, possibly cope with another child. She asked, 'I won't have to have this baby will I doctor? Can't you give me anything to bring my period on?'

1. What do you understand by the rhythm method of contraception?

2. What are the laws governing the therapeutic termination of pregnancy?
3. What are the common presentations of anxiety?

T. A. I. Bouchier Hayes, Camberley, UK

MRS. L.H.   AGED 35   HOUSEWIFE   209

Mrs. L.H. presents at 14 weeks gestation requesting termination of the pregnancy. She has three boys, aged 13, 10, and 7. She states that her 40 year old husband has been angry with her for 'falling in' and has demanded that she has an abortion.

1. What are the real issues behind this request?
2. Should the doctor comply with this request?
3. How would you manage this problem?

J. E. Murtagh, Melbourne.

MRS. A.T.   AGED 39   HOUSEWIFE   210

Mrs. A.T. was happily married with two children, aged 12 and 10 years. She presented because she feared she was pregnant, being 3 weeks overdue, the pregnancy arising as a result of failure of the rhythm method. Clinical examination revealed that she was in good physical health and confirmed a normal pregnancy.

She wanted to have the pregnancy terminated as she did not feel she could cope emotionally with another child. Her husband was aged 49 years, an engineer, and while not keen to have another child, would 'leave it up to her'.

Despite wanting the pregnancy terminated, she had some misgivings as she felt it morally wrong but did not feel able to talk to the minister of her church about it. She felt it was the right thing to do for herself and her family.

1. How do you confirm a pregnancy?
2. What are the risks of pregnancy in this case?
3. How would you manage this case?
4. What are the legal requirements which have to be met before termination is justifiable?
5. What are the long term effects of termination and the risks involved to the mother?
6. What form of contraception would you advise subsequently?

H. C. Watts, Perth, Australia

Complications of pregnancy

---

211 **MRS. N.L.** **AGED 23** **SCHOOL TEACHER**

Mrs. N.L. is a nullipara whose normally regular period is now 2 weeks overdue. Her nephew, who had stayed with her 5 days before, has developed a rash which his GP has confidently diagnosed as German measles.

Not unnaturally she is worried that this might affect her pregnancy as she has never had German measles before.

1. What factors need clarification before accurate advice can be given?
2. How would you interpret the possible rubella antibody results that might be revealed by serological testing?
3. If she has caught rubella how would you explain the risks of pregnancy?
4. Under what circumstances is abortion legal?

A. J. Moulds, Basildon, UK

212 **MRS. D.** **AGED 30** **TEACHER**

Mrs. D. was referred by another general practitioner to the radiologist for an intravenous pyelogram because of recurrent urinary tract infection. Her last menstrual period was on the 4th August and the intravenous pyelogram was performed on the 26th August.

She subsequently missed her period and you confirmed her pregnancy at 8 weeks maturity.

1. What would be your approach to her problem?
2. Her infuriated husband wishes to take legal action against both the general practitioner and the radiologist and wants you to testify. Do you pacify and attempt to talk him out of it or express willingness to testify?
3. How could such a situation be prevented?

F. E. H. Tan, Kuala Lumpur

213 **SARAH P.** **AGED 32**

Five years ago Sarah had had her first pregnancy which resulted in the normal delivery of a male infant. Eighteen months later she had a second pregnancy which this time resulted in a child with a severe meningo-myelocoele. After discussion with the doctors, it was decided not to operate and the child died about 10 days later. Tests done during the first half of the third pregnancy indicated that this foetus was probably affected and a prostaglandin termination, carried out at 21 weeks, confirmed the diagnosis.

Sarah visited her doctor to say after much thought she and her husband had decided to try once more and her period was now 3 weeks overdue. A pregnancy test was positive.

1. How might the doctor manage the consultation?
2. By what methods can meningomyelocoele be detected in a foetus?
3. What kind of problems does the birth of a baby with meningo-myelocoele present?

J. C. Hasler, Oxford

MR. J.M.   AGED 27   MEDICAL STUDENT   214

J.M. is a 27 year old white male medical student married to R.M., a 27 year old white female teacher. At their third visit, J.M. expressed the wish for his wife to become pregnant with their first child. However, before even considering pregnancy, he wanted to be assured that his doctor would get an amniocentesis on his wife during pregnancy. He wanted a karyotype of the foetus early enough to legally abort if the child was detected as 'defective'. R.M. expressed the same wish but not so strongly.

1. What important family history would need to be obtained?
2. How would you explain the benefits vs. risks and indications for amniocentesis to this medical student and his wife?
3. How would you counsel them if they had **no** risk factors in their family and personal history?

P. Boiko, Charleston, SC, USA

MRS. B.   AGED 21   HOUSEWIFE   215

I was called at 4.45 p.m. on a hot summer afternoon by the husband of a young woman seen by me only once previously. He was somewhat inarticulate and all that I could understand from what he said was that his wife was not feeling well and that she fainted twice after attempting to sit up and was feeling unwell while lying down in bed. She had been completely well up until 3 hours prior to the call. He was unable to bring her to the office because he was afraid she would faint again. Her address was within several blocks of the office and in fact I was aware that it was a dilapidated old building which probably was very hot. I was tempted to suggest that he sponge bath her with cool water and phone back if she did not feel better. However, because of the lack of information I decided to make a house call.

On entering the very hot building I found the woman lying on a cot in a poorly lit, dishevelled and dirty room. She was very pale and breathing rapidly with shallow respirations. Her pulse was 135 and her blood pressure was 80/0. She was definitely in shock. She complained of vague abdominal pain, but on examination of her abdomen there was board-like rigidity. Her last menstrual period had been about 6½ weeks previously but she had paid little attention to having missed her last period. She had not been using any birth control method. She did complain of vague abdominal cramps for the preceding two days, which she had attributed to the greasy food that she had eaten at that time. An immediate ambulance call had the woman transported to the emergency department of our hospital.

1. What is the most likely aetiology of this problem?
2. What were the risks in moving this woman to the hospital?
3. How might this situation have been prevented?

W. W. Rosser, Ottawa

216   MISS LOIS D.   AGED 23   SALES ASSISTANT

At 7.15 a.m. on a Friday morning you are phoned by the father of a family who are patients of the practice. He is extremely agitated and concerned about his 23 year old daughter Lois, who has been experiencing excruciating abdominal pain for 20 minutes. You can hear her terrified cries of agony in the background over the phone.

Ten minutes later, on arrival at the home, you find the daughter in a state of near emotional collapse, in great pain, sitting on the toilet. She is in the process of 'delivering' a 20 week foetus. Blood loss appears to be minimal.

1. What are the major obstetrical risks at this stage?
2. What history do you need at this point?
3. What family and social dynamics need to be considered?

M. W. Heffernan, Melbourne

217   MRS. J.W.   AGED 35   HOUSEWIFE AND PART-TIME TEACHER

Mrs. J.W. is pregnant for the second time. During her first pregnancy 6 years previously she lost liquor intermittently from 20 weeks gestation onwards. She spent the rest of that pregnancy in bed at home as ordered by a consultant obstetrician. This first pregnancy ended with a forceps delivery after a long labour 1 week over term. The baby boy was well after delivery and has remained so ever since.

After the pregnancy Mrs. W. became depressed and required care from a psychiatrist who prescribed various tranquillizers and anti-depressants until her second pregnancy.

She has also suffered from intermittent backache. Her husband is a tutor who has spent a long time doing his doctoral thesis. It has been suggested that a wooden board be purchased and placed under the mattress to make their bed firmer and so help the backache. This has not been done.

The second pregnancy is proceeding uneventfully until the 20th week when a painless loss of liquor occurs. Mrs. J.W. is well otherwise. She can feel foetal movements but is depressed about the recurrent loss of liquor.

1. What is the cause of post-partum depression?
2. What complications of pregnancy can be treated at home?
3. How is it possible to balance the needs of the husband and wife when counselling a married couple?

B. H. Connor, Armidale, Australia

MRS. B.S.   AGED 29   HOUSEWIFE   218

Mrs. B.S. is in labour after an uneventful pregnancy. She is a primigravida and at term. A consultant obstetrician has seen her on several occasions and has stated that she should have no problems in labour. The consultant is now on leave and unavailable.

A message from the maternity ward sister states that the cervix is 4 centimetres dilated with an unusual presentation. You confirm that this is a breech presentation. It is a weekend and the nearest consultant help is 100 kilometres away.

1. Should confinements be conducted in isolated country hospitals?
2. What special assistance might be available to help with this unexpected emergency?
3. How should this delivery be conducted?

B. H. Connor, Armidale, Australia

MRS. H.B.   AGED 26   FILM CLERK   219

Mrs. H.B. is 18 weeks pregnant and in for her fourth pre-natal visit. This first pregnancy has been progressing normally and she and her husband have both been exceedingly happy. She has no concerns. On examining her you find her uterus to be only about 12 weeks in size (smaller than the last visit) with no evidence of a foetal heart. You discover that all of her symptoms of pregnancy disappeared 2 to 4 weeks ago. Close questioning reveals that she has had slight brownish vaginal discharge on three occasions in the past 3 weeks. She becomes quite upset when you express your concern about the pregnancy to her.

1. What are the diagnostic possibilities?
2. What investigation might be carried out?
3. Who else might you wish to talk to?

G. G. Beazley, Winnipeg

220 MRS. DENISE S. AGED 25

Denise S. has had two normal confinements. Last year she had a missed abortion at about 14 weeks which required evacuation. The consulting gynaecologist told her that there was no obvious cause for this and no reason to suppose that it would happen again. A scan in the twelfth week of the present pregnancy showed a normal 'very active' foetus. At your first examination she appears to be small for her estimated maturity of 22 weeks but the pregnancy test is positive. A fortnight later the uterine size is unchanged and the pregnancy test is now negative.

1. What is your further management?
2. What reasons can you suggest for this and the preceding intra-uterine death?
3. What advice would you give about further pregnancies?

J. A. Stevens, Ulverstone, Australia

221 MRS. P.M. AGED 26

Mrs. P.M. is 40 weeks pregnant in her second pregnancy. Her present and first pregnancies have been completely normal. She goes into hospital at 4.00 a.m. in early labour. Sister phones you and tells you she can't hear the foetal heart.

1. As she is only in early labour is there any point in getting up to see Mrs. P.M.?
2. If you can't feel movements and can't hear the foetal heart what will you say to the mother and her husband?
3. The labour results in a stillbirth and baby and placenta show no obvious pathology. What matters are there to discuss with the parents?

F. Mansfield, Perth, Australia

222 MRS. X.Y. AGED 32 HOUSEWIFE

You are managing her second pregnancy and she is now 16 weeks having been seen for her first physical a month ago. At that time all was normal, but today she states that in the last 2 days her right calf has become swollen and painful to walk on. On examination there is slight localized tenderness mid-line at the mid-calf level.

1. Could this condition be serious?
2. How would you determine if any pathology existed?
3. What would be considered optimal management?

T. D. Manthorpe, Port Lincoln, Australia

MRS. A.B.   AGED 18   HOUSEWIFE

223

Mrs. A. B. is an 18-year-old married woman who is 5 months pregnant during her first pregnancy. She has been married for 5 months. Her husband is a trainee in the Coast Guard. She comes to the office with the chief complaints of fever, rigors and pain in the right knee, ankle and foot for 24 hours.

Ten days before being seen, the patient had noted a sore throat which had persisted for several days. She first noted several shaking chills beginning during the late afternoon the day she was seen. This was followed by rapid onset of malaise, fever to 102 °F and, 12 hours before being seen, pain on movement and swelling in the right knee. About 6 hours before being seen, the patient noted swelling and pain in the right ankle and in the third and fourth toes of the right foot. She was unable to get around her apartment and was accompanied to the office by her mother.

Her husband had returned to camp after leave at home.

1. What physical findings would you anticipate?
2. What are the essential problems in the problem list?
3. How would one proceed to obtain efficient use of the laboratory in this case?
4. What epidemiological and therapeutic measures would be helpful?

L. H. Amundson, Sioux Falls, SD, USA

MRS. MARTHA M.   AGED 35   LAWYER

224

Mrs. M. who is a long term patient of yours came to see you looking very agitated. She had been playing with her 2 year old son the day before when he bumped her in the breast. Last night she noticed a lump where she had been hit. She is very worried that it might be cancer. She is 7 months pregnant. On examination the lump feels hard and craggy. There is no indentation of the skin.

1. What are some of the important issues you would be thinking about?
2. What would you do?
3. What are the effects of pregnancy on breast cancer?

M. D. Mahoney, Brisbane

Neonatal problems

225   **MRS. NERIDA C.**   **AGED 41**   **HOUSEWIFE**

You have just delivered Mrs. C. of her third baby. She has two other children aged 8 and 6. Prior to her having her first child she had had difficulty in becoming pregnant and had been trying for several years to have a baby. It is the day after the delivery and you have come in to talk to Mrs. C. about her baby who has a severe spina bifida deformity.

1. What are the most important issues to be considered at this stage?
2. How are the parents likely to react at this stage?
3. What are the legal, moral and ethical issues involved with a baby with spina bifida?
4. What are the facilities for children with spina bifida in your state/country?

M. D. Mahoney, Brisbane

226   **NEWBORN BABY GIRL**

This baby is born normally but prematurely in a country hospital. Her birth weight is 1.9 kg and she is an estimated 32 weeks gestation. Immediately after delivery her respiratory rate increases until she is quite distressed and a little cyanosed.

A decision is made to seek help from a neonatal specialist team in a major city centre. However, the only available air ambulance is 250 kilometres away transporting a 4 year old boy suffering from a head injury which occurred as a result of being hit by a brick which fell from a passing truck.

1. What emergency services should be available to help isolated rural communities?
2. What can be done immediately to help the baby?
3. What important preparations can be made before the trip by air ambulance?

B. H. Connor, Armidale, Australia

227   **R.T.**   **AGED 2 WEEKS**

R. is a 2 week old white male born to Mr. and Mrs. T. and was seen by Dr. P. for 'yellow eyes and skin'.

Prior to her pregnancy with R., Mrs. T. had a spontaneous abortion at 7 weeks gestation. At 5 months gestation of R., Mr. T. became ill with hepatitis B and Mrs. T. was found to be a carrier.

While their primary doctor, Dr. C. was on vacation, the baby became jaundiced. He was brought in to see Dr. P., who was Dr. C.'s newly hired, young, female partner.

During the examination of the baby, Dr. P. noted Mrs. T. to smell of alcohol. She asked Mrs. T. directly if she took any drugs or drank during her pregnancy or while she was breast feeding. Mr. and Mrs. T. replied very strongly, 'No', and added, 'I didn't even take an aspirin, maybe I'll have a cup of alcohol a month, that's all!

The baby indeed had scleral and mucosal icterus and the parents were told that blood for a hepatitis B surface antigen needed to be drawn by venepuncture. To this, Mr. T. responded (speaking directly to the baby), 'Go ahead and cry real hard so that the doctor feels guilty about poking you full of holes'.

No blood was obtained during the first venepuncture by Dr. P. and Mr. T. continued to state with more and more fervor, 'Look what they're doing *to* you'. During the second venepuncture the parents refused to leave the room and in the middle of positioning the needle, Mr. T. demanded, 'Are you a doctor or a student? I don't want you experimenting on my baby! What's wrong with you, why can't you get the blood?'

1. How would you feel if you were in Dr. P.'s place? How would you feel if you were Mr. and Mrs. T.?
2. What causes of jaundice in a 2 week old would you want to investigate by further history, physical examination and/or laboratory data?
3. How can you ask about alcohol history without putting a patient (in this case Mrs. T.) on the defensive?

P. Boiko, Charleston, SC, USA

Other problems of pregnancy
---

228   MISS M.T.R.   AGED 18

Miss M.T.R. is a new patient. She gave birth to a healthy live male infant 3 weeks ago. She presents with a painful left breast of 2 days' duration. The upper two quadrants of the breast are red, indurated (well defined) and tender. There is no associated adenopathy. Temperature 37.5 °C. She admits to smoking 20 cigarettes daily and looks grossly overweight (exceeding her ideal weight of about 60 kg by 13.5 kg).

1. What is the probable underlying pathology in the breast?
2. What possible anxieties have assailed this patient's psyche in the last month?
3. What potential for health education/preventive medicine exists in this consultation?

D. Levet, Hobart

229   MR. & MRS. ANTHONY A.   AGED 40 AND 45 RESPECTIVELY
MR. A. STOCKBROKER   MRS. A. JOURNALIST

Mr. and Mrs. Anthony A. are waiting in your office one evening when you return from a house call. They both come into your room looking very excited. You have been treating Mrs. A. in conjunction with her gynaecologist for several years for infertility problems. She and Mr. A. have been married 15 years and have been unable to have children. They are now too old to adopt and have been reading in the popular magazines lately about 'surrogate' mothers. They want your advice about what they should do.

1. What are 'surrogate' mothers and what are the implications of using surrogate mothers.
2. What are the legal, moral and ethical issues that need to be raised with the parents.
3. What are some of the issues that need to be considered with 'test tube baby' research.

M. D. Mahoney, Brisbane

CHAPTER 12

Headaches

The cases and questions in this chapter illustrate the diagnostic dilemmas which headache can pose for the family physician. Migraine, tension headache, headache of musculoskeletal origin, headaches arising from intracranial conditions and hypertension, headache accompanying infection, and other causes of headache are exemplified.

230   STEPHEN G.   AGED 14

Stephen comes alone to see you. His family is well known to you. His father left his mother, Stephen and a younger brother some years ago. A man-friend has been living with his mother in the home for some months but there are recurrent rows and fights after alcoholic excesses.

Stephen comes because he has been suffering attacks of frontal headaches with nausea. More recently he has noted 'shimmering lights and blurred vision' before the headache.

1. What significance would you place on a 14 year old boy coming to consult you alone?
2. Why has Stephen come to consult you at this time?
3. What diagnosis would you make?
4. How would you manage the case?

J. Fry, Beckenham, UK

231   MRS. C.D.   AGED 55   HOUSEWIFE

For many years Mrs. D. has been getting what she says are 'migraine' headaches. These have always been worst pre-menstrually, but since the menopause they have occurred more frequently. They are usually only on one side of her head around and behind the eye. They are constant, not throbbing, aggravated by bright light and they make her nauseated and occasionally vomit. She does not have any visual disturbance and they are helped by the early taking of a combination of codeine and ergotamine with bed rest in a dark room. There are many reasons for her to suffer tension.

1. Why has she presented at this time with these headaches?
2. Is there anything else you would like to know about Mrs. D. or her headaches at this stage?
3. How far should one investigate such a patient?

W. F. Glastonbury, Adelaide

232   MRS. E.B.   AGED 52   HOUSEWIFE

Mrs. E.B. is married with three adult children. As well as caring for her husband, she has the responsibility in the home for her elderly parents, both of whom are senile and have serious chronic medical problems. She insists on looking after them at home. She has a 10 year history of migraine. She also requires treatment for mild essential hypertension with hydrochlorothiazide and she has also required psychotherapy with intermittent drug treatment for bouts of depression secondary to the home situation.

1. What distinguishes migraine from other common types of headache?
2. How do you treat migraine headache?
3. Can migraine be prevented?
4. What are the cross-relationships of migraine?

R. L. Perkin, Toronto

MISS ANGELA T.   AGED 18   NURSE

233

Miss T. comes to see you looking rather sick. She is a nurse at the local hospital and does not appear to be her usual bright self. She has been having a bad headache for a couple of days and when she came off duty the day before, she felt some numbness down the right side of her face, right arm and right leg.

She has had headaches on and off in the past 3 to 4 months and has had a similar episode of numbness on two occasions in the past 3 weeks. On examination, she has no neck stiffness and no papilloedema, her blood pressure is normal but she has definite weakness of her right upper and lower limbs. There are no other abnormal findings apart from her lassitude and she is rather vague in answering questions.

1. What sort of conditions would you be considering?
2. How urgent are her symptoms and signs?
3. What are the next steps after she has been admitted to hospital?
4. All the investigations were done, no pathology found. The numbness and weakness had disappeared in a couple of days. What would you do now?

M. D. Mahoney, Brisbane

MISS MARIE W.   AGED 27

234

Marie complains of headaches. These are apparently of two types, one occurring infrequently being of a one sided variety preceded by a visual migraine aura, and the other coming on in response to stress. The second type originates around the occiput and spreads all over her head and comes on frequently. She is a highly intelligent girl holding down a responsible position in a computer company, but feels she is losing her grip, and flying into rages unnecessarily. She lives in her own house with a man who is a security official in the same company.

Further questioning elicits the fact that she earns much more than he does and that what drives her 'up the wall' is his drinking.

1. Who is the patient?
2. What is the problem?
3. How can it be resolved?

R. M. Meyer, Johannesburg

235 MR. P.M.   AGED 52   SENIOR RESEARCH SCIENTIST

Mr. M. suffers from headaches of increasing frequency and severity. The headaches have prevented him from satisfactorily performing his duties in a government department for over 2 years and it has now been decided that he be prematurely retired from the Public Service on a greatly reduced superannuation pension.

Ten years ago he suffered a whiplash injury in a motor vehicle crash on the way to work. Three years ago he had a cervical fusion performed by a neurosurgeon in an attempt to ease his neck pain which appeared to precipitate the headache.

The headaches have been fully investigated and the consensus of opinion from several consultants is that the headaches have features of migraine, tension headaches and nerve root irritation from the cervical spine. Mr. M. has been treated with every type of migraine prophylaxis, anti-depressant medication, beta-blockers, relaxation therapy, physiotherapy and cervical nerve root blocks – all to no avail.

He is otherwise physically well and when the headaches are not present he helps with the organization of the local Search and Rescue Squad. He has seven very intelligent sons including one who is a doctor and another who was a drug addict. His wife is a trained nurse.

The headaches are now almost constant and quite disabling.

1. How extensively should headaches be investigated?
2. What sort of tensions could be contributing to this man's headaches?
3. How can migraine be prevented?

B. H. Connor, Armidale, Australia

236 B.F.   AGED 5   PRE-SCHOOL

This child presented with a complaint of recurrent attacks of headache over the past 2 months. Mother stated that the headaches were worse in the morning, relieved by soluble aspirin temporarily.

Physical examination (including central nervous system) was normal.

1. What is the differential diagnosis?
2. What would be your next step?

R. W. Roberts, Ravensthorpe, Australia

237 MARY S.   AGED 15

Mary complained of headaches on and off for about 3 months. She was a rather dull girl and a poor historian but it seemed that the headaches were frontal, quite severe and accompanied by nausea and vomiting. She did not have a headache when seen. Her mother, who came to the office with her, said she had noticed the headaches occurred only during the premenstrual week. She thought they might have something to do with school work, as she was not expected to do well in the forthcoming examinations. On examination, there were no abnormal physical signs in the CNS, including the retinae. The BP was normal. The doctor concluded that the headaches were probably due to premenstrual syndrome, exacerbated by anxiety over the examinations.

Two months later, the headaches became increasingly severe and prolonged, were worse on bending and accompanied by persistent vomiting. On examination she was found to have papilloedema and was admitted to hospital where a meningioma was removed.

1. How did the doctor arrive at a diagnosis of premenstrual syndrome?
2. What features might have alerted the doctor to the diagnosis at the initial consultation?
3. Why did the headaches occur only premenstrually?
4. What would you have done in this case at the first consultation?
5. What are the likely effects of stress such as anxiety about examinations on a girl of 15?

G. Strube, Crawley, UK

MR. C.H.   AGED 70   RETIRED   238

This old gentleman comes in to see you while your partner is on holiday. He complains of a frontal headache for the last month for which he has been prescribed tranquillizers, nasal drops and a course of antibiotics. He has no previous history of headache and, on examination, the only abnormal finding is slight tenderness on palpation over the left temporal area.

1. What are the likely diagnoses?
2. What are the possible risks in this situation?
3. How do you cope with the likelihood of error by a colleague, especially if the patient is aware of the implications?

E. C. Gambrill, Crawley, UK

MRS. VERA U.   AGED 38   239

Mrs. Vera U. was having an argument with her neighbour about a new fence which encroached on her property. In the midst of the argument a headache suddenly came on. She was so disabled by it that she literally crawled on all fours back to the house.

1. What is your differential diagnosis?
2. What pathology are you worried about here?

D. H. Johnson, Toronto

240   J.M.   AGED 14   SCHOOLBOY

Following a football match, when he played poorly and took some heavy knocks, he developed fever and was off his food. He went to bed early and next morning had a headache. He had discomfort eating his breakfast and there was a swelling in front of and below his left ear.

1. What conditions should be considered?
2. How would you manage this case?

E. J. H. North, Melbourne

241   MR. F.O.   AGED 35   DAIRY FARMER

F.O. had headache and fever and I was asked to call in to see him at home by his wife, who said she could not remember her husband being sick before. They were in a desperate plight milking just on 100 cows and harvesting just prior to Christmas. He had photophobia, neck stiffness and generalized muscle soreness. A lumber puncture showed some increase in pressure. The initial blood tests were negative.

1. What are the likely causes?
2. How is the disease contracted?
3. Are there any complications to be expected?

E. J. H. North, Melbourne

242   MR. LELAND G.   AGED 52   SCHOOL PRINCIPAL

This primary school principal awakened with a high fever, headache, myalgia and mild nausea. About 12 hours later, he notices that his left wrist is swollen and warm and a few spots of rash are seen about his right elbow. You see him a short time later. He alerts you that he is allergic to penicillin. His wife says that her throat is becoming sore.

1. What is your differential diagnosis?
2. If Gram negative diplococci are found on scrapings from the rash, what treatment would you institute?

D. H. Johnson, Toronto

243   MISS M.N.   AGED 27   NURSE

Miss M.N. said she had seen another doctor at her home 2 days ago when she was feeling very 'crook', hot, sweating, headache and vomiting with some diarrhoea. She had arrived home 3 days previously from a holiday in South Africa via a weekend stopover in Mauritius when she had spent one or two hours sunbaking. The previous doctor had diagnosed 'sun burn'. The symptoms persisted.

1. What else might you have thought about if you had been the first doctor?
2. What are the common causes of a PUO acquired on travel?
3. This patient nearly died of cerebral malaria – she had over one in eight red cells parasitized. What could have been done to prevent her getting to this state?

A. J. Radford, Adelaide

MR. A.B. AGED 50 BUS DRIVER **244**

Mr. A.B. has not seen a doctor for 10 years. He attends because, since he had a road traffic accident in his own car 4 weeks ago, he has had a headache which is present on waking and worse on bending forward. His blood pressure is 180/110. On systematic questioning he admits to nocturnal frequency ($\times 2$) present for about a month.

1. What are the possible diagnoses, and on which would you focus in the first instance?
2. What problems does this consultation present in terms of the doctor's responsibility to the community?
3. What significance do you attach to the patient's not having consulted for 10 years?

P. Freeling, London

ELIZABETH C. AGED 17 SCHOOLGIRL **245**

Elizabeth C. had been a frequent attender for 'something for my headache'. She had been a bit of a 'headache' to her doctor since the age of 9 – and had been referred for exhaustive specialist investigation which had resulted in a number of nebulous suggested diagnoses such as tension headache, atypical migraine, and even 'Could the headaches be due to sinusitis? Note the slight clouding in the left antrum.' She responded to 'How's the headache?' with 'No problem with that since I couldn't see you 6 months ago and your partner manipulated my neck. Actually I've come today to see if I'm pregnant.'

1. Are some headaches due to undemonstrable pathology in the neck which is amenable to resolution by manipulation?
2. What is the rational place of tranquillizers in 'tension headache'?
3. How does the doctor react to being put on the spot?

R. T. Mossop, Harare, Zimbabwe

246   ELIZABETH C.   AGED 23   (NOW ELIZABETH G.)   HOUSEWIFE
       SAME PERSON AS IN 245

Elizabeth had married and had her baby in another town. She came home on holiday 6 years later and decided to look up her old doctor for a prescription for the antihypertensives she had forgotten to bring.

She looked thin, old, and had a slate blue colour, twitches and a nervous manner. It transpired that she was in renal failure. From the age of 9 when she fell out of a tree she had had headaches. When she complained her parents gave her codeine compound tablets. These seemed to have little effect, but were just as good as anything prescribed by the doctor on the occasions she had complained to him. Eventually she was spending all her pocket money on them and was buying tins of 100 every few days.

After the manipulation she had no more headaches to speak of but could not bear to be without the codeine compound. A stormy medical and social history during the past 6 years was described.

1. How was it possible that she could hide from a number of doctors that she was taking drugs for so long?
2. Why would she continue taking analgesic drugs after her headaches had gone?
3. What is the place of chronic dialysis?

R. T. Mossop, Harare, Zimbabwe

CHAPTER 13

Fits, Faints and
Funny Turns

This chapter begins with a number of illustrative cases of febrile convulsions and epilepsy, the problems these conditions create, their management and the complications of anti-convulsant therapy. Thereafter follows a number of diagnostic challenges, where the presenting symptom is blackout or dizziness. The cases illustrate that such symptoms may herald the presence of the most benign or the most serious of conditions. The remainder of the cases illustrate transient ischaemic attacks, stroke and other serious neurological problems.

Fits
---

247 **MR. RONALD B.**   **AGED 20**   **INVALID PENSIONER**

Ronald B. is accompanied by his older sister. He has been an epileptic since early childhood, but is well controlled on phenobarbitone and Dilantin. He usually lives with his parents in another city, along with a mentally defective younger brother. He has been grossly overprotected throughout his life but has managed to complete 12 years at school satisfactorily. However, he dropped out of an apprenticeship as an electrician and now lives on an invalid pension. His sister is deeply concerned about his future and has brought him to stay with her hoping to break his seclusion and dependency.

1. What general attitude should you adopt to this young man?
2. What prohibitions and precautions are necessary in an epileptic?
3. Are there any community facilities which could help him?
4. He complains that his current medications make him drowsy. How would you deal with this?
5. Ronald tells you he fears female entanglements, because he is afraid to marry with his disability. How would you counsel him?

K. C. Nyman, Perth, Australia

248 **MRS. JOAN M.**   **AGED 36**   **HOUSEWIFE**

Joan M. is a bright, garrulous farmer's wife, who has three children, ages ranging from 14 to 9 and takes an active part in running the farm. She has radiologically demonstrated gall stones which she intends to keep.

Four years ago she 'collapsed' and found herself prone in the sprout paddock with no memory of how she got there. By the time you saw her she was vomiting copiously but rational and with no abnormal physical signs. No diagnosis was made.

Two months ago she had a similar episode and a neurologist elicited a history of an aura ('odd tastes and funny feelings') and that she 'took fits' until the age of 7. CT scan and EEG were both normal but he labelled her as an epileptic and started her on phenytoin.

Four days later she appeared with a temperature of 38 °C and a florid morbilliform rash which subsided in 3 days after withdrawing the phenytoin.

Later we discussed the problem.

1. Have I really got epilepsy? How do you know?

2. Would the drug have cured me? What should I do now; a friend who has epilepsy tells me that some drugs are very dangerous.

3. We live four miles out of town, how am I going to get the shopping or the children to school? Can I still drive the tractor on the farm?

J. A. Stevens, Ulverstone, Australia

MASTER A.L.   AGED 15 MONTHS   **249**

A. L. is brought to the office by his agitated parents with a high fever, and a 'peculiar' appearance similar to that which preceded his febrile convulsion 3 months previously.

His temperature is 40 °C, and he has mild otitis media.

While he is being examined he has a severe convulsion, becomes rapidly cyanosed, stops breathing and appears 'dead'. This state lasted 5 minutes during which oxygen was administered and intravenous diazepam given.

1. What is the significance of this episode?
2. How would you manage this problem?
3. What advice would you give to the parents?

J. E. Murtagh, Melbourne

MRS. J.S.   AGED 27   UNIVERSITY TEACHER OF A FOREIGN   **250** LANGUAGE

Mrs. J.S. has a 6 week old baby girl, and had trouble in convincing her husband James, a senior social worker, that she wanted a baby more than she wanted a successful academic career. At her post-natal examination she tells you that she is breast-feeding and is taking a progestogen-only contraceptive pill. Mrs. J.S. says, also, that her baby Natalie has been having episodes lasting only a few seconds during which her arms and legs twitch.

1. What are the pros and cons of progestogen-only pills for contraception in a nursing mother?
2. What conditions may be represented by mother's description of Natalie's twitching?
3. What do you understand by the term 'role' as it is used in psychology and sociology?

P. Freeling, London

251

MR. W.H.   AGED 28   DUSTMAN

This man has a history of bizarre behaviour since childhood. When he was 10 years old, he underwent neurological tests for headaches, but no cause was found, and it was thought he had neurotic tendencies. He has several times attended the emergency department of the local hospital, alleging that he has diabetes, but tests have always been negative. He is of low intelligence, and a year ago married a retarded girl; they have no children.

His wife complains that he has become depressed, and will not get out of bed. He is so lazy, he even wets himself. When visited he is found in bed, drowsy but rousable, and unwilling to converse. No gross signs of disease are found, and a psychiatrist is called in. On arrival at the flat, the psychiatrist and general practitioner are met by Mrs. W.H., who says her husband was taken to hospital by ambulance that morning, having had a 'fit'.

1. What are the likely causes of uncooperative behaviour in general practice?
2. What does the wife mean by a 'fit'?
3. Could this dramatic episode have been prevented?

J. Grabinar, Bromley, UK

252

MRS. V.L.   AGED 58   HOUSEWIFE

Mrs. V.L. is an alcoholic who has been a patient for 6 years. Three years ago she was hospitalized for jaundice which was eventually diagnosed as alcoholic hepatitis. One and a half years ago she was hospitalized for anaemia and rectal bleeding which was found to be related to a colonic cancer for which she underwent left hemicolectomy. She presents now indicating that she has been very weak for 1 month and 2 weeks ago had a generalized seizure. She has never admitted to abuse of alcohol.

1. What would be your strategy for further definition of the problem?
2. What might be the cause of the weakness?
3. What might be the cause of the seizure?

G. G. Beazley, Winnipeg

253

CHERYL M.   AGED 30   HOUSEWIFE

Cheryl is epileptic. Her first attack occurred when she was 28 years old during a hospital admission for a threatened premature labour. She is reported to have 'gone stiff, passing out and shaking all over'. Neurological examination and EEG confirmed the diagnosis of 'centri-cephalic epilepsy' and she was prescribed a combination of phenytoin and diazepam which was changed to phenytoin and carbamazepine after the birth of the baby.

She remained well and had no further fits till 5 years later following a motor vehicle accident when, despite exhaustive neurological investigations, no cause for the fits could be found.

1. What explanations might have been suggested as a cause for these fits?
2. Cheryl continued to be a problem. She complained of 'feeling awful', of experiencing sexual difficulties with her husband, of not being able to do her housework and of falling about the house. She frequently presented to the surgery with facial bruising which she said was due to hitting the wash basin when she 'passed out in the bathroom'. How could these symptoms and signs be best explained?
3. Cheryl's continuing ill health and the recurrence of seizures 8 years after she began effective therapy led to the discovery that her serum phenytoin and carbamazepine levels were homeopathic and that she was not taking her drugs regularly. What is the likely explanation of her behaviour?

W. L. Ogborne, Sydney

MRS. F.P. AGED 34 NURSE 254

Mrs. F.P., a fully trained nurse, height 5′2″, 92 kg, mother of obese Lynette, aged 8, and Daryl aged 6, has the habit of not listening; about obesity, about contraception, about her husband's severe, but controlled, hypertension. She is vague, and a poor historian, and does not confide, often masking or distorting the truth. For 3 years she has had attacks of grand mal fits, now completely controlled with carbamazepine 200 mg tds. At the onset of these symptoms, all investigations were found to be normal; X-rays, brain scan, angiograms and EEG were repeated six months later and no changes discovered.

Initially she was treated with phenytoin sodium, but was changed to Tegretol because she suffered a severe generalized rash. Occasionally she took herself off medication, and would find herself bundled to hospital by ambulance following a fit. She became pregnant much to her delight, though taking oral contraceptives at the time. The baby was born with severe spina bifida and lived only four weeks. This caused great family distress.

Four months later she became pregnant again. At 16 weeks gestation she underwent amniocentesis, was found to be carrying a Mongol and a termination was performed by hysterotomy. She is now back at work, in charge of a ward. There has been discussion of a ligation of her tubes, but this has not been pursued by the patient.

1. What are the hazards of anti-convulsant therapy seen in this patient?
2. What is the most likely cause of this patient's grand mal attacks?
3. What genetic counselling is necessary for this patient?
4. What psychological history would throw light on this patient's behaviour?

G. M. Dick, Hobart

255 MISS C.　　AGED 16　　UNEMPLOYED

Miss C. has vomited five times this morning. At midday you visit her at home. She has been vomiting in the morning for 6 weeks. She suffers from idiopathic epilepsy and takes phenytoin 100 mg t.i.d. and carbamazepine 200 mg t.i.d. She has had two fits in the last 2 weeks. Four months ago she was put on the pill 'to regulate her periods'. Her pill has been changed four times from 'weak ones' to Anovlar but she still has erratic bleeding most of the time (present on the day you see her). She has no abdominal pain, dysuria or diarrhoea. Examination is non-contributory. Her parents seem anxious and both were present most of the time. Father left when she was examined.

1. What questions is it necessary to ask?
2. What are the reasons for her menstrual problems?
3. Why is she suffering from nausea?
4. Why is she still having epileptic fits?

A. L. A. Reid, Newcastle, Australia

Faints

MISS PAULINE V.   AGED 36   SALESWOMAN   256

Miss V. brought a letter of introduction from her last doctor in another State. She explained that she had to leave because of malicious and wrongful accusations of lesbianism, having lived with a female companion for 10 years since the end of a short marriage. Her letter contained reports from a neurologist reporting inconclusive investigations of blackouts, a urologist reporting investigations of left renal colic with normal IVP but repeated haematuria and serum uric acid of 0.52 mmol/l (8.8 mg%), and a psychiatrist reporting neurotic personality and bisexuality.

She related a convincing story of frequent blackouts and renal colic and queried eligibility for an invalid pension. She correctly stated that one cerebral angiogram had reported a possible space occupying lesion, although not confirmed by further tests. Whilst walking to the couch to be examined she clutched her left side crying out in pain and fell to the floor apparently unconscious.

1. What possible problems are present in Miss V's case?
2. How can Miss V's case be assessed?
3. How should Miss V. be treated?

D. G. Chambers, Clare, Australia

MR. X.Y.   AGED 32   PRIMARY SCHOOL TEACHER   257

In a small remote country town you have been called to the hospital to see the patient who has been transported from the school in a colleague's station sedan. The history revealed that following a game of softball with the children he could not use his right arm which quickly went numb and useless. Then the whole body went stiff with some minor shaking and he appeared to become unconscious.

When seen he had heavy breathing with eyes closed, but the eyelids were flickering a lot and the eyelash blink appeared to be responsive. There was no response to painful stimulus anywhere on the trunk or limbs or to questions. All reflexes appeared normal but the muscles appeared to resist passive movements. There was no neck stiffness.

There was a history of a domestic crisis at home recently and considerable tension at work. (Offered by the colleague who transported him to the hospital).

1. What additional information should be sought?

2. Is this condition a medical emergency?
3. How would you manage this condition using only the resources of the country hospital and yourself?

T. D. Manthorpe, Port Lincoln, Australia

258 MR. J.S.   AGED 47   JEWELLER

Mr. J.S. presented with a story that last night he woke at about 3 a.m. with a desire to empty his bladder. On completion of voiding he suddenly felt dizzy and passed out in the toilet hitting his head on the floor.His wife heard the noise, found him recovering consciousness, and assisted him to bed. He refused to call a doctor then, but agreed to come for a check-up in the morning even though he had had a previous check-up by you three months before when no abnormalities were discovered. His general health is normally excellent.

1. What is the likely diagnosis?
2. What investigations would be appropriate?
3. How would you manage the problem?

T. D. Manthorpe, Port Lincoln, Australia

259 MR. CLAUDE K.   AGED 65   RETIRED FISHERMAN

This patient, who was normally well apart from moderate hypertension, was seen at 9 p.m. after complaining of having fainted. He had a poorly localized pain in the back in the upper lumbar region. His blood pressure was 160/90 and his pulse was 80/minute. He fainted briefly again while recumbent. No abnormality was found, no treatment was given, and the patient told to report if further worried. At 6.30 a.m. the following morning the patient was seen again. He was collapsed, BP 44/20, pulse fast and thready. He was alert, bathed with sweat, and still complaining of back pain. A provisional diagnosis of ruptured aortic aneurysm was made and he was sent 20 miles to hospital, where the diagnosis was confirmed at successful surgery.

1. What significant fact was overlooked at the time of the first examination?
2. Often syncope may be confused with an epileptic seizure. What are the implications of an error in diagnosis by the general practitioner?

J. G. P. Ryan, Brisbane

MRS. M.W.   AGED 55

Mrs. M.W., a heavily built, pale, 55 year old, said her usual doctor was to be away for 2 weeks, but he had given her some tablets which made her feel faint and should she continue taking them? She presented a bottle of chlorothiazide from her handbag. She and her husband were due to go on holiday next week to see her daughter – a long flight.

Immediate assessment showed very pale mucosae, and, on questioning, her periods used to be heavy, but there had been none for three months. She had no gastrointestinal symptoms, except troublesome haemorrhoids. She ate well. She had had no previous operations or illnesses.

A full examination showed no abnormality except a soft systolic murmur at the apex. BP 140/85. Breasts normal, abdomen normal, PV normal, cervical smear cytology normal. PR normal except for pendulous haemorrhoids. Urine normal. Blood test revealed a haemoglobin of 5.1 g/dl and hypochromic microcytic red blood cells.

1. What other investigations are necessary, now or later?
2. How should this situation be managed?
3. Are there any obligations to her original doctor?

G. M. Dick, Hobart

MR. A.H.   AGED 62

This man came to see the doctor complaining of blackouts. For the previous 4 weeks he had experienced attacks of unconsciousness. These started with a burning sensation in the limbs and up the back of the neck: he then became shaky, his vision became blurred and he lost consciousness for 5–10 minutes during which he was quite limp and motionless. He would then stir and wake with a headache. Earlier in the year he had had an episode of hysterical aphonia which appeared to be a reaction to his daughter's behaviour. More recently he had had an attack of torticollis which lasted over a month. In the past he had had pulmonary tuberculosis treated successfully and a gastrectomy for duodenal ulcer 10 years before.

The doctor thought that this might be reactive hypoglycaemia due to his previous gastrectomy and arranged a glucose tolerance test. This showed a sudden fall in the blood sugar from 7.9 to 2.3 mmol/l an hour after a 50 g glucose load and seemed to confirm his suspicions. He explained the biochemical events causing the symptoms and advised the patient on his diet. There was no improvement, and after 2 weeks the attacks were as troublesome as ever. On further discussion it appeared that he had misunderstood the doctor's explanation and advice about carbohydrate intake and increased instead of reduced his sugar intake. As he worked in a factory with high speed machinery and dangerous chemicals, it was felt that he could not be allowed back to work. He was referred to a consultant for further investigations.

1. What is the biochemical mechanism of reactive hypoglycaemia following partial gastrectomy?
2. What other conditions could have caused attacks of unconsciousness in this man?

A. G. Strube, Crawley, UK

262   MR. ROBERT J.   AGED 46   MECHANIC

Home visit 7 a.m. Monday. Mrs. J. tried to wake Mr. J. but was unable to get any sense out of him. His health is generally good, although he takes occasional antacid tablets and sometimes gets diarrhoea and frequently vomits.

A domestic upset over the weekend was precipitated by the wife's frustration at his increasing loss of libido. He had then drunk a lot of alcohol and eaten little food.

She described Mr. J. as a moderate drinker with occasional binges. On questioning Mr. J. his answers were unintelligible. Dextrostix blood sugar level was 2.2 mmol/l (40 mg%). Glucose mixture was administered by mouth and Mr. J. rapidly recovered full consciousness.

1. What problem could Mr. J. have had?
2. What are the possible roles of his wife in his illness?
3. What treatment does he require?

D. G. Chambers, Clare, Australia

263   MRS. O.H.   AGED 78   WIDOW

Mrs. O.H. was found in a semi-conscious state in bed early one morning while staying with her daughter following discharge from hospital where she had a total hip replacement complicated by a wound infection. Her daughter called her mother's general practitioner who refused a home visit, so she phoned her own doctor who agreed to travel 8 kilometres to the home.

When he arrived he found a semi-conscious patient who responded irrationally to painful stimuli but there were no abnormal neurological signs. There was a small discharging sinus over her hip. Three bottles of tablets were by her bedside – glibenclamide (Daonil), diazepam (Valium) and chlorothiazide (Chlotride).

1. What is the likely cause of her problem?
2. Who should take responsibility for this home visit?
3. Who should take responsibility for the patient's ongoing management?

J. E. Murtagh, Melbourne

Funny turns

MR. E.S.B. AGED 21 UNEMPLOYED UNSKILLED

264

Mr. E.S.B. presented complaining of feeling 'unwell' and 'dizzy'. On further questioning he admitted to a similar episode 1 month ago when he noticed 'vague loss of balance' for 1 day following an argument with his brother. He is unemployed since losing his only job 4 years ago. He has no training, few prospects, looks depressed, and complains of the noise and tension of living in a cramped housing commission flat with his pensioned mother and four siblings.

1. Is the diagnosis likely to be functional or organic?
2. Examination reveals a sweaty, febrile patient with scattered rhonchi, crepitations and a degree of bronchospasm throughout the chest. Does this change your earlier diagnosis?
3. What further investigations are indicated in this case?
4. Is counselling of any use here?

D. U. Shepherd, Melbourne

MR. WILLIAM L. AGED 59 CHEMICAL ENGINEER

265

Mr. L. was retrenched at work 18 months ago; as a result, he lost considerable income and status within the firm. During the months of his re-adjustment to these circumstances he began to suffer dizzy spells and thought his eyesight may have been responsible, especially in view of the fact that his dizziness was only apparent when he was wearing his bi-focals.

Physical examination reveals only mild hypertension of 160/100 but a paired quadrantic defect is detected on testing his visual fields. Closer questioning discloses the fact that he has had difficulty backing his car and has twice narrowly avoided accidents when he failed to see other motor vehicles on his right.

1. What is the most likely cause of this patient's symptoms and of the physical findings?
2. What is the overall management plan for this patient?

W. L. Ogborne, Sydney

266 MRS. M.S.   AGED 72

This elderly lady called the doctor as she had felt weak and dizzy for a few days. Her companion commented that she had seemed confused at times, complained of headache and had vomited occasionally. Three weeks previously she had fallen over on the ice outside her home and had struck her head on the pavement but had recovered completely from this incident. In the past she had suffered with depression severe enough to require ECT but eventually this was recognized as a manic-depressive illness and had responded to lithium.

The doctor, who knew her well, found her rather withdrawn; there was slight weakness of the right arm and hand and the right side of the face. In view of the recent head injury, he considered the possibility of subdural haematoma and arranged her admission to hospital. On arrival she was bright and cheerful but still with right sided weakness and the medical staff felt that she had suffered a minor stroke. She was treated with physiotherapy in an attempt to rehabilitate her. However, the next day she became more confused and could not co-operate with treatment. A CT brain scan was arranged and this showed a subdural haematoma overlying the left parietal area. This was evacuated and she made a complete recovery.

1. What is the differential diagnosis of this condition?
2. How important was the doctor's previous knowledge of the patient in arriving at the correct diagnosis?

A. G. Strube, Crawley, UK

267 MR. C.G.   AGED 80   RETIRED CIRCUS AERIALIST - WIDOWER

Mr. C.G. complains of attacks of unsteadiness lasting 2 to 3 seconds, occurring several times a day. He has a heart rate of 70 with atrial fibrillation. He is not on any drugs. Past illnesses include a stroke 5 years ago with no residual paresis, but he has an aphasia for names of objects and an homonymous hemianopia. BP is 190/90.

1. What causes of his attacks should be considered?
2. How would you attempt to determine the cause?
3. Would you treat his hypertension?

C. T. Lamont, Ottawa

268 MR. COLIN H.   AGED 45   BANK OFFICER

Colin holds a senior position with a major bank. He gives a 2 month history of momentary bouts of unsteadiness associated with lack of concentration and feelings of 'woolly headedness'. On two occasions this feeling has occurred when motoring and he has pulled his car off the road. The attacks are more frequent at present during a very stressful period at work. Conversely when he was on holidays a month ago, he had little trouble.

After an exhaustive physical examination and investigation, a diagnosis of transient ischaemic attacks (TIAs) was made.

1. You are asked directly whether he should consider early retirement. What factors would influence your advice?
2. Colin asks what activities he should avoid?
3. What treatment would you recommend?

K. C. Nyman, Perth, Australia

MRS. Y.B.   AGED 63   ACCOUNTANT   269

Mrs. Y.B. presented with transient episodes of numbness of her right face and weakness of her right arm that lasted less than ½ hour. There was some minor disturbance of her speech but no symptoms in her leg. The patient was married with two adult children. She had diabetes mellitus for 20 years controlled on 30 units of Lente insulin and 10 units of regular insulin each morning. She was also being treated for hypertension with hydrochlorothiazide, methyldopa and clonidine.

These episodes continued for several days, and each time the patient was left completely normal. She was admitted to hospital where cerebral angiography was done. No surgery was performed. The patient was treated with dipyridamole (Persantin) and aspirin.

1. What is the most likely diagnosis?
2. How would you confirm the diagnosis?
3. How would you treat this patient?
4. What is the prognosis?

R. L. Perkin, Toronto

MR. G.S.   AGED 46   UNIVERSITY PROFESSOR   270

An active, fit (5'9", 150 lb) university professor, a former rugby team mate, presents with painful knees. His wife is a nutritionist. He has a history of bilateral medial and lateral meniscectomy and cruciate ligament repairs. X-rays of his knees reveal extensive calcification of his popliteal arteries. You discuss the significance. Next month he returns complaining of dysarthria, loss of ability to concentrate and fears a stroke.

1. What is causing the pain in his knees?
2. What advice do you give regarding exercise at work and recreation?

3. How do you feel about referral to a specialist?
4. What nutritional advice do you give?

P. R. Grantham, Vancouver

271   MRS. C.D.   AGED 52   HOUSEWIFE

Mrs. C.D. was in a supermarket on her weekly shopping outing. It appears that she suddenly collapsed and had, in the opinion of witnesses, an epileptiform seizure. This was her first such attack. She was rushed to the hospital and was treated and fully investigated. No cause was detected and no definite diagnosis was made. Approximately 6 months later she suddenly developed a second fit followed by a left hemiplegia.

1. What could be the cause of this epileptiform seizure?
2. What investigations and diagnostic procedures would you advise?
3. What would you advise the family and patient?

B. M. Fehler, Johannesburg

272   MR. W.C.   AGED 81   RETIRED GOLDMINER

The patient lived by himself, assisted by neighbours, in a remote seaside village. He was brought to see the doctor by the district nurse because he had become vague and complained of weakness. Questioning revealed increasing weakness and deterioration in vision as well as occasional confusional attacks over the previous few days. Examination was unrevealing apart from the presence of glycosuria. He was admitted to the local cottage hospital for further investigation. Twenty four hours later he developed a profound right hemiparesis.

1. What morbid processes are involved?
2. What investigations are warranted in this case?
3. What is the most appropriate treatment?

R. W. Roberts, Ravensthorpe, Australia

273   MRS. W.H.   AGED 37   MOTHER (EX NURSE)

Mrs. W.H. was a former nurse, married and the mother of seven children. She had chronic asthma all her adult life, reasonably well controlled on medication. For 3 years she had been taking desensitization injections for allergy. She came into the office one evening complaining of numbness and paraesthesiae in both feet but more pronounced in the right foot, and this had been present for 6 days. It had reached a point where she had difficulty walking for the previous 2 days. Also, 2 days before she had suddenly developed loss of vision in the lower half of the visual field of her right eye.

On examination there was decreased sensation to light touch, pin prick and hot/cold sensation on the dorsum of her right foot. Vibration and position sense were intact. There was no motor weakness. The right ankle reflex was absent and the left plantar response was extensor. There was a large scotoma occupying the lower half of her visual field in the right eye and the temporal half of her optic disc appeared pale.

Without anything other than supportive treatment, her symptoms resolved over a 6 week period. The consultant neurologist suggested that her allergy injections be discontinued. Three years later despite advice to the contrary, the patient had her eighth child without any complications, and then consented to a tubal ligation.

1. How do you proceed when presented with a patient who has alarming symptoms?
2. What are the important skills for managing patients with chronic incurable disease?
3. How do you deal with the family and home situation?

R. L. Perkin, Toronto

GAIL M.   AGED 22   PHARMACIST'S ASSISTANT   274

Gail first presented 2 years previously with numbness and weakness of the left arm. She was fully investigated neurologically and by the time the workup was completed her symptoms had completely disappeared. She now presented with severe vertigo and was unable to walk, complained of double vision and became very tearful when questioned and examined. Neurological examination showed diminished tendon reflexes in the lower limbs, and she developed a squint over the next few days. X-rays, CT scan, lumbar puncture, blood tests were all negative, and within 10 days she had recovered apart from a rather strange foot-slapping gait.

1. What would make you suspect that the first incident was physical disease?
2. Are there any further investigations that would assist you in resolving this case?

R. M. Meyer, Johannesburg

MR. C.D.   AGED 45   PROCESS WORKER   275

Mr. D. presented with inability to concentrate at his work and a tremor in his hands. He denied heavy alcohol consumption. He went to school until 14 years and has been in only two jobs since then. He is vague about his family history, but knows his father died at 50 years.

Over the next six months, both symptoms become more exaggerated. He has been asked to leave his job. He developed some bizarre grimacing. He now walks with a dancing gait.

1. What diagnosis is most likely?
2. What iatrogenic causes could present like this?
3. If the patient's father had the same symptoms prior to his death, what advice would you give the patient's son?

A. Himmelhoch, Sydney

276 MR. J.H.   AGED 103   SPANISH AMERICAN WAR VETERAN

Mr. J.H. has a complete heart block which has been present for at least 3 years. Heart rate is 48–52. He has advanced senile dementia and requires assistance in all activities. He takes frusemide 20 mg daily. The chief of the geriatric service has recommended a pacemaker to improve his cerebral circulation and, hopefully, his mental confusion.

1. Do you agree with this recommendation?
2. What type of myocardial infarction is most likely to cause complete heart block?

C. T. Lamont, Ottawa

CHAPTER 14

Eye Problems

This chapter illustrates eye infections, eye injuries, the diagnostic challenges of the red eye, loss of vision and blurred vision, and exemplifies a number of serious eye conditions.

The red eye

277 **MR. ANDREW G.**   **AGED 22**   **UNIVERSITY STUDENT**

Andrew presents complaining of an uncomfortable gritty feeling in his left eye for the last 2 days, and crusting of his eyelids in the morning. You notice his left eye is red.

1. What are the diagnostic possibilities?
2. How will you distinguish between these possibilities?
3. What management is appropriate for each cause of the unilateral red eye?

W. E. Fabb, Melbourne

278 **HARRY L.**   **AGED 40**   **SCIENTIFIC OFFICER**

Harry is yet another victim of influenza, there being a moderately severe epidemic in the practice area. Partly because of the clinical severity of Harry's attack and partly because he is a neighbour, the doctor revisits 2 days later. He finds Harry still confined to bed, but feeling a bit better. Though it is broad daylight, the bedroom curtains are drawn. 'The light hurts my eyes,' says Harry, and examination reveals blepharospasm, epiphora and ciliary injection confined to the left eye.

1. What constitutes an epidemic?
2. What factors influence the doctor's decision to follow up a patient?
3. Does Harry suffer from a potentially serious eye condition?
4. What needs to be done to help Harry?

J. D. E. Knox, Dundee

279 **MR. GEOFFREY B.**   **AGED 24**   **MOTOR MECHANIC**

Mr. B. presents with a painful, red right eye, which he has had for 6 hours. He thinks he has something in it. He works as a motor mechanic in an automotive workshop.

1. What specific enquiries would you make concerning the possibility of traumatic injury?
2. If he revealed that he had been using an emery wheel to take the rough off a weld, what would you specifically look for?
3. How do you manage a ferrous foreign body in the cornea from an emery wheel?

W. E. Fabb, Melbourne

Visual disturbances

MR. DARRYN E.   AGED 38   SHEETMETAL WORKER
280

Mr. E. is brought in because he has been struck in the left eye with a piece of metal whilst hammering a piece of heavy gauge sheetmetal half an hour ago. He was not wearing goggles. He complains of pain and blurring of vision in his left eye.

1. What is the likely diagnosis?
2. How would you assess this patient?
3. How would you manage this problem?

W. E. Fabb, Melbourne

MRS. JESSICA F.   AGED 63   HOUSEWIFE
281

This 63 year old woman presents with marked pain in her right eye for 3 hours, accompanied by blurring of vision in that eye. She is nauseated and has vomited several times.

1. What diagnostic hypotheses would you entertain?
2. What steps would you take to investigate this problem?
3. What emergency measures would you be anticipating may have to be carried out?

W. E. Fabb, Melbourne

MR. T.C.   AGED 28   PROOFREADER
282

This 28 year old black proofreader was referred to the office by an insurance company physician who had found an elevated blood pressure. An examination 2 years earlier had shown his blood pressure to be normal. Additional history revealed that he had sustained a 14 pound weight loss in the past 3 months, a noticeable decrease in vision, particularly in the left eye in the last 2 months, and a decrease in sexual function during the last month.

He gave a family history of diabetes and stated that his mother had died of a stroke; he knew nothing about his father. Review of systems was essentially negative. He did not smoke; however he did drink 4 to 5 beers daily.

Physical examination revealed his weight to be 185 pounds with a blood pressure of 230/150 in all positions. Ophthalmoscopic examination revealed spasm of the retinal arteries with a vein-to-artery ratio of 6:1. Flame haemorrhages, cotton wool exudates, and bilateral papilloedema were noted. The heart was enlarged to the left with a pre-systolic gallop. The peripheral pulses were all palpable; there was no oedema.

1. What main types of hypertension should be considered in this case?
2. What compliance factors will be important in the management of this case?
3. What are the feared complications of sustained non-malignant hypertension?

L. H. Amundson, Sioux Falls, SD, USA

283 MR. JONATHON J. AGED 23 BOOKKEEPER

Mr. J. presents because yesterday he noticed that when he closed his right eye, the vision in his left eye was quite blurred. He has never noticed this before.

1. What conditions would you be thinking about which might have caused his blurred vision?
2. How would you investigate this problem?
3. If he told you that he had noticed some clumsiness in his gait whilst walking to work a couple of weeks ago, which cleared up in a few days, what would you suspect? What would you do to confirm or rule out your suspicions?

W. E. Fabb, Melbourne

284 MR. D.W. AGED 25 SOCIAL WORKER

Mr. W. hobbles into your surgery on crutches with one leg encased in plaster. He reports that 2 weeks ago he fell at football with an opponent across his leg. This caused him extreme pain in his knee. He was taken to hospital and found to have ruptured ligaments in his knee, which were sutured under a general anaesthetic. About 1 week later, while still in hospital he noticed some blurring of his vision, particularly the upper part of his visual field. He reported this to the intern, but he could find no abnormality in his left eye. Mr. W. was discharged 2 days ago and has now come to see you because he feels his vision is getting worse. He has virtually no vision in the upper half of his field, as though his upper lid is drooping over the eye. Everything that he can see has a blurred edge.

1. What is the most likely cause of his visual loss?
2. What other conditions could cause these symptoms?
3. Mr. W. is entitled to compensation for his leg injury. What about his eye injury?
4. Knee permitting, will Mr. W. be able to return to football?

W. F. Glastonbury, Adelaide

MRS. J. AGED 27 MEDICAL SECRETARY

285

Mrs. J. presented to the office with sudden impairment of vision in the right eye of 6 hours' duration. Vision testing was 20/200 in the right eye and 20/30 in the left eye. Crude visual field testing was difficult to assess in the right eye and normal in the left eye. Fundoscopic examination revealed some evidence of retinal haemorrhage. The patient was referred to an ophthalmologist who diagnosed a retinal detachment secondary to a congenital retinal degenerative condition.

She was admitted to hospital for management of the problem by surgical intervention (laser therapy was not practicable in 1973). Post-operatively she was very nauseated and was given 5 doses of 10 mg of Torecan (thiethylperazine) to control the vomiting. She recovered some vision but realized within two weeks that she had been amenorrhoeic for the previous 2 or 3 weeks. A pregnancy test revealed that she was indeed pregnant and had been during the hospitalization. She was very anxious to have the baby and sought advice as to the risks of teratogenic effects on the foetus. The other major problem was the risk of further retinal detachment during labour and delivery from pushing and straining.

1. What are the signs and symptoms of acute retinal detachment?
2. How can the risk of giving women undesirable drugs very early in pregnancy be reduced?
3. How would you propose to manage labour in this situation?

W. W. Rosser, Ottawa

MRS. H.J. AGED 58 HOUSEWIFE

286

Mrs. J. has essential hypertension and has been on therapy from your practice for 6 years. She is a compliant patient and has been ordered chlorothiazide 1 g per day and propranolol 40 mg b.d.

She presents today with a request to have her eyes checked. She had new glasses fitted 6 months ago, but during the last month her vision has deteriorated and she cannot see figures on the television screen. Examination reveals she has lost 10 kg in weight in 3 months and now weighs 58 kg. Her blood pressure is 140/95 sitting and standing and her pulse rate 60/min. Examination of the ocular fundi reveals no cataract, no exudate, but with her new glasses on one cannot see the vessels in focus clearly.

1. What is happening?
2. What side effects can occur with chlorothiazide and propranolol?
3. What other side effects can occur with anti-hypertensive therapy?

A. Himmelhoch, Sydney

287 MR. G.H. AGED 75 RETIRED

Mr. H. had no significant illnesses until 3 weeks ago when he suddenly became unwell with fever, muscle pain and morning stiffness. Appetite had diminished. Generalized headache began two days ago. Today he complains of mistiness of vision.

1. What points are you looking for when examining the patient?
2. What investigation might give you the diagnosis?
3. What is the management of the case?

A. Himmelhoch, Sydney

288 LISA P. AGED 9 MONTHS

Lisa is the second child of a pleasant, middle-class couple, and had a normal delivery at the local hospital. She attends the baby clinic regularly, and one day the health visitor happens to note an odd appearance in one eye. There is a white reflex, replacing the black pupil, and with an ophthalmoscope all that can be seen is a pink-white mass obscuring the fundus. The other eye is normal.

Uncertain as to the diagnosis, you refer her to the ophthalmologist next week. A month later, she is discharged from hospital, having had the eye enucleated. She is fitted with a realistic glass eye, but has a sticky discharge in the socket.

1. What eye conditions merit such drastic treatment?
2. What reactions are possible from her parents?
3. How should her present problem be treated?

J. Grabinar, Bromley, UK

CHAPTER 15

Upper Respiratory Problems (Including ENT Problems)

This chapter comprises a series of ear problems, with emphasis on the recognition and management of otitis media; nasal problems, including epistaxis, sinusitis and nasal allergy; mouth and throat problems, including a number of cases of sore throat of varying aetiology; several cases of cough resulting from a variety of causes; and the problem of a bone in the throat. These cases represent some of the most common conditions seen by the family physician.

Ear problems

289 **MATTHEW B.   AGED 2**

Matthew B. had had a cold for the past 24 hours. He had had no previous ear trouble but an hour before being brought to the office, had developed an intense earache affecting his right ear. He was crying and distressed by pain.

1. What clinical examination would you make and how would you do it?
2. What is the most likely diagnosis?
3. What predisposing conditions might be associated with this disorder?
4. What is the most likely causative organism?
5. What medications would you prescribe?
6. What advice would you give the parents?

H. C. Watts, Perth, Australia

290 **M.N.   AGED 3**

The patient presents with a coryza for 4 days, cough for 2 days and pulling at the ears with disturbed sleep in the previous night. He has had two similar previous attacks. On examination, the temperature is 38 °C, throat slightly red, chest clear. Ears: left drum – shiny, slightly full and injected, right drum – red around the handle, dull drum and bulging a little.

1. What are this child's problems?
2. What immediate treatment is indicated?
3. What advice would you offer to the parents about future management?

T. D. Manthorpe, Port Lincoln, Australia

291 **JOHN F.   AGED 6**

John is brought by his mother. He awoke last night with earache. He has had earaches before. He is chirpy and not in pain. Examination shows a red left ear drum. There is no fever.

1. What is the diagnosis?
2. What would you do?

J. Fry, Beckenham, UK

DAVID M.   AGED 3

292

Doctor M. had built a small cottage at a remote beach. It was about 50 miles over a poor road from the nearest doctor. He had had a busy few weeks and decided not to take his medical bag as he wanted to get away from it all and not be disturbed by medical work.

As they approached the cottage David M. began to complain of a pain in the cheek. He was about 3 years old and his father thought he might be cutting a tooth. Presently the pain worsened and David was very miserable and cried a great deal. Dr. M. had a look as best he could in the mouth but that seemed quite normal. The nose was a little congested but otherwise in the absence of medical equipment, nothing could be found. Eventually a visit to the general store produced an aspirin and David was made sufficiently comfortable to go off to sleep.

In the morning, to his horror Dr. M. discovered a small patch of moisture on David's pillow and there was some pus in the aural canal. David felt much better.

1. Why was the cause not recognized?
2. What treatment would you have recommended if the diagnosis had been made in the first instance?
3. Do you regard otitis media as a medical emergency?
4. Would you wish to follow up the child?

J. G. Richards, Auckland

JAMES H.   AGED 7   SCHOOLBOY

293

James H. developed fever, running nose and cough 4 days ago. The night before last he was very restless and complained of earache and the next morning there was discharge from the right ear and he felt better. This morning he has been vomiting, the earache has returned and he is feverish. He looks sick and the ear is still discharging. He has marked tenderness over his right mastoid.

1. What problems have occurred?
2. How would you manage this problem?
3. Discuss the infection process in this case?

E. J. H. North, Melbourne

MASTER J.R.   AGED 3

294

Master J.R. is brought to you by his mother because of a high temperature last night and today crying incessantly, pulling at both ears and with a rattling chest cough. He has been seen many times over the last 2 years with infections of both ears in association with tonsillitis, and has been hospitalised on a number of occasions at the Children's Hospital for 'bronchitis'.

1. Is this just another attack of otitis media and 'bronchitis'?
2. What do you want to know about the social situation?
3. What long term effects are taking place?

W. F. Glastonbury, Adelaide

295 MRS. S.K.   AGED 29   SCHOOLTEACHER

Mrs. S.K. is happily married to an ambitious bank accountant, six years her senior. They have two children: Ronnie aged 3 years, and Susan aged 6 months. She is obviously worried. 'I am sure that Ronnie is partially deaf, doctor' she says.

1. How would you clarify this problem?
2. What are the implications on the family, of a child suffering from permanent hearing impairment?
3. What facilities in the community can assist the family to cope with a child suffering from impaired hearing?
4. Could Ronnie's hearing disorder have been diagnosed at an earlier age, or perhaps been prevented?

M. R. Polliack, Tel-Aviv, Israel

296 MR. C.K.   AGED 50   ENGINEER

Mr. C.K., aged 50, is a 'resident engineer' who has recently moved to the practice area to supervise a construction project. He is living on his own in a hotel. He consults with a 10-day history of bilateral deafness associated with an acute upper respiratory catarrh.

When he reports a week later, it is obvious that the medical measures which were instituted have effected no improvement – his deafness is worse than ever.

Physical reassessment gives no reason to alter the original diagnosis, but he now confesses to feeling generally unwell; it is agreed to put him on the sick list.

He wishes to take the opportunity to convalesce at his own home where his wife resides on her own; but this is 400 miles away and he would like to make the trip by air.

When he returns a week later, his deafness is even more marked. It is decided to seek specialist advice.

1. What measures do general practitioners take to enable patients, who are new to a practice, to make the best use of the services they have to offer?

2. Deafness is a relatively common presenting symptom in family medicine. In general, what are common causes of bilateral deafness?
3. Putting a patient on the 'sick list' is a common doctor activity. Viewed in sociological terms, what does this activity entail?

J. D. E. Knox, Dundee

MR. G.   AGED 54   COMPANY DIRECTOR   **297**

Mr. G. presents complaining of an upper respiratory infection. He has not been overseas for the past 5 years and is currently about to fly to Malaysia on business in two weeks. He wants to know what he should do about immunizations. He is particularly worried about the possibility of getting malaria.

1. What advice will you give him related to his current infection?
2. What will you advise him about immunizations in general?
3. What is your advice about malaria prophylaxis?

J. R. Marshall, Adelaide

Nose problems

298   **MR. GERALD M.   AGED 71   RETIRED SCHOOLTEACHER**

Mr. M. is brought into your office with a bleeding nose. He has tried to stop it for the last hour. He has had several previous episodes of epistaxis, but all have stopped quickly when he held his nose. He is on treatment for moderate hypertension.

He has his nose covered by a very blood-stained towel and spits out blood clots as you examine him.

1. What are the likely contributing factors to his epistaxis?
2. How would you manage this situation?
3. What follow up will be needed?

W. E. Fabb, Melbourne

299   **G.P.   AGED 2½**

G.P. transferred from another practice when the family moved house. Past history of severe nose bleeds with one packing (GP) and two cauteries (ENT specialist) and said to have been fully investigated. The child presented with a severe nose bleed and was said to bruise easily.

1. Why is the above history unsatisfactory?
2. What would your next move be toward effective management?
3. What are your intuitive feelings about this story?

W. D. Jackson, Launceston, Australia

300   **MR. C. CHAN   AGED 46   CHINESE RICE MERCHANT**

Mr. Chan complained to the doctor that he had noticed a lump in his neck a few weeks ago. He attributed this lump to his recent bout of late nights and heavy smoking. In the last 2 weeks he has also been having recurrent nose bleeds. However, his main worry is the fact that he has been coughing up some dark, bloody sputum. He does not know whether the blood is coming from his nose or from his lungs. He also has a persistent smelly, post-nasal discharge.

Physical examination revealed a firm mass, size 3 cm × 2 cm in the mid-cervical chain; other lymph nodes were normal. Chest X-ray and peripheral blood smear were normal.

1. What further examination and investigation are required to establish a diagnosis?
2. What is the treatment of choice?
3. What is the prognosis?

N. C. L. Yuen, Hong Kong

MR. N.M.   AGED 41   SAW MILLER

301

This man has a 10-year history of non seasonal recurring 'colds', blocked nose, operation on sinuses and nose by an ENT specialist 3 years ago, an antral wash out 1 year ago and a lack of response to nose drops, antihistamines, and Rynacrom (sodium cromoglycate). The ENT specialist feels no more can be done, but this patient is still dissatisfied and often in considerable discomfort with a blocked, snuffly nose.

1. Is another referral advisable and if so, to whom?
2. Do simple radical antrostomies have a high success rate in chronic sinusitis?
3. Are there any simple measures that may be helpful?

T. D. Manthorpe, Port Lincoln, Australia

MR. F.M.   AGED 42   INSURANCE AGENT

302

Mr F.M. was seen in the office by appointment complaining of nasal stuffiness for several weeks. Following a cold, several weeks previously, there has been continued nasal congestion and a feeling of fullness in the face. There is no significant nasal drainage. A proprietary antihistamine-decongestant helped a little, briefly, a few weeks previous to the appointment.

Past medical history revealed no previous similar symptoms and no allergic history. The only medications have been occasional aspirin for URIs.

Physical examination revealed a 'nasal' speech. On examination of the nose, there was mild redness of all nasal mucous membranes with some mucopurulent drainage from the inferior right nasal passage, mild to moderate tenderness over the right malar region and equivocal transillumination of the right maxillary sinus. Examination of the heart revealed a grade III left precordial systolic murmur and normal rhythm.

1. What would constitute an appropriate differential diagnosis of this man's respiratory symptoms?
2. What are the ramifications of this man's heart murmur?
3. What laboratory procedures would be of most value in assessing this patient's respiratory infection?
4. What are the expected outcomes of a general type screening examination, even for seemingly well-defined, localized problems such as upper respiratory infection?

L. H. Amundson, Sioux Falls, SD, USA

Mouth and throat problems

303 BETTY R.   AGED 2

This child presented with a history of fever and anorexia for 2 days. On examination her temperature was 39.9 °C. She had an offensive breath, ulceration of the tongue, mucous membranes and gums, and enlargement of the cervical lymph nodes. She was drooling saliva and was obviously distressed. Her mother said that she absolutely refused to eat and it was very difficult to persuade her to drink anything.

1.   What was the most likely cause of her illness?
2.   If this condition were due to an infective agent, what other clinical manifestations could be produced by it?

J. G. P. Ryan, Brisbane

304 MR. Q.R.   AGED 65   RETIRED ENGINEER

Mr. R. consults his doctor for the second time about an ulcer on his tongue. On looking at the ulcer, the doctor feels quite certain it has undergone malignant change and he is perturbed about the status of a small lump beneath the mandible. Before he can think what to say next, the patient proceeds to tell the doctor how grateful he and his wife are that the doctor had previously pursued the occurrence of his chest pain to the diagnosis of myocardial vascular insufficiency, and how fortunate it was that the doctor persuaded him, almost against their wishes, to agree to by-pass surgery. He never has angina and has been able to do most of the things he wishes in the 20 months since the operation.

1.   What is the doctor thinking?
2.   What does he say next to the patient?
3.   What does he say to the patient's wife, whom he knows will be ringing up after the consultation?

P. L. Gibson, Auckland

305 DR. P.F.   AGED 32   UNIVERSITY LECTURER

Dr. P.F. presents with an acutely painful throat which reveals a marked tonsillar exudate. He has recently arrived from overseas to take up a new position. His wife is pregnant and due to be confined in 6 weeks time. They have two other small children. He has a heavy work load and has heard about the debilitating effects of infectious mononucleosis which is endemic in the area.

1. How specific can a general practitioner be when diagnosing viral respiratory infections?
2. What viral infections cause concern during pregnancy?
3. How does a nuclear family cope when the only wage earner in the family is ill?

B. H. Connor, Armidale, Australia

S.P. AGED 5

306

S.P., a 5 year old male, gives a 2-day history of sore throat and fever. There has been some trouble swallowing, especially solids. The mother reports that the child has been lethargic. An 8 year old sister had a similar problem one week previously, and a 10 year old sister a similar problem two weeks previously. None of the children have had any immunizations.

1. What would be key diagnostic elements in the history and physical examination?
2. What factors would be helpful in making a positive diagnosis?
3. What other physical findings might help confirm or exclude a streptococcal tonsillo-pharyngitis?

L. H. Amundson, Sioux Falls, SD, USA

TRACEY N. AGED 4

307

Tracey has had up to ten attacks of follicular tonsillitis in the past 8 months. Her appetite is poor, with consequent weight loss. She plays with her friends, but tires easily. The mother says she snores frequently and has marked halitosis. Today she has a severe attack of follicular tonsillitis, temperature 39.6 °C with large cervical glands.
There is a history of a previous convulsion as an infant.

1. How would you manage the present complaint?
2. What advice would you give the parents?
3. Would you refer the patient to an ENT surgeon?

B. M. Fehler, Johannesburg

MASTER A.T. AGED 8

308

Master A.T. is brought to your office because of a fever and sore throat of 24 hours duration. He is normally quite well. His family are well known to you, and Anthony is rarely sick. Physical examination reveals acute tonsillitis only.

1. What immediate treatment is necessary?
2. When should antibiotics be prescribed in an otherwise healthy child?
3. What signs of complications would you look for?
4. At this age, and with this history, what other diagnoses are likely?
5. Is tonsillectomy indicated? If so, when?

D. U. Shepherd, Melbourne

309   DICK THOMSON   AGED 8   SCHOOLBOY

Dick's mother brings him along saying 'He's got a sore throat again doctor'. Before you can say anything she is demanding antibiotics to fix it quickly and asking about taking his tonsils out. You notice on the card that Dick has had two episodes of sore throat this winter, the second of which was diagnosed as tonsillitis and treated with penicillin.

This time in fact, the main symptoms (and signs) are a runny nose and cough. He is afebrile. His throat is injected with only slight tonsillar enlargement and no pus. There are a few non-tender cervical lymph nodes. Chest, ears and sinuses are clear.

1. Would you prescribe an antibiotic?
2. Would you arrange a tonsillectomy?
3. What other factors are there in managing this case?

R. P. Strasser, Melbourne

310   DAVID P.   AGED 10   SCHOOLBOY

David is brought in by father having had high fever, headache, muscle pains and sore throat for four days.

David was seen two days ago by a partner and was prescribed salicylates and the father was told he had 'flu'.

The father is angry and demands that something more definite is done.

1. What two problems face the doctor?
2. What could be a differential diagnosis of David's condition given the few facts above?

F. Mansfield, Perth, Australia

311   MR. A.J.   AGED 25   UNIVERSITY STUDENT

It is Sunday morning during the local summer holiday. You visit Ahmed J., a 25 year old Middle Eastern postgraduate university student, living with his wife (from the same country) and 2 year old child in their flat. The reason for the visit is Mr. J., who is lying in bed, looking sorry for himself, and complaining of a sore throat. He does not look ill.

You remember a previous visit for a similar situation some 6 months ago, when you felt that Mr. J. was rather introspective. You note a profusion of patent medicines on the dressing table and at his bedside.

The salient positive physical findings are: pulse rate 82/min; temperature 37.8 °C; a diffuse faucial injection, and palpable tender cervical lymph nodes on both sides.

1. What physical diagnoses would you consider to be likely?
2. What problems, real or imaginary, may be inherent in this situation?
3. How would you manage this situation?

J. D. E. Knox, Dundee

MASTER J.R.   AGED 6   SCHOOLBOY   312

J.R. is in his second year of primary school. He presents with a 2 day history of high fever, sore throat and tender enlarged cervical nodes. He had several similar episodes during his pre-school years, but since starting school has been averaging 3–4 attacks per year. He often has an associated earache and on a number of occasions has been noted to have acute otitis media. His mother also reports that he is a mouth breather and often snores while sleeping.

On examination his tonsils are large with pus in the crypts. The anterior triangle cervical nodes are tender and enlarged. The ears and chest are clear. The oral temperature is 39 °C. A throat swab was taken and oral penicillin and an antipyretic prescribed. The child was given a return appointment for three weeks.

1. Is it possible to determine the aetiological agent of an acute upper respiratory infection on the basis of your physical examination?
2. What are the indications for tonsillectomy and adenoidectomy?
3. What is the role of allergy in the hypertrophy of tonsils and adenoids?

R. L. Perkin, Toronto

MASTER Y.L.   AGED 4   ATTENDS NURSERY SCHOOL   313

A four year old boy, Y.L., comes in to see the doctor with a sore throat. This is his third attack within 9 months. He is pyrexial, 37.6 °C, and has enlarged tonsils and palpable tonsillar glands. The tonsils appear to have pus on them. The doctor initiates a 10-day course of penicillin VK.

The mother brings the patient back 4 days later and if anything, the child looks worse but he is not complaining of his throat. The throat looks unchanged on examination. This failure to respond is unlike the previous attacks.

The doctor tells the mother to come back with the child a week later.

He persists with penicillin and analgesics. The mother is distressed and says that 'It's about time the tonsils were taken out'. The doctor explains his conservative approach to tonsillectomy and what he feels may be the diagnosis here. He also says that he will do blood tests then if the child is still 'ill'.

1. What do you understand by the 'problem solving method', 'hypothesis forming', 'hypothesis testing', 'probability diagnosis', 'testing a hypothesis by treatment' and 'time as a diagnostic tool'?
2. What are your indications for tonsillectomy?
3. Why did the doctor prescribe penicillin VK and for the length of time he did?

J. H. Levenstein, Cape Town

314 MRS. J.A.   AGED 26   HOUSEWIFE

Mrs. J.A. was a working class wife in her twenties with four children between the ages of 2 and 8. She had frequently caused problems in the practice by being abusive towards the receptionist and the nurse and by shouting and swearing at her children in the waiting room. She did her best to see each of the three doctors in turn, always referring to the others by their surnames only and attempting to play off one against the other. Each consultation began aggressively and, if it did not result in a prescription, ended equally aggressively. A source of contention was 6 year old Dawn who had frequent upper respiratory tract infections. Each of the partners in turn reassured Mrs. A. about Dawn's symptoms and the fact that they would diminish as she grew older. Mrs. A. was unconvinced. She had had her own tonsils removed in childhood and was of the firm opinion that her daughter would require the same treatment. The doctors stuck to their guns. Mrs. A. frequently travelled with the children to a nearby city to stay with her mother. On one such occasion Dawn developed a sore throat and was taken to the casualty department of a nearby teaching hospital. There she was treated for tonsillitis and arrangements were made for her to be admitted for tonsillectomy. Mrs. A. returned to the practice in triumph with Dawn minus her tonsils.

1. What is the likely nature of Dawn's problems?
2. What are the indications for tonsillectomy?
3. What are the possible reasons for aggression in a patient?
4. What ethical principles govern relationships between medical practitioners?

T. A. I. Bouchier Hayes, Camberley, UK

315 MRS. FLORENCE A.   AGED 71   HOUSEWIFE

Mrs. A. presents rather distressed an hour after having choked on a fish bone. She feels it is stuck in her throat. She persistently tries to cough it out as you examine her. She tells you she has eaten dry bread in an attempt to remove it, without success.

1. How would you assess this patient?
2. How do you examine a patient with a suspected foreign body in the throat?
3. If the symptoms suggest a foreign body in the throat, but none can be detected, what would you do?

W. E. Fabb, Melbourne

Respiratory problems
---

316 KUMBURAI M.   AGED ?   TODDLER

Mrs. M., previously not known, chubby and obviously pregnant, carried Kumburai into the office. She complained he had been coughing for 3 days and wanted an injection to make him better.

On examination the chest was clear, the temperature was 37.4 °C at 10 a.m., and a crusted discharge could be seen about the nostrils. Kumburai weighed 9 kg but Mrs. M. did not know his age. On questioning it turned out that he had been born at the beginning of the rainy season the year before last, which put his age at about 20 months. He looked normally nourished for a year old baby, and his mid arm circumference was 12.5 cm.

Mrs. M. had walked 9 km to bring him to the office.

1. What treatment should Kumburai have?
2. Is Kumburai suffering from anything of extreme danger to him?
3. What should Mrs. M. be told?

R. T. Mossop, Harare, Zimbabwe

317 JOHN W.   AGED 5   SCHOOLBOY

This 5 year old boy is brought in by his mother because he has a high fever, is irritable and crying, and is refusing food and fluids.

The child is restless, crying loudly, flushed and sweating.

1. What are the likely causes of his condition?
2. How would you assess this child?
3. What general advice would you give mother?

W. E. Fabb, Melbourne

318 WILLIAM ANDREWS   AGED 2   INFANT

William's mother has brought him to see you because from time to time he has bouts of coughing, especially at night. This has been particularly bad over the last 3 days and nights. He has seemed otherwise well and has been sick only once before with croup when he was 8 months old. There is no specific family history although his mother had bronchitis frequently as a child. Physical examination is completely normal.

1. What possible diagnoses are you considering?
2. What investigations would you do?
3. How would manage this problem?

R. P. Strasser, Melbourne

MRS. O.R.   AGED 46   HOUSEWIFE

319

Mrs. O.R. who has never had a day's illness in her life develops a flu-like illness with a high temperature and a dry, harsh cough.

After 2 days in bed taking aspirin and patent cough medicines a visit is requested as she still feels unwell. Her cough is productive of only scanty sputum but is becoming painful.

She does not look seriously ill but has a temperature of 38 °C, a pulse rate of 90 and some scattered fine crepitations at the right lung base.

1. What is the diagnosis?
2. Is it either desirable or possible to determine the actual infecting agent?
3. Which, if any, antibiotic is indicated?

A. J. Moulds, Basildon, UK

E.P.   4 YEAR OLD GIRL

320

E.P. has just entered kindergarten. Previously she has lived in the country with her parents. They now live in a suburban area.

E.P. has had a dry cough and fever for five days. The fever comes and goes – at times she is very sick, but may be bright two hours later.

She has been given only an occasional dose of paracetamol in the last week.

1. What diagnostic hypotheses would be in your mind?
2. How would you test your hypotheses?
3. How would you manage the situation?
4. E.P. has a sister, aged eight months. Mother asks if you can prevent her getting the same condition. What would be your reply?

A. Himmelhoch, Sydney

MR. D.E.   AGED 18   COLLEGE STUDENT

321

This lad is a member of a visiting football team. There is an epidemic of influenza at this time. He feels a bit cold and has muscle aches. He plays football today. You are called to see him tonight because he has aches and pains in the muscles, cannot get warm and has a dry cough.

You confidently make a diagnosis of influenza and order aspirin 600 mg, four times a day. You are called again 24 hours later – he is much worse.

1. Is your first diagnosis correct?
2. On the second visit, what do you think has happened?

A. Himmelhoch, Sydney

322 DEREK B. AGED 40 CIVIL SERVANT

Derek B. presented with a variety of symptoms, including fever, malaise, and muscular aches and pains which had been present for a few days. Ten days previously he had returned from a holiday in the Mediterranean. On examination he had a temperature of 39 °C, but nothing else of significance.

Derek was well known to the doctor and had consulted him frequently over the years. He held an important position in the civil service but found it difficult to make decisions. There were problems in his marriage for many years and after much hesitation he finally divorced his wife some months ago.

1. What are the main diagnoses that you would consider for this pyrexial episode?
2. What investigations might you order?
3. How does a patient's past history influence the doctor's approach and management?

J. C. Hasler, Oxford

323 MR. D.C. AGED 40 COMPANY EXECUTIVE

Mr. D.C. consults you because of a dry cough for 3–4 weeks. He is embarassed at coming, and only did so to please his wife. He feels well and has lost no weight. He has had no significant past illnesses. He has a wife and two small children, is a rising company executive, and smokes intermittently when he is under stress, up to 30 cigarettes per day. He drinks socially. He feels his wife is ambitious. He suspects he is being groomed for a senior company position, and is trying to improve his performance at work.

1. Should you discuss his obvious embarrassment?
2. What are the likely physical findings in this case?
3. If the physical findings are negative, should a chest X-ray be performed?
4. Should the management include a cough suppressant?

D. U. Shepherd, Melbourne

MR. A.C.   AGED 32   STOREMAN

324

Mr. A.C. presents because of a persistent dry cough which has been present for over 2 months. He is apparently otherwise well with no previous illnesses of any significance. He works in a warehouse containing machinery and building supplies. He thinks he has lost some weight recently. He smokes 30–40 cigarettes per day, and is trying to give them up.

1. If your physical examination indicates no specific abnormal findings, with the exception of possible weight loss, what are the most likely diagnoses?
2. What investigations are indicated in this case?
3. What would you prescribe for this cough?
4. If the cough proves to be simply related to excessive smoking, how would you handle this problem?

D. U. Shepherd, Melbourne

CHAPTER 16

Breathing Problems

This chapter begins with a series of cases of dyspnoea due to cardiac, respiratory, allergic, haematological and psychological conditions. Then follows a number of cases of asthma of varying origin, respiratory infection and occupational lung disease. Respiratory problems are among the most common conditions seen by the family physician and often provide him with a challenge in diagnosis or management. The latter is especially true with chronic conditions, such as asthma.

Dyspnoea

325 **MR. JOHN J.   AGED 75**

A 75 year old man presented to his doctor with increasing shortness of breath on exertion and vague pain in the left upper chest for 6 weeks. Otherwise he felt well. The doctor found an area of bronchial breathing in the left upper zone and arranged a chest X-ray.

1. Why should the doctor arrange a chest X-ray?
2. The chest X-ray showed a carcinoma of the bronchus. What would be the doctor's immediate course of action?
3. The chest specialist recommended no treatment. How would the doctor manage the case now?

J. C. Hasler, Oxford

326 **THOMAS R.   AGED 62**

He is an old friend of the practice. In 1952 you arranged for him to have a partial gastrectomy for a troublesome chronic duodenal ulcer. He is very grateful for the complete relief from pain and dyspepsia.

In the past 3 months he has noted breathlessness on exertion with a tightness in his chest.

He is a relaxed, ungrumbling person but today he complains of general weakness, pins and needles in his feet and a sore mouth.

1. What are the long term complications of partial gastrectomy?
2. Give your assessment of his new symptoms.
3. How would you manage the likely conditions that you discover?

J. Fry, Beckenham, UK

327 **MR. & MRS. S.   AGED 64 AND 62   PENSIONERS**

Mrs. S. had consulted the GP several times in recent months complaining of body pains, headaches and dizziness. She seemed convinced that there was something seriously wrong with her physically, but investigations all proved negative.

Mr. S. presented several months after his wife had first consulted the GP. He complained of severe effort dyspnoea. Examination, including ECG, was normal except that he looked pale and his Hb was found to be 4 g/dl. He was admitted to hospital where he was found to have G.I. bleeding.

1. What was the best way of managing Mrs. S.?
2. What was the cause of Mr. S's symptoms?
3. Was there any connection between Mrs. S's symptoms and those of her husband?
4. How are Mr. and Mrs. S. likely to present in the future?

S. Levenstein, Cape Town

MR. J.G.   AGED 76   328

This elderly gentleman had been treated for hypertensive heart disease and late onset asthma. His dyspnoea increased for no very obvious reason. Blood examination revealed significant anaemia. In searching for a cause of this a filling defect was found in his caecum during a barium enema.

1. Should surgery be performed?
2. Would you discuss the whole problem with the patient?
3. How could he be offered the best hope for successful surgery if that is the chosen option?

W. D. Jackson, Launceston, Australia

MRS. I.S.   AGED 45   329

This mother of 3 teenagers, who works with the local Crisis Centre and currently has a contractual arrangement with her husband (who is also your patient) that allows each of them significant extramarital relationships, presents with a cough of 2 months' duration and dyspnoea on exertion. Physical examination reveals a regular tachycardia at 125, gallop rhythm, no murmurs, normotensive, raised JVP and hepatomegaly. Chest X-ray reveals evidence of pulmonary congestion. She asks you not to discuss her medical condition with her husband.

1. What is the most likely diagnosis and the initial management?
2. Extensive cardiological investigation later establishes a diagnosis: idiopathic congestive cardiomyopathy. Now what is the management?
3. You and the patient here face a rare and fatal illness, of unknown cause, with an uncertain natural history. What general principles of management do you establish?

P. R. Grantham, Vancouver

MR. CHARLES B.   AGED 48   FARMER   330

Charlie B., who seldom consults a doctor, presents complaining of increasing dyspnoea, which is impairing his capacity to work his dairy farm, which he manages with the help of his wife. He says this has 'crept up on him' over the last 2 or 3 years. He has smoked 30 cigarettes per day for the last 30 years and has a 'smoker's cough', mostly in the morning, when he coughs up about an egg cup full of clear sputum.

He is a thin, slightly-built man, with tanned, wrinkled skin. He looks older than his chronological age. He is breathless after walking into the room and for the first few minutes after sitting. He breathes through pursed lips. His colour is pink.

1. On this evidence, what diagnostic hypotheses would you be entertaining?
2. What further information would you seek?
3. What plan of action would you develop if your most probable hypothesis is verified?

W. E. Fabb, Melbourne

331 MISS D.R. AGED 70 RETIRED SECRETARY

Miss R. has a long history of chronic obstructive pulmonary disease which has progressed to the point where she needs supplemental oxygen especially during exercise. She has been on prednisone 20 mg daily prior to admission to hospital and has steroid side effects including muscle weakness and osteoporosis.

1. How would you adjust her steroid dosage?
2. How would you treat her osteoporosis?
3. What other measures would be indicated in her rehabilitation programme?

C. T. Lamont, Ottawa

332 MR. J.A. AGED 28 PLUMBER

At 2 a.m. you are called to see a male at home who cannot get his breath. He had been getting worse for the last hour or so. He was a plumber, aged 28 with no relevant past history. He had chest discomfort, some cough with frothy sputum and some wheeze. He had tachycardia, increase in jugular venous pressure, creps at both bases and some ankle oedema.

1. What disease process is occurring?
2. How would you manage the patient?
3. What is the prognosis?

E. J. H. North, Melbourne

MR. W.G.   AGED 72   RETIRED SHOPKEEPER

333

Fit and active with no past history of any significance, Mr. W.G. was seen during the night with an attack of acute pulmonary oedema. At that time his pulse appeared regular and he responded well to treatment.

When revisited the next morning he complained of palpitations and was found to be fibrillating (160 plus). Apart from fine basal creps there were no other abnormalities on examination.

Although home circumstances were good the GP thought that he needed admission to hospital for cardiac monitoring and treatment of his arrhythmia. He said as much to the anxious relatives then phoned the hospital to arrange a bed. Unfortunately the admitting physician did not feel the case warranted hospital care and advised digitalization at home.

1. What is the treatment of acute pulmonary oedema?
2. Was the decision to admit the patient a correct one?
3. What consequences are likely to flow from the refusal to admit and how can they best be coped with?

A. J. Moulds, Basildon, UK

MRS. N.   AGED 72   WIDOW

334

Mrs. N. who had a lifetime history of a heart murmur developed congestive heart failure 10 years prior to this time and had a diagnosis of idiopathic hypertrophic subaortic stenosis made by ultrasound 3 years previously. She had been on digitalis and diuretics for about 10 years. She presented complaining of acute shortness of breath, swelling in her ankles that had slowly developed over the preceding 1½ months and had reached the point where she was unable to walk more than half a block. There was no other contributory history.

The physical examination revealed a woman in left congestive heart failure. Diffuse rales were heard over both lung fields most marked at the base, with some oedema in her ankles. She was very careful about taking her digitalis and diuretics and on further questioning did mention that the pharmacist had substituted a new brand of digitalis about 3 months prior to this visit.

1. What causes of congestive heart failure must be ruled out in this woman?
2. Are different brands of drugs interchangeable?
3. What steps may be necessary because of variable bioavailability of drugs?

W. W. Rosser, Ottawa

TIMOTHY S.   AGED 9

335

Timothy had accompanied his parents to a Chinese restaurant with his sisters and brothers. During the meal he suddenly complained of difficulty with breathing. His lips and eyes had began to swell. The swelling of the lips had occurred 6 months previously, cause unknown.

He was brought to the doctor who made his diagnosis and treated him as an emergency.

1. What is the diagnosis?
2. What therapy was instituted?
3. What advice should be given to the parents?

B. M. Fehler, Johannesburg

336 MADAM P.L.H. AGED 57

Madam P.L.H. a spinster has been under your care for the last year. Her main complaints are tightness of the throat, with poor appetite and weight loss. She also complains of associated flatulence and epigastric discomfort, and at times of sore throat.

Prior to seeing you she has had full investigations by a physician. Barium meal and follow through, oesophagoscopy, gastroscopy and blood tests were all normal. A tonsillectomy done by an ENT surgeon did not relieve her symptoms.

At the age of 35, she had a partial thyroidectomy for thyrotoxicosis. Last week you were called to her house because she developed difficulty in breathing. On arrival you notice hysterical over-breathing which settled with your management. You also noticed that she has been taking care of an aged, partially blind mother and obtained the history that she has been doing this for the past 10 years. In the last week her mother has been having frequency and dysuria and has been very demanding and difficult to manage.

1. To what extent has the house call helped you reappraise the diagnosis of your patient's complaints?
2. How would you now manage your patient?
3. How could your management of her mother's problems assist your patient?
4. What resources are available for the care of the elderly in your community?

F. E. H. Tan, Kuala Lumpur

337 MRS. F.B. AGED 59 WIDOWED OFFICE WORKER

Mrs. F.B. complains of recurrent feelings of choking and difficulty in breathing accompanied by palpitations of the heart. The doctor notes a flush above the sternal ridge, extending into the supra-clavicular fossae and up the anterior surface of her neck. The symptoms have been present intermittently for 4 weeks.

1. What is your approach when there is a need to distinguish between the emotional and organic origin of symptoms?
2. If these symptoms prove to be emotional in origin what methods are available for Mrs. F.B.'s treatment?
3. What are your views on the label sometimes given to patients of 'suffering from mixed anxiety and depression'?

P. Freeling, London

MARION B.   AGED 15   SCHOLAR   338

You have known Marion for only about a year. She and her sister aged 16 have come to live with her mother whose first marriage broke up some years ago after which she married one of your patients 5 years ago. Marion had been living with her father and his new wife. She and her sister were unhappy and they decided to move in with their mother.

She comes in an anxious state because, for the past 3 days, she has been 'unable to get her breath'.

1. What questions do you ask her?
2. How do manage the situation?

J. Fry, Beckenham, UK

Wheezing

339 ROBERT S. AGED 18 MONTHS

Robert was the second child in the family. His father was a carpenter, who suffered from asthma and they lived in their own home.

As an infant, Robert had atopic eczema which was now well controlled.

He had had no previous respiratory problems until 9 a.m. that morning when he developed a cough, wheeze and dyspnoea which had increased in severity over the following 2 hours, so that he was very breathless when mother brought him to the office.

1. What diagnostic possibilities would you consider?
2. What physical signs would suggest he had a serious disorder?
3. What treatment would you give him?
4. If he were not ill enough to require hospitalization, what advice would you give to the family?
5. How do you manage atopic eczema?

H. C. Watts, Perth, Australia

340 S.B. AGED 3

Simon, an only child, has presented several times in the past 6 months with increasingly severe bouts of wheezing, lasting for several days, sometimes accompanied by fever and considerable malaise. Between attacks he is well but often has a muco-purulent nasal discharge. The parents, mother in particular, are very anxious.

1. What is the probable basis of Simon's condition?
2. What additional history might be of value?
3. What tests could be of value in diagnosis and treatment?
4. What would you tell the anxious parents?
5. How is treatment going to influence his condition?
6. What is the long-term prognosis and what is your long-term advice?

K. C. Nyman, Perth, Australia

341 MEHMET G. AGED 10

Mehmet's family are Moslems; His father is a head waiter, and they live in a small, modern home. Despite ill health, his father manages to send both his sons to good private schools. Mehmet's brother has had asthma for years, but needs only occasional treatment. Now his mother brings Mehmet, saying that he has a cough and is breathless. You observe a slight wheeze on expiration, with some use of the accessory muscles of respiration. His mother is obviously concerned, although the patient is cheerful; she asks if this is asthma too.

1. What does the word 'asthma' mean to patient, mother and doctor?
2. How can further attacks be prevented?
3. Should this case be managed at home, or referred?

J. Grabinar, Bromley, UK

MARK A.   AGED 19   STUDENT

342

Mark, a well built athletic engineering student, complains that recently after training for sport or playing football, he cannot get enough air and feels quite distressed for some time afterwards. You examine him and find no abnormal signs.

1. What is the probable diagnosis?
2. What diagnostic tests could be helpful?
3. Having established your diagnosis, how would you treat Mark?
4. What are Mark's chances of eventual cure?

K. C. Nyman, Perth, Australia

KATHERINE J.   AGED 10   SCHOOLGIRL

343

This 10 year old girl, with a past history of asthma, is brought to you in the evening by her parents because they have been unable to control her asthma, which has been present all day. She uses a Ventolin (salbutamol) inhaler.

The child is sitting up, has moderately severe bronchospasm, and appears anxious. The parents too look worried.

1. What are the possible causes of the child's condition?
2. What action would you take first?
3. What therapy would you consider? What are the indications for each form of therapy?

W. E. Fabb, Melbourne

MISS S.G.   AGED 14   PENSIONER

344

This girl is the eldest child of a large family. Her parents are separated with the mother caring for the children. She is a known asthmatic and her current therapy is Intal qid (for 4 months of the year), Ventolin inhaler 2 puffs qid p.r.n., Nuelin (theophylline) nocte. She has been well for the previous 4 months and you last saw her 2 months earlier when you reinstituted her Intal for the 'allergy season'. She presents to you one spring morning with an acute episode of asthma.

Examination reveals a pale girl with tachycardia and tachypnoea. She is using her accessory muscles of respiration and auscultation of her chest reveals high pitched inspiratory and expiratory rhonchi in all areas. She last used her Ventolin inhaler 3 hours earlier.

1. What are the possible aetiological factors in this attack?
2. What would be your short and long term management of this problem?
3. What is the significance of your examination findings?

D. S. Pedler, Adelaide

345 MRS. F. AGED 40 HOUSEWIFE

Mrs. F. has suffered from bronchial asthma for the past 2 to 3 years. Her condition has necessitated several admissions to hospital in the past, usually in 'status asthmaticus'. She is currently on prednisolone, 5 mg b.d. with salbutamol and beclomethasone by inhaler.

Mr. F. telephones at 6.30 requesting a home visit 'because the wife's a bit wheezy tonight'. He tentatively suggests a 'look-in tomorrow, when you're passing' will meet the situation.

1. In contacts with patients, family doctors usually accord some kind of priority in grading their responses: why do they do this?
2. What clinical phenomena constitute 'status asthmaticus'?
3. What might the doctor carry in his emergency bag to be ready to deal with this situation?

J. D. E. Knox, Dundee

346 JAMES P. AGED 15

James P. came when his usual doctor was on holiday, for a further prescription of his bronchodilator aerosol inhaler for asthma. It transpired that he had been wheezy most days intermittently for the last year or two – particularly in the morning, when it often woke him from sleep at 6 a.m. Other triggering factors were exercise and pollen sensitivity.

He was on no other drugs and his mother appeared to be unwilling to consider further therapy. The doctor detected an apparent general reluctance by both James and his mother to take his asthma seriously.

1. What would be the best way of assessing James' asthma?

2. How might the doctor handle the apparent unwillingness to take the asthma seriously?
3. What drug therapy might be considered for this patient?

J. C. Hasler, Oxford

MICHELLE V.   AGED 16   SCHOOLGIRL

347

Michelle has had bronchial asthma since early childhood when she was 'always in hospital'. Although she has coped better in her teens she has a perpetual wet cough and suffers from recurrent bouts of severe wheezing. Her effort tolerance is poor and, as a consequence, she plays very little sport. Her current medication is theophylline with salbutamol aerosol p.r.n. to relieve severe wheezing. On the advice of a friend, who is a patient at the practice, she seeks a second opinion.

1. What are the factors critical to the clinical assessment of this patient?
2. What factors will influence the doctor's management plan?
3. What are the important issues to be addressed in the education of this patient regarding long term management of her asthma?

W. L. Ogborne, Sydney

MRS. S.   AGED 70   PENSIONER

348

In your morning's mail is a note from Mrs. S., who writes: 'I would so much like for you to send me my sleeping pills and Ventolin inhaler. I have been very tired of late. I hear of a new drug to help my trouble – it's made by (pharmaceutical company): it's for all chest troubles. If possible, could I get this?'

You remember reading in the newspapers about a recently released antibiotic, hailed as a 'major breakthrough'. Mrs. S., aged 70, is housebound, suffering from chronic obstructive airways disease, chronic bronchitis and emphysema, the latter of which is now the main impairment. You saw her last at home about a week ago, when she was depressed and complaining bitterly of her shortness of breath.

1. What are the pro's and con's of issuing prescriptions to patients without seeing them at the time of issue?
2. What is the role of antibiotics in 'secondary prevention', i.e. preventing exacerbations of chronic bronchitis?
3. Patients' needs are not synonymous with patients' demands. What factors govern the creation of patient expectations?

J. D. E. Knox, Dundee

349 MR. C.C.E.   AGED 28   UNEMPLOYED

Mr. C.C.E. is single. He has attended for 4 years and has suffered from asthma since childhood. He has a personality problem with low self esteem and confidence (certainly contributed to by his asthma) resulting in:

- abuse of alcohol in the past.
- current abuse of sympatheticomimetics (aerosol).
- an inability to make friends (resulting in a tendency to promiscuity and several attacks of urethritis).
- poor compliance.

He presents with a history of coughing up green-yellow sputum and insomnia. There is poor air entry, prolonged expiration and musical rhonchi all over. Pulse 120; physique good although somewhat overweight.

1. What determines someone's personality?
2. What constitutes patient compliance?
3. What prognostic factors are evident in this case?

D. Levet, Hobart

350 MR. H.D.   AGED 49   BUSINESS EXECUTIVE

This 49-year-old business executive with long-standing asthma arrived at the hospital with cough and fever of 2 weeks' duration. The illness, he tells you, began with fever, chills, cough, and muscle pain. Three days after the onset of his illness he was much improved, as was another member of his family with a similar illness. On the fourth day, however, when he awoke, he was sweating profusely and his cough became productive. His temperature rose to 103 °F.

1. What salient physical findings should be sought?
2. What laboratory aids might be expected to offer positive diagnostic information?
3. What are the most likely aetiological causes for secondary or post-influenzal pneumonia, more likely with underlying pulmonary disease such as asthma?

L. H. Amundson, Sioux Falls, SD, USA

351 MR. L.S.   AGED 62

This man's wheezing and breathlessness became worse and feeling that he had another chest infection he went to his doctor for antibiotics. For many years he had been subject to attacks of cough and breathlessness but recently the wheezing had become continuous and the breathlessness was now so marked that he was finding difficulty in keeping his job as an engineer. The doctor concluded that he had another chest infection and prescribed a course of tetracycline, 250 mg q.d.s. and Ventolin 4 mg q.d.s. The patient improved slightly but remained unable to return to work.

1. Does this patient suffer from bronchitis or asthma?
2. Discuss the management of late onset (intrinsic) asthma.

A. G. Strube, Crawley, UK

MRS. T.   AGED 23   BANK CLERK

352

Mrs. T. presented with a severe attack of bronchitis, her third in 6 months. There was marked accompanying bronchospasm. Initial response to treatment was poor, but eventually the symptoms subsided. On questioning, the patient admitted to smoking 40 cigarettes per day. Her peak expiratory flow on testing in the rooms was well below the normal range for her age and height. On being asked whether she felt she could give up smoking she replied that she had had a 'nervous breakdown' the last time she attempted to do so. She said she also gained a great deal of weight when she stopped smoking and that she had had nervous breakdowns on two other occasions.

1. Why was the patient's illness initially refractory to treatment?
2. How would you manage this patient further?

S. Levenstein, Cape Town

MR. L.B.   AGED 52

353

This man presented with a productive cough, wheezing and breathlessness. Three months previously he had suffered a myocardial infarct, but had apparently made a complete recovery and returned to work as a taxi driver. On examination there were signs in the chest and the doctor concluded that he had a chest infection and prescribed antibiotics and an expectorant cough mixture. Three days later another doctor was called in at night as Mr. B. was choking and could not get his breath due to the copious sputum he was coughing up. Again he had signs of congestion in the chest and the doctor concluded that the infection was resistant and so changed the antibiotic. As there was little improvement the patient came to the office and saw a third doctor who questioned him carefully about his symptoms: it seemed that although he was breathless on exertion in the day, with a tiresome cough and wheeze, it was not until night time that the breathing was really bad, when he was forced to sit upright in order to cough up the frothy sputum. If he lay down the difficulty in breathing became even worse. There was no chest pain. The doctor thought this sounded like the nocturnal dyspnoea of heart failure and with this in mind he examined the patient carefully. The pulse was 100 regular, blood pressure normal. There was some left ventricular enlargement but heart sounds were normal. Venous pressure was not raised and there was no ankle oedema. ECG showed the old posterior myocardial infarct. The chest X-ray report read: 'Extensive consolidation is present, particularly over the right lung field. A small effusion is demonstrated at the right base with bilateral enlargement of the heart.' He was admitted to hospital for treatment.

1. How could the diagnosis have been made earlier?
2. What is meant by the term 'congestion'?

A. G. Strube, Crawley, UK

Other respiratory problems

MR. G.   AGED 32   FARMER   **354**

A 32 year old single farmer had been seen by three physicians prior to seeing me. He presented with a history of fever, chills, cough, shortness of breath and generalized weakness. He had lost 25 pounds in the preceding 3 months. He had several physical examinations and diagnostic tests including sputum cultures, chest X-rays and four courses of antibiotics. He has been diagnosed as having recurrent influenza, acute bronchitis and chronic bronchitis. His condition was continuing to deteriorate.

On physical examination he was somewhat pale, and slightly febrile with a temperature of 38.5 °C. The only physical finding was a slightly elevated pulse rate of 90 and sharp crackling rales over both lung fields. There were no rhonchi heard in the lungs.

1. What further historical information is necessary to confirm the diagnosis?
2. What further investigations would be helpful at this point in time? Even though a chest X-ray was done one month previously would a repeat chest X-ray be of benefit?
3. Why have previous efforts to treat this man failed?

W. W. Rosser, Ottawa

MR. PETER Z.   AGED 57   STOREMAN   **355**

Mr. Z. was admitted to hospital with classical signs and symptoms of a right lower lobar pneumonia. This was confirmed on X-ray, and all other investigations fitted the diagnosis except that he was found to have a haemoglobin of 6 g/dl. He was treated with antibiotics and blood transfusion followed by parenteral iron and made a rapid recovery.

1. What investigations would assist in diagnosis?
2. If all your investigations regarding the cause of the anaemia were negative, how would you manage the patient in the future?

R. M. Meyer, Johannesburg

356   MRS. BETINA A. & MR. HARRY A.   AGES: BETINA 42, HARRY 44
BETINA: HOUSEWIFE   HARRY: PANEL BEATER

You notice in your afternoon appointments that Betina and Harry A. have a joint appointment. You used to look after them 10 years ago when you were the doctor in a small rural community. You remember them as a pleasant, happy couple. Harry owned the local panel works.

Today they are coming about Harry's heavy head cold.

On meeting them you are struck by several things within the first minutes of the consultation.

- Harry looks physically unwell, with speech and breathing patterns that suggest he has obstructive lung disease.
- Both appear much older than their chronological age. This is particularly marked in Harry's case.
- Both appear to be unhappy, within themselves and with each other.

1. What are some common causes of accelerated biological ageing?
2. What diagnoses are you considering at this stage?
3. Given that you have limited time available, how will you manage the consultation from this point onwards?

M. W. Heffernan, Melbourne

357   MR. R.S.   AGED 38   TRUCK DRIVER

Mr. R.S. a 38 year old truck driver for a small bulk chemical company, was seen by his family physician complaining of a 3 day history of chills, cough, fatigue and lower abdominal pain. He was tender in the left lower quadrant, his lungs had left basilar creps and his chest X-ray demonstrated consolidation in that area. His white cell count was 6000 per cmm. Ten days later, he showed little improvement in spite of a course of antibiotics and his physician changed the antibiotic to erythromycin. R.S. improved slowly over the next 2 weeks and then returned to work.

Six months later, R.S. presented again to his physician with a similar complaint and reported that he had had one more episode between this and his last visit, which was similar, but of lesser intensity. On this occasion the patient mentioned that his wife had noted that these episodes seemed to come on each time he hauled nitric acid in his truck. Further questioning indicated that he filled his truck through an opening in the top of the tank and determined when it was full by watching through this opening.

The patient was referred to a respirologist with a special interest in occupational health, who confirmed the diagnosis.

The driver requested that his physician not report this case to the Workman's Compensation Board lest he lost his job. The chemical company was a small one, which was not required to pass government inspection and had no union, and the driver was due to be moved to an office job with the company.

1. What does the family physician suspect as the aetiology at the first visit?
2. How commonly do patients suffer from occupational related diseases?
3. What are the issues – ethical, moral and legal, relating to this man's concerns about reporting his disease?

C. A. Moore, Hamilton, Canada

CHAPTER 17

Chest Pain

This chapter begins with the diagnostic challenge of a series of cases of central chest pain in patients ranging from the adolescent through to the elderly. Then follow cases of right or left sided chest pain, a number of cases of actual or potential cardiac neurosis and some illustrations of work problems related to cardiac disease. Chest pain is one of the most common symptoms presenting to the family physician and often carries with it serious connotations. Patients often present fearing they have heart disease. The way in which the family physician manages these problems is of the utmost importance to the outcome. Failure to diagnose serious heart disease can result in the patient losing his life; failure to positively reassure the patient when no heart disease exists can result in the development of life-long disabling cardiac neurosis.

Central chest pain

358 **MR. B.P.**   **AGED 18**   **FARM LABOURER**

You have been asked as a rural practitioner to see a youth after hours with a story of having developed severe chest pains radiating to both shoulders and through to the back associated with sweating, shortness of breath and vomiting while playing football that day. It lasted about ½ hour and then recurred 4 hours later at rest. There had been several similar but less severe previous attacks over the last 6 months. There was no apparent relationship of the pain to respiration or posture. On examination he appeared pale, sweaty with an occasional irregular heartbeat and BP of 105/70; heart sounds normal; chest and lungs clinically clear.

1. What additional information is required to reach a diagnosis?
2. What possible causes should be considered?
3. How should this patient be managed?

T. D. Manthorpe, Port Lincoln, Australia

359 **JOE SMITH**   **AGED 33**   **ELECTRICIAN**

You know Joe Smith, although you haven't seen him as a patient for many years. He is known as the town's best electrician and is also very active as a coach with the local junior football team.

It's 1 p.m. Sunday and Joe has been brought in to see you because of an episode of central tight chest pain and headache which he developed at midday soon after getting up. The pain lasted about ½ hour, was associated with some light headedness and resolved spontaneously. There was no radiation and no other associated features. Until today he has generally felt well.

Last night Joe was out celebrating until 3 a.m. after the football grand final. He smokes 20–30 cigarettes per day and drinks on Saturday nights only. Over the last few years, he has been working 18 hours per day, 6 days per week because he says he needs to meet loan repayments and wants to 'get ahead'. All his clients want him to do the work (rather than his partner) and it's always urgent. He feels he has to oblige them. His wife and two children (aged 6 and 8) rarely see him and when they do he is cranky and irritable. This is beginning to worry him.

Physical examination is completely normal.

1. What are the possible causes of his chest pain?

2. What investigations are indicated?
3. What is this patient's main problem?
4. How would you manage this problem?

R. P. Strasser, Melbourne

MR. M.T.   AGED 31   CLERK   360

Whilst on call one evening you receive an urgent call to this patient because of an acute pain in the chest. On arrival you find him pale and hyperventilating, with incipient tetany. His wife is extremely anxious and upset.

Subsequent history and examination lead to the conclusion that the chest pain was caused by a muscle injury following lifting a heavy car battery.

1. What diagnostic possibilities would you consider whilst driving to the patient's home?
2. Why might he be hyperventilating?
3. What factors tend to make relatives particularly anxious about a patient's condition?

E. C. Gambrill, Crawley, UK

JOHN ROBERTS   AGED 48   COMPANY MANAGER   361

John, a visitor to your district, has been rushed in to see you by his cousin with whom he is staying. You notice John is pale, sweaty and tremulous. He tells you that 10 minutes ago he was sitting watching television when he noticed his heart thumping fast in his chest. After this he felt a tightness across the chest (no radiation) and a light headed feeling. He put an Anginine tablet under his tongue but it made no difference to his pain, although soon after he developed a thumping headache. The chest tightness subsides while you are talking with him.

Six months ago he had a similar episode and his doctor sent him into the local public hospital casualty department for a cardiograph. At the hospital, the doctors admitted him for observation, took blood tests several times and attached him to the cardiac monitor for 24 hours. He had returned to the hospital a week later for a test where he rode a bicycle. The doctors said all the tests were normal, but gave him the Anginine in case it happened again.

Apart from that one episode, John has no significant past history or family history. He mentions that his best friend and business colleague dropped dead last week from a heart attack.

Physical examination is essentially normal. ECG is within normal limits.

1. What is the problem in this case?

2. Are any further investigations indicated?
3. How would you manage this problem?

R. P. Strasser, Melbourne

362 MRS. S.S.   AGED 45   CLERICAL WORKER

Mrs. S.S. had a hysterectomy for fibroids 5 years ago. Since then she has complained persistently of pain in the left iliac fossa. Laparoscopy, 3 years ago, showed a small ovarian cyst and this was later removed without relieving her pain. Sigmoidoscopy and barium enema were normal 1 year ago and neither the prescription of bran nor dicyclomine hydrochloride have relieved her pain. Mrs. S.S.'s father died 6 months ago and she remained severely depressed so that 4 weeks ago the doctor prescribed imipramine. You are called to see Mrs. S.S. in an emergency complaining of pains across her upper sternum, palpitations, and feeling cold and faint.

1. What is your differential diagnosis for the emergency consultation?
2. What is your problem list for Mrs. S.S.?
3. What are your criteria for giving antidepressant medication?

P. Freeling, London

363 MR. M.F.   AGED 59   RETIRED CLERK

You receive a phone call at 6 a.m. from Mr. F's wife. M.F. is a very active man who retired because of moderate hypertension. Since his retirement his blood pressure has been well controlled on beta-blockers (140/90).

His wife, who sounds very worried on the phone, explains that her husband has had severe lower chest and upper abdominal pain for over one hour and that he is sweating profusely. When you see him shortly afterwards he is pale and very sweaty with a pulse of 90 and blood pressure 100/70. The remainder of the examination is normal. You perform an ECG which shows a pattern of a full thickness inferolateral infarct.

1. What are the aetiological factors in this man's myocardial infarction?
2. What is your management of this situation?

D. S. Pedler, Adelaide

364 HAROLD O'HALLORAN   AGED 85   PENSIONER

The last time Harold was sick (3 years ago), he had pneumonia and your partner put him in hospital for intensive physiotherapy. In hospital he rapidly deteriorated becoming agitated and confused.

Today his daughter has brought him to see you because he was woken during the night by a severe central crushing chest pain that had lasted for about an hour. He says the pain was 'pretty bad' and he was very 'short winded' with it. His wife rubbed his chest with a hot ointment and eventually the pain went away. Harold says he wouldn't let his wife or his daughter call you because 'you young people need your sleep'. Physical examination reveals mild CCF and ECG shows signs of a recent inferior myocardial infarction.

Together with his 80 year old wife, Harold has lived in the same house for the last 30 years. His daughter and her family live next door. Apart from the bout of pneumonia, his general health has been pretty good, although Harold has been becoming more forgetful over the years.

1. How do you explain the episode of agitation and confusion three years ago?
2. Is hospital admission indicated this time?
3. Could you manage this patient at home?

R. P. Strasser, Melbourne

MR. M.S.   AGED 42

365

Mr. M.S. was happily married with 3 young sons. He was a non-smoker who had been under considerable stress at work. He had a cold and a productive cough for the last 2 weeks and on the morning he presented, he had developed chest pain, a feeling of dull tightness across the lower chest, not related to respiration or exertion.

He was concerned that he might have heart disease as a colleague at work had had a heart attack 3 months ago.

1. What are the diagnostic possibilities you would consider?
2. What other information would you wish to obtain to arrive at a more precise diagnosis?
3. How do you exclude a diagnosis of ischaemic disease in a young man?
4. In a patient with proven ischaemic heart disease, when do you refer him to a consultant?

H. C. Watts, Perth, Australia

MR. K.W.   AGED 38   BUSINESSMAN

366

Mr. W. presents with a history of central chest pain intermittently for the last 18 hours. He describes it as a burning tightness behind his sternum, it does not radiate, is not altered by food or liquids but seems a little worse with exercise. Pain began last night during intercourse, but at that stage it was not sufficiently severe to terminate the act, although the pain did keep him awake afterwards.

On examination he has a BP 140/95 (the same as on several previous occasions). The remainder of the examination is normal, as is the ECG. He has a family history of sudden death of his father aged 40 from heart attack, and his mother aged 51 from a CVA. He is known to have a slightly raised fasting serum cholesterol, about which he has done nothing despite advice. 18 months ago Mr. W. took over a neglected business, and with hard work, long hours and much worry he has built up a successful business. He smokes 40 cigarettes and drinks 4 whiskeys a day.

1. What is the significance of his chest pains?
2. What are the most important risk factors in cardiovascular disease?
3. What should you do about his other risk factors?

W. F. Glastonbury, Adelaide

367 MR. L.P. AGED 54 CLERGYMAN

Mr. L.P. presented with three episodes of substernal tightness over a 3 day period. One occurred after the exertion of gardening and lasted a few minutes. The second was related to tension at work and was also transient. The third appeared to be precipitated by a bout of coughing at bedtime and lasted intermittently all night. There was no radiation of the pain and there were no associated symptoms.

The patient is a non-smoker and physically active. He is married with three adult children. Six months previously he left an administrative job with the Church and took over as minister of a suburban congregation. There was a strong family history of coronary artery disease with the patient's father and several uncles all dying of this disease in their 60's.

The initial physical examination was normal. The cardiac rate was 74/minute and regular; blood pressure was 120/80. The initial electrocardiogram showed inverted T waves in the anterior chest leads V1–4 and two days later the ST segments were slightly depressed in the same leads. The electrocardiogram reverted to normal within a few days and there were no changes in the cardiac enzymes done serially over 4 days. The patient was treated with bed rest, nitroglycerine sublingually for the pain, isosorbide dinitrate and a beta-blocker.

1. How do you decide if chest pain is serious?
2. What diagnostic tests help?
3. What counselling do you give to the patient with coronary artery disease and to his family?

R. L. Perkin, Toronto

Lateral chest pain

MRS. C.D.   AGED 55   HOUSEWIFE

368

Mrs. C.D. presents with left anterior chest pain of recent onset. There is an unusual feeling in the skin associated with this pain. She has a past history of myocardial infarction and a left mastectomy for carcinoma of the breast. She smokes 20 cigarettes per day and has chronic bronchitis.

1. What is the cause of the pain?
2. What place have corticosteriods in the treatment of this patient?
3. How much of this patient's illness has been due to cigarette smoking?

B. H. Connor, Armidale, Australia

MR. A.W.   AGED 31   CLERK

369

Mr. A.W. complained of left parasternal pain which he first experienced carrying some heavy furniture when he moved into his new home with his wife and two children. The pain was at first acute and stabbing in character but it subsided to a persistent dull ache. A resting ECG was performed and found to be normal. An analgesic prescribed didn't prevent the recurrence of the stabbing pain when he again lifted heavy objects. A stress ECG revealed myocardial ischaemic changes.

1. How would you manage his clinical problem?
2. How do you prevent the patient from becoming a cardiac invalid?
3. How would his problem affect his family and his community?

F. E. H. Tan, Kuala Lumpur

WALTER M.   AGED 45   STOREMAN

370

Walter M. presented to his family doctor complaining of an acute right sided chest pain while lifting at work. He looked tired and pale and admitted to a loss of 13 kg weight over the past 6 to 8 weeks.

On examination his right chest cage was painful to pressure in the mid axillary line, suggesting rib fracture.

1. What diagnostic suspicions should these findings arouse in the doctor's mind?

2. What is the most likely cause of Walter M's rib fracture?
3. What matters should the family doctor discuss with the patient and his family?

W. L. Ogborne, Sydney

371 MR. T.S.   AGED 45   BUSINESS EXECUTIVE

Mr. T.S. had not attended the office for years. He was married with two grown-up children and held down a demanding job with a firm in the city. When he arrived to report his chest pain, he had just returned from a trip to Canada. He described a sharp localized pain on the right side of his chest. It was exacerbated by movement and inspiration. He admitted to smoking 20 cigarettes a day and to having a 'smoker's cough'. There was little to find on examination apart from some localized tenderness at the site of his pain, heavily nicotine-stained fingers and some bruising on his left upper arm which he attributed to horseplay with his young grandson.

A chest X-ray was arranged and showed two newly fractured ribs on the right and three healed rib fractures on the left. When Mr. S. returned for the X-ray results 2 days later he was at a loss to explain how the fractures might have occurred. On this occasion the doctor noticed a distinct smell of brandy on his patient's breath.

1. What is your differential diagnosis?
2. Which one diagnosis would most logically explain all the features of this patient's history and examination?
3. To what aspects of the history and examination would you pay particular attention in carrying out a routine check-up on a 45 year old man?

T. A. I. Bouchier Hayes, Camberley, UK

372 MISS P.C.   AGED 25   OFFICE CLEANER

Miss P.C., who works mainly in the evenings, consults you because of chest pain. She states she developed a cold about 10 days ago. A cough started 2 days ago, and she developed overnight a pain in the right side of her chest on deep breathing. She does not smoke. Her father, a heavy smoker, died of lung cancer. Your examination reveals a female, normal on physical examination, except for a slighly elevated temperature, and a friction rub audible at the site of her pain in her right chest. She can produce no sputum for examination.

1. What are the likely diagnoses here?
2. What investigations would you undertake?

3. Does a negative chest X-ray alter your diagnosis?
4. What is the significance of her statement that her father died from lung cancer?

D. U. Shepherd, Melbourne

MRS. J.P.   AGED 51   HOUSEWIFE   373

Mrs. J.P., the wife of a clergyman, still had two of her six children living at home. She was a cigarette smoker and worked part-time outside the home. She had head cold symptoms for 10 days which seemed to be getting better when she suddenly experienced over a 3 hour period chills and rigors, fever up to 39.5 °C, and a sharp pleuritic pain in the right lower chest posteriorly. She had a cough with purulent sputum but no blood or rusty sputum. There was a history of pneumonia on three previous occasions.

She was seen as an emergency on a house call. At that time she appeared acutely ill and had a friction rub over the right lower chest posteriorly and laterally with associated dullness and decreased air entry. She was immediately admitted to hospital where an X-ray showed consolidation of her right middle lobe. Her white cell count was 23,000. Sputum culture subsequently confirmed the diagnosis. Because she was allergic to penicillin, she was treated with erythromycin.

1. What is the pathogen?
2. How would you treat the patient?
3. What preventive measures would you advise for the future?

R. L. Perkin, Toronto

MR. B.F.   AGED 44   PLANT WORKER   374

This 44 year old male developed spontaneous chest pains which were associated with cough and dyspnoea but not with hemoptysis, vomiting, or wheezing. This recurrent chest pain had been occurring for 2 or 3 days with no previous history of chest pain. He had a history of hypertension for the past 8 years for which he had received intermittent oral therapy.

The history revealed one episode of thrombophlebitis of the left leg 3 years earlier; treated with bed rest, hot packs and stretch bandages. He was treated at home. The leg cleared in 7–10 days and he had suffered no recurrence.

Physical examination revealed a blood pressure of 160/110 and a pulse of 100. He was slightly dyspnoeic sitting in bed. Fundi showed grade I hypertensive changes, consisting of some arterial sheen and early AV nipping. The heart was slightly enlarged and a grade II systolic murmur was heard over the lower left sternal border. The extremities reveal 1 + peripheral oedema bilaterally. There was a negative Homan's sign.

1. What are the essential problems and their differential diagnosis?
2. What are the possible risk factors to be considered in this case?

L. H. Amundson, Sioux Falls, SD, USA

Other chest pain

MR. K.   AGED 45   BANK CLERK

375

Mr. K., currently being treated for hypertension with beta-blockers, saw the GP's partner just before he went on leave, complaining of chest pain. He was told that his pain was probably not of cardiac origin, but advised him to spend 3 days in bed and report back.

On coming to see the GP he said he had not had much pain over the past 3 days, but was clearly highly anxious. He wanted to know what the other doctor had thought the trouble was, and asked if he could go back to work. An ECG was performed which was normal. The patient was told this, and allowed to go back to work the next day. He was clearly much relieved. He was asked to return in a week's time for another BP check. His hypertension appeared to be adequately controlled.

1. What was the first GP's diagnosis?
2. Why was the patient so anxious at the consultation with the 'locum' GP?
3. Why was the patient relieved after the consultation with the 'locum' GP?

S. Levenstein, Cape Town

MR. C.H.   AGED 57   LABOURER

376

Mr. C.H., a skilled labourer, attended the office for the fifth time in 3 weeks. Once again he gave a graphic description of his chest pain which was sharp, situated just beneath the left nipple, unrelated to exercise and usually momentary. 'Do you think it could be my heart, doctor?' He was reassured, as he had been many times before, that the pain was nothing to do with his heart and that the tests which had been done had all been completely normal. Yes, he understood that, but still did not seem completely satisfied. The doctor checked his pulse and blood pressure. Mr. H. was not yet ready to leave the surgery. Despite being ½ hour behind time the doctor asked him to take off his jacket. He clamped his stethoscope over the site of the pain, listened intently and pronounced everything fine. Beaming broadly, Mr. H. left apparently happy.

1. What syndrome does Mr. H.'s story illustrate?
2. What are the reasons for frequent office attendance by a patient with no evidence of physical disease?
3. What resources are available for the health education of patients?

T. A. I. Bouchier Hayes, Camberley, UK

377 MRS. S.H.   AGED 40   HOUSEWIFE/SOCIAL WORKER

Mrs. S.H., a social worker by training and work experience, is a rather anxious happily married mother of three healthy children. She has presented six times in the past 3 to 4 years complaining of intermittent chest pain and numbness of her hands and has indicated each time that she is quite concerned that it is her heart. On each occasion she has appeared extremely distressed. Extensive investigation by the family physician and two different cardiologists has revealed no evidence of heart or other organic disease.

1. What investigations might be indicated at this most recent visit?
2. What referral(s) might be indicated at this most recent visit?
3. What is the most likely cause of this patient's symptoms?

G. G. Beazley, Winnipeg

378 MR. J.P.   AGED 53   EXECUTIVE

He complains of two pains:

One present for 2 months and located in the centre of the chest – quite severe and worse under stress – seems to be relieved by bringing up wind – may last 15–30 minutes – occurs several times a week – it feels tight and makes him feel rotten.

An upper abdominal discomfort which seems worse before meals and has woken him at 2 a.m. on several occasions. This has been present off and on for 2 years and is getting worse.

1. What would be your strategies for dealing with such an obviously complex problem in a busy consulting session?
2. How can you distinguish between the various causes of retrosternal and epigastric pain?
3. What would you do if you're not sure of the diagnosis even if you have sought another opinion?

F. Mansfield, Perth, Australia

379 LES B.   AGED 32   SALESMAN

Les B. is a fit looking man recently discharged from the navy after 10 years of active service. He complains of aching discomfort in the anterior chest around the left breast often associated with a prickling sensation. He first noticed this in Singapore after loading 2000 × 50 lb artillery shells on his ship. Full investigations, including stress ECG, failed to reveal a cause at that time.

The chest pains and discomfort have recurred several times since but, despite numerous medical consultations and various tests, the problem persists undiagnosed.

1. What is the single most likely process by which Les B's symptoms will be diagnosed?
2. Why have so many doctors failed to diagnose the cause of Les B's chest pain?
3. During physical examination the spinous processes of T3 and T4 are very tender when firm pressure is applied with the thumb. What relationship, if any, does this finding have to Les B's chest pain?

W. L. Ogborne, Sydney

DESMOND K.   AGED 58   FACTORY MANAGER   380

This slightly obese patient with a history of attacks of gout presented 3 months ago complaining of transient retrosternal pain when playing the first hole of a round of golf. His blood pressure was 180/95 and the ECG was relatively normal. The pain responded to sublingual glyceryl trinitrate. He now complains that the pain has become much more troublesome over recent weeks. He has to take a tablet during his playing of every hole and he is experiencing pain when he takes his dog for a walk.

1. What are the characteristics of the pain of angina pectoris?
2. What action should the general practitioner take in relation to the patient's complaint at the most recent consultation?

J. G. P. Ryan, Brisbane

MR. M.N.   AGED 41   FORK HOIST DRIVER   381

Mr. N. consults Dr. Y. during Dr. Y.'s weekly visit to the factory. Dr. Y. is a GP in an industrial area, has many associations with industry, and attends clinics in two of the larger firms.

Mr. N. has been sent to the medical section by his foreman, who is concerned that Mr. N. seems to have had chest pain lifting some materials and on getting on and off the fork hoist. Mr. N.'s own doctor is thought to be treating him for obesity and anginal pain, and the foreman does not think Mr. N. should operate the fork hoist until Mr. N. has seen a specialist at the hospital outpatient clinic. Mr. N. is indeed overweight and has significant hypertension, despite the stated treatment regime. He is indignant about the foreman's attitude because he gets higher rates as a fork hoist driver, as well as better chances of overtime. His own doctor is overseas for two months and he refuses to visit the old doctor who is acting as locum tenens.

1. How should Dr. Y. advise the patient?

2. How should Dr. Y. advise the employer?
3. What should Dr. Y. do with regard to the patient's own doctor's locum?

P. L. Gibson, Auckland

382 THOMAS D.   AGED 52   COMPANY EXECUTIVE

Thomas D. had been a senior executive with an important company but had been forced to retire owing to the development of angina and transient ischaemic attacks. Shortly before his consultation he had been informed that the Driving Licence Authority had informed him he was no longer eligible for a driving licence on medical grounds.

1. How would you manage the continuing care of his angina and transient ischaemic attacks?
2. How would you react to the decision preventing him from driving a car?
3. What responsibility does the general practitioner have in the prevention of arterial disease?

J. C. Hasler, Oxford

383 MR. W.R.   AGED 65

Mr. R. had a coronary bypass operation at age 59 for intractable angina. He did well, requiring only chlorothiazide 0.5 g daily and propranolol 40 mg t.i.d. for treatment of mild hypertension (180/95 mmHg sitting).

At age 64 he developed intermittent claudication although his peripheral pulses were all palpable. This did not improve significantly when another beta-blocking drug was substituted, and withdrawal of this produced tachycardia. He was finally controlled on chlorothiazide and prazosin and is without adverse symptoms.

1. Are coronary disease and peripheral vascular disease related?
2. What is the basis for this patient's hypertension?
3. Is it rational to treat this patient's blood pressure?

A. L. A. Reid, Newcastle, Australia

CHAPTER 18

Abdominal Problems

This chapter comprises a series of diagnostic challenges – indigestion, epigastric pain, central and lateral abdominal pain, lower abdominal pain, abdominal pain with diarrhoea, diarrhoea, sometimes with vomiting, and jaundice. Abdominal problems present commonly to the family physician, who needs to be able to diagnose and manage a wide variety of conditions, varying from those of psychogenic origin to those resulting from the most serious disease. To miss a serious abdominal condition, such as appendicitis, is a tragedy; on the other hand, to over-investigate abdominal discomforts of psychogenic origin often does more harm than good.

Upper abdominal pain

384 **MRS. P.M.**   **AGED 65**   **HOUSEWIFE**

Mrs. P.M. is the wife of a general practitioner who has been treating her for gastro-oesophageal reflux for the past 3 years. She was referred to a colleague because her indigestion had become severe and persistent. She had one episode of severe burning epigastric pain that lasted for 2 hours, and was unrelieved by antacids. She has had no energy for several weeks and develops burning epigastric pain and dyspnoea on any exertion. On examination she looks pale and frail. A barium meal taken 3 years ago and repeated recently showed marked gastro-oesophageal reflux.

1. What are possible causes of her problem?
2. What are the next steps in the management of this patient?
3. What principles in overall management are embodied in the management of this patient?

J. E. Murtagh, Melbourne

385 **MR. A.P.**   **AGED 27**   **DEPARTMENT STORE SUPERVISOR**

Mr. A.P. presents because of abdominal pain. On questioning, the pain is a burning feeling in the epigastrium. It is episodic and is relieved by food and antacids. Mr. A.P. has been otherwise well, and has had no serious illnesses in the past. He is single, and shares a flat with a friend.

1. What further information would you elicit in relation to food?
2. What further information would you elicit in relation to habits?
3. What family history would be of help?
4. What investigations are indicated in this patient?
5. What advice would you give to this patient?
6. Is surgery preferable to medical management in this case?

D. U. Shepherd, Melbourne

386 **MR. A.H.**   **AGED 55**

This man had a long history of indigestion for which he took antacids from time to time. He worked hard in his own printing firm and was a heavy smoker. He came to see the doctor as his attacks of pain were becoming more frequent and his self medication less effective.

The doctor found that the pain was burning in character and situated in the epigastrium. It came on after meals and would frequently extend a little way into the chest. It was worse when he lay down and would often wake him when he lay flat in bed at night.

Antacids provided some relief. Mr. H. was overweight with blood pressure of 160/100. Chest X-ray and ECG were normal. There was some tenderness in the epigastrium and the doctor concluded that he suffered from reflux oesophagitis. He advised the patient to reduce weight, stop smoking, avoid stooping down, and at night to sleep on a slight incline by putting a pillow under his shoulders. He prescribed Gaviscon mixture, 10 ml to be taken after meals and again at night. Mr. H. seemed unable to modify his way of life and his symptoms continued. He was persuaded to take a holiday and while he was struggling to hitch his caravan onto his car he had a severe attack of pain in the chest, collapsed and died.

A coroner's post-mortem revealed a large myocardial infarction as the cause of death.

1. Could these long-standing symptoms of 'indigestion' have been due to cardiac pain?

A. G. Strube, Crawley, UK

MR. A.R.   AGED 22   UNEMPLOYED LABOURER   **387**

Mr. A.R., complaining of indigestion, consults the doctor. He was in trouble with the police 2 years ago for taking and driving away a car. He was recently arrested for breaking and entering a liquor shop. He is now out on bail, guaranteed by his widowed mother, his father having died when Mr. A.R. was 10 years old. He has been a known poorly controlled asthmatic since he was twelve.

1. What are the possible sources of Mr. A.R.'s indigestion?
2. What is your approach to the management of asthma in young people?
3. What is your response to the information that a patient has a criminal record?

P. Freeling, London

TONY C.P.W.   AGED 15   HIGH SCHOOL STUDENT   **388**

Tony was presented to the doctor by his mother for advice. Tony has been having stomach pains for 2 years, almost continuously. He has consulted many doctors and has received medication which he has taken constantly. In the last 12 months he has had three episodes of 'bleeding ulcer'. A month ago he lost so much blood he was admitted to hospital and was transfused. During the last admission, after investigations, the consulting surgeon advised Mrs. W. that surgery should be considered then.

However, Mrs. W. was reluctant for Tony to have the operation. Tony, being the eldest son in a Chinese family, shoulders the heaviest family expectations and has to maintain his already good scholastic achievement.

1. What is the treatment of peptic ulcer?
2. Why is Tony suffering from this condition?
3. What is child abuse?

N. C. L. Yuen, Hong Kong

389   MRS. M.   AGED 63   WIDOW

Mrs. M. has been a patient for 33 years. She was widowed 2 years ago when her husband died suddenly. She lives alone. Her only close relative is a daughter but she has shunned contact with the daughter and grandchild. Mrs. M. had a very unhappy childhood compensated by a very happy marriage. However, she never adjusted to the death of her only son who was killed in a motor vehicle accident 20 years ago.

In the past 20 years she has had a series of surgical operations which, in retrospect, have achieved nothing. She has been found guilty of shoplifting on three occasions. She has been jointly managed by her general practitioner and a psychiatrist. Attempts to modify her medication (tranquillizers and sleeping tablets) have usually led to the onset of symptoms which closely resemble organic disease and have led to numerous nonproductive investigations when she visits other practitioners. Recently the general practitioner and psychiatrist agreed that no attempt would be made to change her treatment and any symptoms that manifest themselves were probably better treated symptomatically without further investigations. At her next to last visit she appeared with persistent dyspepsia, anorexia and loss of weight.

Symptomatic treatment failed to produce any relief and a barium meal was subsequently performed. This showed the presence of a duodenal ulcer.

1. How much can a doctor rely on previous experience and pattern of behaviour in a patient?
2. Why is this woman a kleptomaniac?
3. Should this patient's medical problem be given priority over her psychiatric condition?

P. F. Gill, Hobart

390   MR. G.P.   AGED 29   SCHOOLTEACHER

For the last 4 months Mr. P. has had recurrent bouts of epigastric pain. These pains are central about 5 cm above his umbilicus. They do not appear to be related to meals. On several occasions the pain has woken him. Mr. P. admits that his smoking has increased to more than 30 cigarettes a day and his alcohol intake to at least 2 bottles of beer per day. On examination the only significant finding is very mild tenderness in the epigastrium.

1. How significant are the negative physical findings?
2. What role could tension play in producing his pain?
3. What does the future hold for him with his current alcohol intake and cigarette consumption?
4. Where do you begin with counselling this man?

W. F. Glastonbury, Adelaide

THE D. FAMILY

391

At 12.45 a.m. Mrs. D. phoned her doctor. She was very worried about her daughter B., aged 12 years who had had upper abdominal pain for 5 hours.

When he arrived about 15 minutes later, Mrs. D. met him at the front door and announced that the pain had now settled, and that B. was quite better. It was noted that the other members of the family were still quite relaxed and apparently enjoying the late television show.

B. confirmed that the pain was better, but indicated that it had been in the epigastrium. It had been constant in nature. She had not vomited, nor had her bowels been open since the onset of the pain. She had had a very large evening meal. No other members of the family were sick.

After examination, Mrs. D. was assured that there was no immediate problem and that they should contact him in the morning if the pain recurred.

Mr. D. then appeared on the scene and said that he had been meaning to come and see the doctor for some time about his 'sinusitis and hayfever'. He said that as the doctor was already there it seemed to be a good idea if he could 'have a look at him' now. The doctor declined to pursue this further on this occasion but suggested an appointment time.

No member of the family has contacted the doctor subsequently.

1. What are the most likely causes of B.'s abdominal pain?
2. How should the general practitioner manage inconsiderate patients?
3. What are the possible reasons for Mr. D.'s request for medical advice for 'hayfever and sinusitis'?

D. A. Game, Adelaide

MARY L.   AGED 11

392

Abdominal pains – mainly central and epigastric – make her want to lie down – come and go over about an hour – worse possibly in the morning – more intense over the last 3 months though probably the pains have been coming and going for 2 years.

Teacher says she often has to lie down at school and has asked mother to take her to the doctor *again*. Father thinks it's her appendix, and wants something done.

1. What do you consider the significance of the pains having been present for 2 years?
2. What pressures face the mother?
3. What examination and investigation would you perform?
4. What is your management of abdominal pain in children which seems almost certainly 'benign'?

F. Mansfield, Perth, Australia

393 MRS. S.T. AGED 30 HOUSEWIFE

Mrs. T. consults you because she has been having pain underneath the rib margin on the right side. It has been affecting her on occasions for about a year, but once or twice lately, always after a big meal with some wine, it has been more severe. Until now, antacid tablets have eventually relieved it.

Some friends have urged her to make this consultation. She likes 'good food', gin and tonic, and wine when they are appropriate, and she smokes 20–25 cigarettes daily. She is 20% above ideal weight and does not have regular exercise.

1. What things are in your mind before you proceed to examination and investigation?
2. If examination was to reveal only a slightly elevated blood pressure (135/90), how would you describe your assessment to the patient?
3. How would you reply to the question: 'I haven't got cancer, have I, doctor?'

P. L. Gibson, Auckland

394 MRS. P.S. AGED 43

This intelligent, obsessive-compulsive nutritionist with two nationally-ranked, athletic, teenage daughters and married to an old school chum of yours, presents with abdominal pain and a palpable epigastric mass. A year ago she had a cholecystectomy for cholelithiasis and biliary colic; exploration of the abdomen had been negative. Laparotomy this time reveals a football-sized solid retroperitoneal tumour which is biopsied and reported malignant-sarcoma.

ABDOMINAL PROBLEMS

1. What do you say to this woman when she has recovered from the anaesthetic?
2. What happens next?
3. How do you respond to questions about the prognosis?

P. R. Grantham, Vancouver

Mid abdominal pain

395 **CHERYL C.   AGED 10**

You have been called at midday to see Cheryl who is in bed at home. After a restless night she has complained of central abdominal pains since early morning. Her temperature is mildly elevated and she vomited once after eating a piece of toast for breakfast. She has had no diarrhoea.

1. What are the most likely diagnoses you would consider?
2. How will the history you take influence your thoughts?
3. What examination will you perform?
4. What will your advice be if the examination is negative apart from some general abdominal tenderness?

J. R. Marshall, Adelaide

396 **MR. J.McN.   AGED 65**

There was a mild epidemic of viral enteritis in the district when a request came to visit Mr. McN., a senior executive, who had abdominal pains. He had come home from a meeting the afternoon before with nausea and had gone to bed, which was most unusual for him. Today, Thursday, he felt better and was annoyed with his wife for phoning. Nevertheless, he had had pains in his abdomen, and was still in bed. His bowels were normal and he had eaten his breakfast.

A diagnosis of viral enteritis was made, for he had a mild pyrexia of 37.8 °C and mild tenderness on deep palpation with minimal tympany over his ascending colon. He was told to contact the office if he became worse or if he was no better the next day.

Two days later, Saturday, he was admitted for emergency operation for a ruptured appendix. He had felt better for 24 hours with no nausea and eating all meals, but a return of the abdominal pain made him ring late on Friday. He was seen by a partner who again diagnosed that he had the current viral enteritis.

1. What might have alerted the doctor to the seriousness of the illness?
2. How could delayed care have been avoided?

G. M. Dick, Hobart

MRS. S.   AGED 58   HOUSEWIFE

397

Mrs. S. was staying at a suburban hotel for the weekend. She lived in the country and was leaving for a 'safari type' holiday in the outback on the Monday morning. She was having this holiday mainly as a badly needed respite from caring for her mother who had been invalided following a motor vehicular accident in which Mrs. S. was the driver. She came to the office at 10 a.m. on Saturday stating that she had woken up at 4 a.m. with central abdominal pain. The pain had persisted and had prevented her sleeping. She felt a little nauseated but had not vomited. She had had one small bowel action. On examination she was apyrexial and slightly tender in the right lower abdomen.

On review at 5 p.m. the same day she stated the pain had moved to the right lower abdomen. She had had no food, felt nauseated and had vomited once. Her temperature was 38.2 °C, her tongue furred and she was very tender in the right lower abdomen. There was no guarding. Physical examination revealed no other abnormality.

A diagnosis was made and operation was arranged for the same evening.

At operation, no intra abdominal pathology was noted. However, in view of the pre-operative diagnosis the organ supposedly implicated was removed. Post operatively she had an uneventful convalescence. She lost her pain and was apyrexial in 2 days. Histopathological examination of the tissue removed was reported as showing chronic inflammatory changes.

1. What diagnosis was made?
2. Was the general practitioner justified in performing the operation?

D. A. Game, Adelaide

JOANNE W.   AGED 11

398

Mr. and Mrs. W. who are separated, have three children, Joanne being the youngest. The children live with Mrs. W. and her unmarried sister. You are called to see Joanne because of severe mid-line abdominal pain, colicky in nature, present for the last ½ hour. She was quite well last night, but has been off her food today and unusually quiet. Joanne was seen 4 days ago by your partner when she complained of a sore throat. He could find nothing wrong and prescribed nothing. When you examine Joanne you find a normal temperature and pulse, ENT examination is normal and there are no glands palpable. However, she doubles up every 1 or 2 minutes with crampy abdominal pains crying loudly at the same time. It is almost impossible to examine her abdomen because every slight touch brings more tears and strong guarding. Bowel sounds are normal. Mrs. W. says she is due to go interstate on business in a few hours time and should be away 5 days. However, she now thinks she will postpone her trip.

1. Is it advisable to seek another opinion at this time?
2. How significant was the consultation 4 days ago?
3. What is the management of this situation?

W. F. Glastonbury, Adelaide

399 MISS D.W.   AGED 12   STUDENT

As a rural practitioner, you are called out to see this child at 10 o'clock at night suffering from central abdominal pain for 2 days moving down to the central lower abdomen over the last few hours. She has been vomiting 2 to 3 times since tea tonight. Bowels normal today, micturition normal, menstrual history – no menarche as yet. Past history: she had a similar attack a month ago which lasted all day. Examination revealed a soft abdomen with no masses, no rigidity, no rebound tenderness and a normal rectal examination. Urine was normal, throat normal, there were no glands present and she has grossly bitten nails.

Further questioning revealed some tension at home between her and mother regarding her 16 year old boyfriend.

1. What would be your immediate management of this problem?
2. What additional information should be sought?
3. How would you undertake long term management of this problem in order to prevent further attacks?

T. D. Manthorpe, Port Lincoln, Australia

400 MISS B.S.   AGED 3   PRE-SCHOOL

This child presents with peri-umbilical abdominal pain and a high fever of 3 hours' duration. She has vomited twice.

She is flushed, has a temperature of 40 °C and a pulse of 144. Otherwise there are no abnormal findings on clinical examination.

1. What is your diagnosis?
2. What investigations would you arrange?

R. W. Roberts, Ravensthorpe, Australia

401 JENNIFER E.   AGED 8   SCHOOLGIRL

Jennifer is brought in by her mother because of fever and abdominal pain. The pain is mid-abdominal (more on the right side than the left), dull, and has been present on and off for 2 days. She has been off her food, but drinking plenty of fluids.

She looks flushed and uncomfortable. Her temperature is 39.2 °C and she is mildly tender over the right mid-abdomen.

1. What diagnostic hypotheses would you entertain?
2. How would you assess this patient?
3. What follow up might be required?

W. E. Fabb, Melbourne

MR. E.   AGED 38   BANK CLERK   402

Mr. E., aged 38, has always been an apparently fit healthy man. He is seen at home at midnight; he is in severe pain, of sudden onset 2 hours previously. Situated in the right loin, the pain is constant and does not appear to be a colic; it radiates into his groin. Aspirin has had no effect. Examination reveals only some tenderness in the right renal angle. He emptied his bladder before going to bed and cannot provide a sample of urine.

1. What conditions should be considered in the differential diagnosis?
2. What should be done to help Mr. E?

J. D. E. Knox, Dundee

MRS. J.S.   AGED 54   HOUSEWIFE   403

Mrs. J.S. presents complaining of recurrent bouts of right sided abdominal pain, colicky in nature. These pains have occurred every few days for the last 18 months. They are not related to meals, she has no nausea, no change of bowel habit and no weight loss. The pain remains on the right side of her abdomen, from the right iliac fossa to the costal margin.

You have known Mrs. S. and her family for some years, although you haven't seen Mrs. S. for some time. About 2 years ago Mr. S. had a bowel resection for carcinoma of the descending colon. Their eldest son, aged 24 has a serious drinking problem.

1. What is the most likely cause of Mrs. S.'s abdominal pain?
2. How would you manage this problem?
3. What will be the most likely course of Mrs. S.'s condition?

W. F. Glastonbury, Adelaide

Lower abdominal pain
---

404 MRS. Q.　　AGED 35　　HOUSEWIFE

Mrs. Q. had laparoscopic sterilization 3 months ago. At 5 a.m. she awoke with lower right abdominal pain which was continual and over 2 hours grew rapidly worse. When seen at 7 a.m. she was writhing with pain and vomiting.

She was afebrile, pulse 82, and had RIF tenderness with no rebound tenderness. PV she was tender in the right fornix but her reactions to the discomforts of the examination were only moderate.

1.　What is your differential diagnosis?
2.　What would you say to the husband?
3.　What would be your management?

F. Mansfield, Perth, Australia

405 MRS. Y.　　AGED 24　　HOUSEWIFE

Mrs. Y. presented with lower abdominal pain and vaginal spotting for 3 days. She has been married for 1 year and is not practising any contraception. Her periods had been regular, but she was then 10 days overdue. Pregnancy tests and pelvic examination were negative.

Ten days later she again presented to her GP telling him that she was admitted to a public hospital in the middle of the night with lower abdominal pain and PV spotting. Subsequently she was discharged from hospital after 3 days' observation, with no definite diagnosis. Her pregnancy tests were still negative. Her GP concluded that she probably had had an incomplete abortion and arranged admission to hospital for curettage.

Pathology of the curettings showed segments of secretory endometrium. No chorionic villi or decidual tissues were seen. She was well and was discharged the next day. One week later she was readmitted with acute abdominal pain and in shock.

1.　What is the diagnosis?
2.　How does one advise the patient regarding the possibility of a future pregnancy?

N. C. L. Yuen, Hong Kong

MISS G.A.   AGED 17   BANK CLERK

406

A pleasant, 'well presented' young Miss gives a history of lower abdominal pain of 2 days' duration, causing sufficient discomfort for her senior work mates to get her off to her doctor.

1. What is the most likely differential diagnosis?
2. Why, if the discomfort is so severe may a young girl not readily seek medical care unprompted?
3. Questioning reveals that she had been treated for a 'bladder infection' 3 months earlier. What might have been missed?

A. J. Radford, Adelaide

MISS M.B.J.   AGED 14   SCHOOLGIRL

407

The patient, brought by her mother, complained of severe colicky lower abdominal pain which began at the right iliac fossa and was later localized over the whole of her lower abdomen. She also could not void any urine for the last 10 hours.

Three months ago, she had three episodes of mild colicky lower abdominal pain accompanied by low grade feverishness. She was seen and treated by another general practitioner with tablets on those occasions.

Examination revealed that she had a temperature of 37 °C and that the lower abdomen was distended up to the level of the umbilicus by a cystic mass.

You have been requested by your colleague to look the patient over. He was about to refer her to the hospital with a provisional diagnosis of acute appendicitis with early perforation.

1. What conditions would you consider in the differential diagnosis?
2. What relevant history and physical signs would you try to obtain?
3. How would you manage this patient?

F. E. H. Tan, Kuala Lumpur

MRS. M.W.   AGED 68   HOUSEWIFE

408

Mrs. W. has been well until the last few weeks when she noticed crampy abdominal pain associated with constipation. She has put off visiting the doctor because her 70 year old husband was recently treated for an abdominal aneurysm and metastatic prostatic cancer. However, for 2 days she has noticed a blood stained discharge per rectum. Pelvic examination reveals a grapefruit size mass and at sigmoidoscopy, a proliferative mass is seen at 15 centimeters.

1. What should the doctor tell her at this point?
2. What are the available treatment modalities?
3. Assuming she has metastatic disease and an inoperable tumour, how could she be managed?

E. Domovitch, Toronto

Diarrhoea

MRS. C.D.   AGED 36   HOUSEWIFE AND SHIFT WORKER   **409**

Mrs. C.D., a tall woman with a determined look on her face, presented with a 2 day history of abdominal pain and considerable diarrhoea. As she was leaving the office she asked if I would recommend some vitamins.

1. What questions need to follow with respect to her abdominal pain and diarrhoea?
2. What management plan would you institute on empirical grounds if further questioning provided no significant positive findings?
3. What line of questioning would you pursue regarding her request for vitamins?

A. J. Radford, Adelaide

MRS. J.C.   AGED 21   STENOGRAPHER   **410**

Mrs. J.C. has been married for 7 months and admits to being an anxious personality. She presents with a 3 week history of variable colicky abdominal pains with loose bowel actions. She had not felt ill, had continued going to work and had used no treatment. There was no weight loss, no blood in the faeces and she had not vomited. Variable headaches; no significant past medical history; admitted that there were pressures at work and had some doubts about her libido.

1. What is the likely diagnosis?
2. How important is further history in this situation?
3. If the patient asked about the possibility of cancer what would you say?

D. S. Muecke, Adelaide

MRS. M.C.   AGED 23   FARMER'S WIFE   **411**

This young mother of two small children presents with an acute onset of offensive diarrhoea and vomiting, associated with abdominal pain.

Examination reveals a sick girl with a temperature of 39.4 °C and a pulse of 124. There is generalized mild abdominal tenderness but no guarding or rigidity. Blood is present in a stool specimen.

Over the next 48 hours the diarrhoea persists; the temperature and pulse rate remain elevated and her two young children develop a similar illness, although less severe.

1. What is your diagnosis?
2. What investigations would you order?
3. What treatment would you institute?

R. W. Roberts, Ravensthorpe, Australia

412 GEORGE TE H.   AGED 6   MAORI SCHOOLBOY

George lives at the Orakei Marae. He has been at school for a year and he is normally a very lively youngster with a ready smile.

Whenever he gets the chance he goes down to the Orakei wharf to fish for piper and occasionally he tries his luck with a schnapper line. Last Saturday after the tide went out George and his friend Stephen thought they would explore some of the rock pools. Later in the sand they discovered some cockles. George loves shellfish and best of all he likes them raw. They smashed the shells open and had quite a feed.

Last night (Sunday) George was not feeling so well. He had some colicky pains in his abdomen and he was nauseated. He went to bed early and woke with a fever. Then came the diarrhoea. It seemed as though George would never get off the toilet. When he did eventually get up to struggle off to bed he felt really faint and only just made it. After his diarrhoea he felt a little better but presently the pain returned as did the diarrhoea and this time his mother who came to help him noticed a little blood with the motion and the smell was terrible. George was very thirsty and his mouth was dry. Mrs. Te H. could see that he was too sick to take to the surgery and so she gave the doctor a ring. Later that morning the doctor arrived and examined George.

1. What is the likely cause of the diarrhoea?
2. What public health measures are needed?
3. How will you manage the diarrhoea?

J. G. Richards, Auckland

413 MR. G.L.   AGED 28   FARMHAND

Mr. G.L. presented with diarrhoea for 4 days. He was having 12–15 bowel motions a day, watery with some mucus and blood spots. He had little pain but felt weak. The diarrhoea began about 20 minutes after he fell on his back from the carry-all on the back of the tractor as it went over a small drain.

He had never had this problem before. Over the next few weeks, the diarrhoea continued. Faecal cultures were NAD. Blood streaks and mucus were frequently observed in the bowel motions. The patient lost weight and became anxious. Various therapies were used with some relief but diarrhoea continued at approximately 8 bowel motions/day.

1. What are the likely causes in this case?
2. How can the condition be treated?

E. J. H. North, Melbourne

MR. GORDON B.   AGED 32   CLERK

41

Mr. B.'s ulcerative colitis had been well controlled by regular medication for 8 years. One week previously he had attended a public health glaucoma screening survey. The sister who tested his eyes told him the pressure in one eye was elevated and he should consult an ophthalmologist. He sought an appointment immediately but the earliest appointment was in 2 weeks. As an uncle had gone blind from glaucoma Mr. B. had been unable to stop worrying about his eyes. His anxiety increased over the week and severe diarrhoea had developed; now passing pure blood and mucus every ½ hour with lower abdominal cramps. On checking with a Schiøtz tonometer he had a normal pressure in each eye.

1. What problems need to be considered in the diagnosis?
2. How can a diagnosis be made?
3. What is the treatment of acute ulcerative colitis?
4. What are the pros and cons of health screening measures?

D. G. Chambers, Clare, Australia

MRS. P.W.   AGED 50   CINEMA USHERETTE

415

Nine years ago, Mrs. P.W. developed ulcerative colitis, which presented originally as diarrhoea and erythema nodosum. Four years later, she underwent a total colectomy and has managed her ileostomy well ever since. She has gained weight and has not needed any prophylactic treatment for years. Her children have grown up, but about 18 months ago her husband left her unexpectedly.

She has come now for advice about the hurtful messages and innuendoes which the BBC have been broadcasting about her, on radio and television. She has complained to them, and even visited an official at Bush House, only to be 'rudely' shown the door. She shows a postcard, printed with an acknowledgement and bearing the BBC 'logo'.

1. What explanation can you offer for her complaint?
2. How relevant is her past medical and personal history?
3. How can she be persuaded to accept treatment?

J. Grabinar, Bromley, UK

416   JASON L.   AGED 6 MONTHS

It is 10.30 p.m. Mr. P.L., whom you have not met before, calls you to his house to see Jason, aged 6 months, who has some vomiting and diarrhoea. You find Jason has been a bit unwell all day, he has had two loose bowel actions and vomited at his last breast feed. After assessing the situation you advise a boiled water routine and Mrs. L., whom you know well, quietly agrees to notify you of progress tomorrow. Mr. L. becomes angry that you haven't done anything and asks to see a specialist!

1. Why do people request 'trivial' calls at night?
2. Why couldn't this baby have been given some 'proper' treatment?
3. How does a doctor feel about advice as treatment?

A. L. A. Reid, Newcastle, Australia

417   WILLIAM P.   AGED 10 MONTHS

Three nights ago William refused to settle, cried a lot and had a fever. His mother noticed that he had a running nose and did not seem very interested in food although he was quite thirsty. In the morning he had two very loose bowel motions and his mother took him to the doctor.

'I think he's got a tummy bug, doctor. He's developed diarrhoea and is off his food.'

The doctor examined the child and found the ear drums to be normal. The nose was congested and the fauces were red, although there was no tonsillar enlargement and no lymphadenopathy. The neck was not stiff, and the abdomen was soft. The doctor said, 'He has a red throat. Give him this amoxycillin three times a day and let me know if he is not improving.'

'But what about the diarrhoea, doctor?'

'Many children with an upper respiratory tract infection have loose motions – when the infection is better that will settle down' replied the doctor.

William started on the amoxycillin, but after 24 hours the stomach had not settled. William was even more miserable and was having a loose motion every 3 hours. Mrs. Pearce brought him back to the doctor.

1. What is the likely cause of the diarrhoea?
2. What treatment would you have prescribed initially?
3. Is it possible that the treatment prescribed influenced the outcome?

J. G. Richards, Auckland

418   MADELINE P.   AGED 4 MONTHS

Madeline Phillips is 4 months old. She has been bottle fed since birth because her mother had an inadequate supply of milk. Her mother is a slim, tense person who worries a lot about Madeline, who is a first baby.

Madeline's growth curve has been a little disappointing but she takes her food well and the district nurse says there is no cause for alarm.

Mrs. P. has been disappointed and feels that she cannot be a good mother because that awful Mrs. Eileen Smith down the road had a baby at almost the same time and her child is almost double Madeline's birth weight already. Mrs. Phillips has been supplementing her baby's bottle with Farex and more recently with banana. She also gives her a lot of orange juice because she has heard that this is very good for babies and helps to prevent colds. To help the baby put on weight she has now started fortifying the Farex and she has increased the amount of fluid she gives Madeline with each feed.

Today she is back at the doctors because, to her shame, baby has developed diarrhoea and she knows that if this persists, baby's weight will fall right back.

1. What is the likely cause of the diarrhoea?
2. What counselling does Mrs. Phillips need?

J. G. Richards, Auckland

MRS. DONNA M.   AGED 53   419

Because she had encountered so many previous difficulties with her health, Mrs. M. was being followed regularly in the office. Her early obstetrical experience included six miscarriages and the delivery of a handicapped infant with major mental and physical defects. Later she had two normal children. At age 45, she developed marked essential hypertension requiring significant medication and monitoring. Soon after, she suffered an occlusion in her right cental retinal vein, ultimately requiring enucleation and an ocular prosthesis. With all this, she is a successful wife and mother, but is an anxious person.

During an office visit for a periodic health assessment, she stated she felt generally well, but noted flatulence and a change in bowel frequency from once to three times daily. She felt her bowel emptied well, but the movements were smaller. She ascribed the change to following advice that she should start eating wheat bran daily. She added that her sister had recently died of carcinoma of the pancreas.

1. How important is a change in bowel habit in a woman of 53?
2. What principles govern the amount of investigation you would order to elucidate a minor complaint in an anxious person?

F. B. Fallis, Toronto

MR. L.C.   AGED 20   4TH YEAR DENTAL STUDENT   420

Mr. L.C. consulted his family doctor for the first time 2 weeks ago with pain in the left hip and back. There was a marked loss of weight and a history of incessant diarrhoea. A fistula in ano, on which he has had four operations by four different surgeons, was present. He has been treated by a psychiatrist for neurosis.

On examination he appears anxious and anaemic. Rectal examination reveals a small bulging area superior to the prostate. Reflexes and power are all normal. He was referred for a number of tests. Barium meal demonstrated a lesion involving the terminal six inches of the ileum. He returned 2 days later and it was found that his reflexes had now increased and he had clonus reactions of knee and ankle with positive Babinski responses. He had become very much weaker and was now grossly anaemic clinically.

1. What is the differential diagnosis?
2. What diagnostic procedures should be advised?
3. What medical treatment would be ordered?
4. What is the prognosis?

B. M. Fehler, Johannesburg

421 MR. C. AGED 45 FIRE OFFICER

Mr. C., aged 45 years, is a sub-officer with the Fire Brigade. Three weeks ago he suffered an acute exacerbation of his known long-standing Crohn's disease, necessitating his emergency admission to hospital.

He comes to let you know he has been discharged from hospital and to let you see a small sinus at the site of an abdominal drain in the right iliac fossa. He tells you that 'a piece of bowel' has been removed at operation 2 weeks ago. The laparotomy wound is healing well.

You have no up-to-date information from the hospital.

1. What are common inter-professional communication problems in 'transfer of care' in either direction across the general practice/ hospital interface?
2. What is Crohn's disease?
3. What management decisions need to be taken in Mr. C's case?

J. D. E. Knox, Dundee

Jaundice

MRS. A.C.   AGED 43   HOUSEWIFE/PHARMACIST

422

Mrs. A.C. had felt nauseous for a week before her consultation. 24 hours ago she developed pain in her right hypochondrium. She was apyrexial, had marked tenderness over the liver which was enlarged to two fingers. Slight icterus was present in the conjunctivae. Urine was a dark yellow and showed that urobilinogen was present.

A tentative diagnosis of infective hepatitis was made.

1. What is the differential diagnosis?
2. What basic diagnostic investigations would you suggest?
3. What advice would you give the patient?
4. Is immunization of contacts necessary?

B. M. Fehler, Johannesburg

MRS. A.J. AND JOHN J.   AGED 55   MANAGER

423

Mrs. Alison J., aged 55 years, consults you. 'It's not about myself, doctor,' she says. 'We have been given a fabulous offer – a very rich friend of John's (her husband) has offered us a month in his holiday house on a small Carribean island next summer. You know John's state, and I thought I should discuss the proposed holiday with you before we go any further. By the way, he doesn't know I've come.'

John, aged 55, suffers from primary biliary cirrhosis. In the last 6 months he has had two episodes of severe abdominal pain. He has a chronic low-grade icterus, and, despite a constant degree of malaise, he has held down his responsible job as general manager of a large electrical business. He has daily vitamin K by mouth, attends monthly for injections of vitamin D. On occasions he takes oral cholestyramine (Questran).

1. What is primary biliary cirrhosis?
2. What is the role of drug therapy in this disease?
3. How would you manage the consultation with Mrs. J?

J. D. E. Knox, Dundee

MR. P.   AGED 68   RETIRED PLUMBER

424

Mr. P. a mild diabetic, presented at the surgery with painless jaundice. Investigations showed this to be obstructive in type and surgery was recommended. At operation a firm mass was discovered in the pancreatic area. A biopsy was not performed but the surgeon was confident from the appearance that the condition was malignant. A palliative operation was performed, and the patient was returned to his general practitioner.

A conspiracy of silence was agreed upon and the patient was not told the diagnosis. His wife however was informed. Over the next couple of years there was no deterioration in his general condition or his diabetes until a further episode of jaundice occurred. This was treated conservatively and resolved spontaneously. Five years later his condition remains good.

1. What is the differential diagnosis of painless jaundice?
2. Was this doctor wise in not informing the patient of the diagnosis?

J. G. Richards, Auckland

CHAPTER 19

Genitourinary Problems

This chapter begins with a series of cases of urinary tract infection in both adults and children, enuresis, incontinence, haematuria, prostatism and renal failure. Then follow examples of vaginal discharge, menstrual problems and uterine cancer, after which a series of cases of sexually transmitted diseases in males is presented. The pros and cons of circumcision are discussed in the last case. The problems presented are frequently seen by the family physician and represent a challenge in diagnosis and management.

Dysuria and frequency

425 MISS A.S.   AGED 19

A pretty girl complains of frequency and pain on micturition for two days, worse today. She looks worried. Office test with Albustix reveals 30% proteinuria.

1. What is your management and treatment?
2. Discuss the necessity for correct laboratory diagnosis.
3. What underlying factors should be discussed with the patient, both for primary and secondary prevention?

G. M. Dick, Hobart

426 JAN H.   AGED 17

Miss H. has cystitis. Her father is an elderly minister of religion and you treat her mother for tension headaches and neck problems.

1. What is the correct management for a first case of cystitis at age 17?
2. In family medicine, how does one decide when to treat an individual and when to look at the family?
3. Is there any relationship between the stiff neck and tension?

A. L. A. Reid, Newcastle, Australia

427 MRS. S.R.   AGED 28   HOUSEWIFE/UNIVERSITY GRADUATE

Mrs. S.R. has had recurrent attacks of frequency and dysuria since the birth of her first child, a boy now 2½ years old. Mid-stream urines have sometimes shown an infection with *E. coli*, but not usually. On the other hand they have often shown a large number of white cells. She has twice had episodes of bleeding PR each of which seemed associated with a fissure-in-ano which responded to conservative treatment.

Mrs. S.R. tells the doctor that she and her husband want a second child. They have used no contraception for the past 8 months. She has a recurrence of her bleeding PR. A fissure-in-ano can again be seen.

1. What is your approach to the management of urinary frequency and dysuria in the long and short term?

2. What, if any, may be the relationship between Mrs. S.R.'s physical problems and her failure to conceive?
3. What is your approach to antenatal care of women with Mrs. S.R.'s history of urinary problems?

P. Freeling, London

SUSAN M.   AGED 10

428

Susan had been suffering from headaches and tummyaches on and off for about 6 months. They did not appear to follow any pattern, although they did not occur during the school holidays. There was no identifiable precipitating factor and no other symptoms apart from occasional nausea. She was an intelligent child, who enjoyed school. She worked hard and would worry if she failed to complete homework in good time. Her father was an intensely conscientious man with a responsible job. He was also a lay preacher. He suffered from a duodenal ulcer. Her mother was a weak, anxious woman. She had a bouncy extrovert sister, 2 years older than herself.

The doctor thought the symptoms were due to stress in an over-conscientious individual but, when on one visit she appeared febrile and unwell in addition to her other symptoms, he arranged an MSU. This showed a urinary infection (400 pus cells and 300,000 *E. coli*) which he treated with a week's course of amoxycillin. A second MSU was clear. Her previous symptoms continued and further MSUs were clear. However, 6 months later she had a further proven urinary tract infection which again resolved satisfactorily. An IVP was normal.

1. Are the symptoms presented by Susan common in children?
2. How do urinary tract infections in girls of this age usually present?
3. What are the dangers of missing a diagnosis of urinary tract infection in a child?
4. How would you manage this case?

G. Strube, Crawley, UK

DOROTHY A.   AGED 3

429

Dorothy A., a healthy 3 year old girl, was seen in the emergency department at 2 a.m. with marked irritability and apparent lower abdominal pain. She was afebrile. Examination and observation over a couple of hours did not suggest an intra-abdominal lesion. Urinalysis revealed many white blood cells, some bacteria, and a trace of protein. Urine culture later revealed *E. coli* with over 100 000 colonies per cmm. She was treated with amoxycillin, but the report on sensitivities showed resistance to ampicillin, and in fact her symptoms recurred. She was then given cotrimoxazole and her symptoms and cultures finally cleared after a second course.

She was referred to a paediatric urologist, who found her normal on examination and she had a normal urinalysis. Intravenous pyelogram was normal and the cystogram showed a normal bladder with no reflux into either ureter. A catheter urine sample obtained at the time of the cystogram was also sterile.

1. What are the common presentations of significant lower urinary infection in young children?
2. Are there hygienic measures to be taken with a young girl with urinary tract infection to prevent recurrences?
3. How would you now treat Dorothy A. if she had a definite recurrence of symptoms?

F. B. Fallis, Toronto

430 MRS. S.E.   AGED 85   PENSIONER

Mrs. S.E. lives alone since the death of her husband 5 years ago. She admits to being lonely and relatives are 'forcing' her to go into a home. For 2 weeks she has felt unwell and noticed an increased frequency of micturition at night only (D/N 4/5–6) – mild stranguary but no pain or burning. There was a fullness in the region of the bladder eased by micturition. Microscopy shows 10–23 WBC/HPF. She also suffers from pernicious anaemia (treatment with vitamin B12 and folic acid).

1. Is she likely to have an urinary infection – if not, why not?
2. Could these symptoms have a psychological basis?
3. List likely possibilities.
4. What investigations are necessary?

D. S. Muecke, Adelaide

431 MRS. J.F.   AGED 34   SECRETARY

Mrs. J.F. presents with a chronic problem of frequency of micturation including nocturia. She has a distressing sensation that 'my bladder feels as though it is about to fall out'. Physical examination is normal.

She directly consulted an eminent urologist 6 months ago and he claimed that stretching her bladder neck under general anaesthesia would solve her problem. However, the problem deteriorated. He did not visit her postoperatively and refused to speak to her on the telephone.

1. What is the likely cause of her problem?
2. What problems confront patients who directly consult specialists about their medical problems?
3. What are the important aspects in total care of this patient?

J. E. Murtagh, Melbourne

SUSAN STONE   AGED 22   STENOGRAPHER

432

This 22 year old stenographer complained of a sore throat. She was afebrile. Cervical lymphadenopathy was not present and examination of the throat revealed mild pharyngitis and tonsillitis. There was no exudate. She appeared tense and slightly tearful. The morning was a very busy one and the patient, who denied any worries at the time, was invited to come back later in the week. This she did. Questioning disclosed some minor marital disharmony since her marriage 18 months before and a history of recurrent mild urinary tract infection over the past few months. Microurine revealed a few pus cells only. However, on examination, her right kidney was palpable and appeared a little enlarged. Intravenous pyelogram was reported on as revealing a cyst of the right kidney. The urologist to whom she was referred considered that investigative surgery should be performed, although the lesion was expected to be benign. Surgery revealed an adenocarcinoma of the kidney, which was removed. The patient had three successful pregnancies subsequently with no evidence of recurrence of her malignancy.

1. What was the sequence of the diagnostic labels applied to this patient as her story unfolded?
2. What sequence should be followed in treating and investigating a recurrent urinary tract infection in a female?

J. G. P. Ryan, Brisbane

Enuresis and incontinence
---

433   **MISS C.L.**   **AGED 6**

Miss C.L. is a very active, talkative little girl. 'Potty' trained at age 2 years but following the arrival of her young brother, 18 months ago, began to wet her pants during day and night though not constantly wet. Taken to several different doctors by her parents. Investigated with X-rays and urine checks. Picture later confused by several episodes of renal tract infection. Some temporary response to imipramine. Paternal grandparents very concerned.

   1.   Would you feel the psychosocial aspects of this child's environment are the key issue to diagnosis and management?
   2.   What do you advise parents about 'potty training'?
   3.   How do you monitor and control renal tract infection in such a case?

W. D. Jackson, Launceston, Australia

434   **DEBBIE**   **AGED 12**   **SCHOOLGIRL**

Debbie was brought to the doctor by her foster mother because she was frequently wetting her pants. Although she had formed a good relationship with her foster parents and their two teenage children, her own mother came to visit her on occasions which made her confused. Her school record was below average.

   1.   What steps should one take to deal with Debbie's enuresis?
   2.   How might the question of her school work be investigated?
   3.   How might Debbie's emotional problems be further explored?

J. C. Hasler, Oxford

435   **N.L.**   **AGED 15**   **SCHOOLBOY**

Mother presented with her sons N.L. aged 15 and R.L. aged 9 at the end of a busy morning to seek advice on bed wetting for both her sons. Both had had normal urine tests some years previously and N.L. had been placed on Tofranil (imipramine) some 3 years ago with improvement. N.L. had hearing problems and had hearing aids in both ears since the age of 4. School mates were prone to ridicule him because of this.

1. What would you do in these circumstances?
2. What other course might the parent/s take?
3. What is the incidence of this condition?

E. J. H. North, Melbourne

MRS. M.P.   AGED 38   HOUSEWIFE   **436**

Over the years, Mrs. M.P. has attended frequently with anxiety, marital difficulties, and her asthmatic elder daughter; she also has young twins. Her husband is a police officer and in the last year they have moved to a comfortable house.

She complains of occasional loss of control of her bladder for the past 6 months. This happens without warning, and consists of small leaks only, mainly by day. Coughing or sneezing do not cause incontinence. There is no pain, and urine cultures have proved negative. Examination shows no loss of vaginal tone, prolapse or urethral disease. She seems surprisingly unconcerned by the symptom.

1. Is the symptom likely to be physical or psychogenic?
2. What are the possible organic causes?
3. What specialist advice would you request, if any?

J. Grabinar, Bromley, UK

MR. A.F.   AGED 77   RETIRED FROM ARMY   **437**

Mr. F. has arteriosclerotic heart disease. He did have congestive heart failure but this is controlled with diuretics and digoxin. He has problems with urinary incontinence at night and recurrent urinary tract infections. A neurogenic bladder has been diagnosed by the GU service. He also has recurrent faecal impactions due to an 'atonic' bowel.

1. How do you manage this patient's incontinence?
2. How would you manage the bowel dysfunction?
3. What support will he need if he returns home?

C. T. Lamont, Ottawa

Haematuria

438 MR. K.V.   AGED 40   BUSINESSMAN

Mr. K.V., a Swiss businessman, in Melbourne for a conference, calls you urgently to his hotel because of 'difficulty' with urine. When you arrive, he appears well, but states that 1 hour before, he attempted to void, had difficulty, and on forcing noticed pain, followed by a sudden rush of blood-stained urine. He now feels well but has noticed his urine is still slightly blood stained, although not painful to pass. He is to leave early next morning for Japan. He sees a Swiss doctor for his annual check-up.

1. What is the **most** likely diagnosis?
2. What important question should be asked in the history?
3. What investigations should be performed?
4. What should be the management of this case?

D. U. Shepherd, Melbourne

439 MRS. BETTY F.   AGED 29   CLEANER

This patient has been referred to you from the local Family Planning Clinic. She has not been to see you before. She has been noted to have blood in her urine on the usual ward test done at each of three attendances at the Family Planning Clinic in the past year and they have referred the patient to you for further investigation. She has no symptoms of renal disease at present and has no past history of renal disease as far as she knows. She had three children whose ages are 11, 9 and 5. However, in her family history, there is a worrying family history of early coronary artery disease. Her father died at 36 of a heart attack and the father's brother also died of a heart attack at the age of 42.

1. There are two main issues here, the one of the family history of coronary artery disease and the second issue of a possibility of renal disease. How would you proceed?
2. You discover that her serum cholesterol and triglycerides are borderline. She had a cholecystectomy in 1975 and hepatitis in 1972. She is 51 kg in weight and 155 cm tall. What advice would you give her about coronary artery disease?
3. What should you do about the renal disease?

M. D. Mahoney, Brisbane

MR. F.R.   AGED 62   STOREMAN

440

Over the last 4 months Mr. F. has had intermittent episodes of painless haematuria. Gradually the haematuria has become more frequent and severe until now every specimen is heavily bloodstained. He has only mild symptoms attributable to his prostate.

3 months ago he was investigated by blood tests and urine examination, (he does not know just what was done). He was told the bleeding was coming from his prostate, and some day he might need it removed but since his tests were normal it was best to ignore the bleeding for the present.

1. Was it reasonable for the other practitioner to accept negative results as indicative of no serious disease?
2. How would you set about investigating this man?
3. What is the likely disease process involved in a patient of this age?

W. F. Glastonbury, Adelaide

Bladder neck obstruction

---

441 | **MR. R.D.**   **AGED 88**   **UNMARRIED, RETIRED CARPENTER**

Mr. D. is referred to the geriatric evaluation unit from the GI service after removal of a benign colonic polyp. He is mentally alert, and looks younger than his stated age. He complains of urinary frequency, urgency and nocturia. Rectal examination reveals a slightly enlarged, smooth prostate. Urinalysis is negative. His haematocrit is 27, assumed to be secondary to GI blood loss from the polyp.

1. How should his urinary problem be investigated?
2. What are the treatment options for benign prostate hypertrophy?
3. What causes of anaemia, other than blood loss, should be considered?
4. What assessment will be necessary prior to his returning home?

C. T. Lamont, Ottawa

442 | **MR. F.C.M.**   **AGED 72**   **PENSIONER**

Mr. F.C.M. has been attending for the past 5 years with chronic renal failure secondary to delayed relief of prostatic obstruction. The failure has been only slowly progressive. Current serum creatinine and urea levels are 291 mmol/l and 11.5 mmol/l respectively (normal ranges 60–130 and 2.5–7 respectively). There is also a mild degree of hypertension and mild generalized osteoarthritis.

The laboratory profile (including haemoglobin, uric acid and electrolytes) is monitored 6 monthly.

He presents feeling that he is going downhill and requests a repeat of tests 2 months early. He is giddy (an old complaint) and his muscle cramps (an old complaint) are worse. His blood pressure is 170/105 sitting, 135/95 standing. His medication (unaltered for years) consists of Chlotride 1 daily, Aldomet 250 mg b.d. and an occasional tablet of paracetamol.

1. How closely should the renal failure be monitored by the laboratory in this patient?
2. What criteria should one use when prescribing medication in a patient with renal failure?
3. What is the likely prognosis in this patient?

D. Levet, Hobart

Vaginal discharge

MISS K.E.   AGED 21   UNIVERSITY STUDENT

443

Miss K.E. has been sexually active on the birth control pill for 3 years. There have been several male sexual partners in the past but she has had a steady boyfriend for the past few months. She presented with a frothy green vaginal discharge of 1 week's duration. The discharge had a disagreeable odour and caused vaginal itching.

1. What are the common causes of vaginitis in women of child-bearing age?
2. How do you treat vaginitis?
3. What are the predisposing factors for vaginitis?
4. How are older women with vaginitis different?
5. How are children with vaginitis different?

R. L. Perkin, Toronto

MRS. X.Y.   AGED 29   HOUSEWIFE

444

Mrs. X.Y. came into the office and, with something approaching desperation in her voice, requesting something for 'recurrent thrush down there'. She had never been to my office before and was embarrassed at having come to another doctor.

1. What pattern of questioning would you use in such cases?
2. What are the indications for laboratory (at the office or central) diagnosis of vaginal infection?
3. What are the standard treatments used for candidiasis of the pudendal area?

A. J. Radford, Adelaide

MRS. C.J.N.   AGED 36

445

Mrs. C.J.N. is a regular patient. You learn today that her marriage is about to break up.

She presents with vaginal discharge and irritation for the last few days, getting worse. She had it once before when she was unsuccessfully treated with tablets by her former GP. (She took herself to a gynaecologist who cured her with a vaginal cream.)

On examination the vaginal walls are red. There is a moderate amount of non-frothy creamy discharge in the vagina, not adherent to the walls.

1. What are the most likely causes of this patient's symptoms?
2. How could her marital state tie in with her symptoms?
3. Does a previous experience of a similar episode help you in your management?

D. Levet, Hobart

446   MRS. L.B.   AGED 35

This patient came to see the doctor complaining of a persistent irritant vaginal discharge. This had troubled her on and off over the years since the birth of her last child 2 years earlier. The doctor remembered this event as she had delivered a baby of 4 kg with some difficulty. She had used the usual fungicidal agents with only temporary relief. She had not felt well recently, had lost weight and was passing urine more frequently. On testing the urine the doctor found glycosuria and ketones to be present.

1. What investigations are necessary to confirm the diagnosis of diabetes mellitus?
2. What treatment is required?
3. Would you refer this patient to hospital or treat her yourself?

A. G. Strube, Crawley, UK

Menstrual problems

MISS A.H.   AGED 20   SECRETARY

447

Miss A.H. is a very thin, attractive girl with sparkling eyes. She complains of 3 months amenorrhoea following two scanty periods. She has missed periods occasionally in the past. She has never taken the contraceptive pill and says that there has never been any reason for doing so.

1. What alternative diagnoses would you consider?
2. What steps would you take to distinguish between them?
3. What is meant by the term 'denial' as used in psychology?

P. Freeling, London

MRS. VERA S.   AGED 27   CLEANER

448

For the last 5 years, since the birth of her second child, Mrs. S. has noticed that 3 to 4 days before her period is due her ankles swell, her breasts tingle and swell and she gets a bloated feeling in the abdomen. She also notices that she is irritable with her husband and children and has feelings of tension and depression. She is not interested in sex during this time. Her mother had similar symptoms.

Physical examination shortly after her period reveals no abnormality.

1. What is she suffering from?
2. What would you do for her?
3. In people who suffer severely from this condition, what is your opinion about their culpability if they exhibit criminal behaviour?

W. E. Fabb, Melbourne

MRS. Y.B.   AGED 36   HOUSEWIFE

449

Mrs. Y.B. is a doctor's wife. Two years ago she had a hysterectomy for menorrhagia. She now complains of dizziness, flushing and dyspareunia.

1. What conditions affect the uterus in a woman of child-bearing age?
2. How would you investigate abnormal uterine bleeding in a 36 year old woman?
3. What are the indications for hysterectomy?
4. What hormonal changes take place after hysterectomy?

T. A. I. Bouchier Hayes, Camberley, UK

450 **MRS. Y.L.** **AGED 52** **WIFE OF COMPANY DIRECTOR**

Mrs. Y.L. is a fairly intimidating lady who is used to getting what she wants. Her periods have become irregular and since her last period 3 months previously she has been increasingly troubled by flushes and sweats. Sleep is disturbed and although she has no early morning waking she feels irritable, exhausted and a bit depressed. Having read many articles on the subject she has decided she wants you to prescribe hormone replacement therapy. As she puts it 'Not only will it stop me feeling awful but it will also help to keep me looking young'.

1. Is the menopause an ovarian deficiency disease?
2. What are the disadvantages of treating flushes with hormone replacement therapy (HRT)?
3. Is it better to submit to, confront or bargain with this patient?

A. J. Moulds, Basildon, UK

451 **MRS. I.F.** **AGED 25** **HOUSEWIFE**

Mrs. I.F. complained of excessive growth of coarse hair on her face and legs in the last 6 months. She has also put on excessive weight from her usual 50.5 kg to 82 kg. In the last year she has had no menstruation.

Examination revealed a grossly obese patient. Her voice was feminine and her skin without striae. Her blood pressure read 150/90 mmHg. On examination of the genitalia an enlarged clitoris was seen. Pelvic examination was difficult in this obese patient. The ovaries were not palpable bimanually.

1. What are the possibilities in the differential diagnosis?
2. How would you carry out your investigations?
3. What further aspect of management is of importance to the patient?

F. E. H. Tan, Kuala Lumpur

Uterine problems

MRS. Q.   AGED 35   HOUSEWIFE

452

Mrs. Q. is an attractive mother of two children. Five years ago she had a Pap smear which was reported as Type 4. The cone biopsy specimen was reported as that of carcinoma of the cervix in-situ with microinvasion.

Her gynaecologist had advised total hysterectomy with bilateral salpingo-oophorectomy. She has without fail come to you for her 6-monthly Pap smear but has refused to undergo the operation as it 'threatens my femininity'.

Her husband was treated for gonococcal urethritis by your colleague last week.

1. Identify the problems presented by the patient.
2. What are the possible reasons for the patient's refusal of operation?
3. How would you manage her?
4. How would you manage her husband?

F. E. H. Tan, Kuala Lumpur

Male urethral discharge

---

453   **MR. S.M.**   **AGED 22**   **MORMON MISSIONARY**

Mr. S.M. is a clean cut, smartly dressed, very pleasant young man who comes to see you for the first time bringing a letter from the local casualty department.

He had presented there 1 week previously with a history of dysuria, frequency and urethral discharge. The doctor had diagnosed a urinary tract infection, sent off an MSU and prescribed a 5 day course of Septrin. He had also advised a check-up with you in a week's time when the MSU result would be available (it showed no abnormalities).

1. What are the likely causes of urethral discharge?
2. Was prescribing Septrin a reasonable course of action?
3. How often does social stereotyping interfere with the making of rational clinical judgements?
4. How would you proceed to manage the case?

A. J. Moulds, Basildon, UK

454   **ALLAN F.**   **AGED 26**   **LONG DISTANCE TRUCK DRIVER**

Allan returned today from a 3 week cross continental haul. He is in great distress because of a urethral discharge following intercourse with a girl he met casually in a hotel bar 3 nights ago. His wife is 6 months pregnant with her first baby and he is most anxious that she know nothing of his problem.

1. What would you advise him about telling his wife?
2. What tests would you perform?
3. What advice regarding resumption of sexual activity would you give to Allan?
4. How would you initiate treatment as he is allergic to penicillin?
5. How would you organize follow up and subsequent testing?
6. What are the dangers to the baby?

K. C. Nyman, Perth, Australia

455   **MR. C.D.**   **AGED 32**   **CAR SALESMAN**

Mr. C.D. and his wife have been your patients for 5 years. They have had marital problems over the past 2 years. You have given them counselling and it appears that the marriage situation is improving. Mr. C.D. returns from a business trip with symptoms of urethritis. A culture confirms he has gonorrhoea. He has had unprotected intercourse with his wife. He insists his wife must not find out about his infidelity.

1. How would you treat his gonorrhoea?
2. How would you investigate his wife?
3. What would you do about the marriage relationship?

E. V. Dunn, Toronto

SAMUEL N.   AGED 47   BANK MANAGER 456

Samuel N. is the manager of the local branch of a large bank. He has been married for 20 years to Dorothy aged 45 years, a housewife. They have three children aged 13, 16, and 17 years. Samuel complains of severe dysuria and urethral discharge of 2 days' duration, 4 days after a casual sexual encounter with a young secretary from another bank branch, at a weekend staff study convention. 'I do not want anyone to know, doctor', is his final remark.

1. What is your clinical management of this patient?
2. What further action would you consider?
3. Can you make any predictions as to the interpersonal family relationships which could have contributed to Samuel's one-time infidelity?
4. What is the role of the family physician in preventing venereal disease in his practice population?

M. R. Polliack, Tel-Aviv, Israel

Penile sores
---

457 **PHINEAS Z.   AGED 22   SOLDIER**

Waiting for discharge from the forces after the cessation of war in Africa, Phineas presented to the MO of a remote bush camp with a penile sore of 1 week's duration. It had failed to heal and had changed its character despite, or because of application of a salve provided by a traditional healer.

He was unable to suggest an incubation period as there were a large number of very cooperative girls near the camp. No meaningful laboratory facilities were available to the MO.

1. How might inguinal adenopathy, if present, influence your diagnosis?
2. Should sexually transmitted disease be notifiable?
3. How can we combat the problems of sexually transmitted disease?

R. T. Mossop, Harare, Zimbabwe

458 **JOE M.   AGED 23   UNEMPLOYED**

This leather-jacketted, tousle-haired, tattooed, ear-ringed male presented with a penile discharge (without dysuria), a small painless dorsal penile sore and tender groin which he informs you if you dare to touch, he couldn't help himself, he'll smash your face in!

1. What was the differential diagnosis?
2. What would be your line of questioning about his illness?
3. What line of questioning would you choose regarding contacts?
4. What clinical follow-up is now regarded as essential for gonorrhoea cases?
5. What are the treatment alternatives for acute gonorrhoea, other urethritides and lymphogranuloma venereum?

A. J. Radford, Adelaide

459 **MR. WILLIAM R.   AGED 77   RETIRED CLERK**

Mr. R. presents rather embarrassed because of a rash on his glans penis under his foreskin, which has been present for 4 days. He now has several ulcerated patches which are sore and there is some exudate coming from the ulcerated areas. Although married, Mr. R. has had no sexual contact for many years.

Examination reveals reddening of the inside of the foreskin, and a number of red papules on the glans penis, several of which have broken down into ulcers 1–2 mm in diameter. There is a small amount of exudate present under the foreskin. The ulcers are mildly tender. There is no inguinal lymphadenopathy and Mr. R. is otherwise well.

1. What are the most likely causes of this condition in this man?
2. How would you deal with this problem?
3. How could this situation be avoided in the future?
4. If the patient was twenty-seven, unmarried and sexually active, what causes would you consider and how would you manage them?

W. E. Fabb, Melbourne

Other male genital problems

---

460 **MR. T.K.** **AGED 28** **WOODWORKER**

Mr. T.K. presents with a complaint of blood in his ejaculate. He has had infrequent intercourse over the last year but has noticed blood in his seminal fluid on three occasions. A biopsy is performed by the local surgeon in this small town. This is negative. The patient's wife complains to her doctor on a separate visit of his lack of libido and of her concern about what his problem may be. Following this, the doctor notices that this man has large hands and feet. He requests pictures of the patient over the last 10 years and X-rays of his heel and his skull. A complicating factor at this point is the fact that the man is a Jehovah's Witness.

1. What is the cause of the haemospermia?
2. What is the simplest way of making a diagnosis in this case?
3. How does the fact that this man is a Jehovah's Witness complicate the case?

J. K. Shearman, Hamilton, Canada

461 **MRS. JANET K.** **AGED 24** **HOUSEWIFE**

Janet is mother of two children, a girl of 3 years and a baby boy born 10 days ago. After the birth she requested that the baby be circumcised, because her husband had been, as had all her brothers. She and her husband had spoken to doctors at the hospital, who had given the idea a cool reception and the baby was discharged uncircumcised.
She has come with a request that you do the operation?

1. Would you speak to both parents in this situation? If so, what points would you make?
2. What are the advantages and disadvantages of circumcision?
3. If you decided to circumcise the baby, discuss what you would tell the parents.
4. Discuss the doctor's role in breaking down parents' prejudices about health matters.

K. C. Nyman, Perth, Australia

CHAPTER 20

Skin Problems

This chapter begins with a series of diagnostic challenges in the form of generalized or widespread rashes, after which a number of cases of eczema are presented. An assortment of other skin conditions completes the chapter. Skin conditions are commonly seen by the family physician, who needs to be able to diagnose their nature and provide effective management, especially in chronic conditions which so often are accompanied by psychological overtones.

Generalized rashes

---

462   **GARRY J.   AGED 18 MONTHS**

It was not yet 8 a.m. and the telephone call was direct to the doctor's house. Mrs. J. sounded anxious, insisting on a home visit because 'Garry has come out in spots'. Garry, aged 18 months, is the youngest of three (Lisa, 7 years and Ian, 4 years).

When the doctor visits, he finds Garry dressed and running about; he is obviously not ill, but he has a diffuse maculopapular rash over arms and legs, and to a lesser extent over the trunk. Both cheeks show a marked confluence of the rash, giving a striking erythema on his face.

Physical examination is otherwise negative; in particular, there is no occipital lymphadenopathy, and Koplik's spots are not present.

1. What factors govern accessibility and availability of doctors to patients in general family practice?
2. What diagnostic processes are used by clinicians?
3. If the doctor diagnoses an infective disease in Garry's case, what are the implications?
4. Might the issue of notification of infectious diseases arise?

J. D. E. Knox, Dundee

463   **M.E.   AGED 8   SCHOOLBOY**

M.E. is normally healthy. Mother reports that he has had a rash since yesterday. He had been unwell for 2 days a week earlier but had been fine since then. On examination there were no general signs. There was a sparse rash on his face, head, trunk and limbs. Elements consisted of small macules, papules, and a few clear vesicles on a red base. The vesicles were 1 to 2 mm across. There were no spots in the mouth.

1. Why has this child been brought to you?
2. What are the most likely causes of this rash?
3. Your record sheet has a space for 'diagnostic plans'. What would you put in there?
4. Your record sheet has a space for 'treatment plans'. What would you put in there?
5. Your record sheet has a space for 'patient education plans'. What would you put in there?

D. Levet, Hobart

A.W.   AGED 15   FEMALE STUDENT

464

Miss W. presents because there are red spots appearing over her torso, none on face or limbs; itch a bit at night. About a week before she had noticed one large spot on her left chest.

1. What other information would you seek from any patient with a skin rash?
2. What are the commonest types of skin rashes you see now in general family practice?

W. D. Jackson, Launceston, Australia

MISS A.   AGED 16   SCHOLAR

465

Miss A. presented with a 2 week history of a circular dry scaly spot on the inside of her left thigh. She had been seen by her doctor 10 days ago and was given some cream. However, there was no improvement and the day before she had noticed the appearance of multiple dry spots of a similiar type on her body (front and back) but none on the face or extremities. She had also noticed a creamy vaginal discharge over the same period.

1. What is the most likely diagnosis?
2. What prognosis can you give the patient?
3. Is there need for notification to health authorities?

D. S. Muecke, Adelaide

MR. F.   AGED 40   TEACHER

466

Consultations with Mr. F. are usually tinged by buried resentment on his part: he is very bitter at the way his two sons have been handled by the medical profession (and the orthopaedic surgeon in particular) in efforts to deal with the talipes equino-varus from which each suffers. Chris (the older boy, now aged 15 years) is attending a 'faith healer'.

The reason for the consultation is a very acute exacerbation of widespread dermatitis: Mr. F. has large areas of moist red weeping eczema round both axillae and across his trunk.

1. Frank resentment is not a common component of doctor–patient relationships: why may it be 'buried'?
2. What is generally implied by 'fringe medicine'? What governs a family doctor's attitude to it?
3. What is eczema?
4. What treatment would help Mr. F. at this stage?

J. D. E. Knox, Dundee

Eczema

467 KAREN M.   AGED 5

Karen is brought to the doctor because she is 'scratching herself to ribbons'. Her mother says that she had a rash on her arms and legs and neck when she was a baby but this cleared up and has only recurred lately in a very aggravated form. During the interview the mother drops the hint that she has 'problems enough already' and closer questioning elicits that she and her husband have been quarrelling for the last few months over projected changes in his job and the financial implications. Karen had typical flexural eczema on her arms and legs and had indeed been scratching herself to ribbons. Questioning the child revealed that she was in a nervous weepy state and upset by her mother's ill temper.

1. What is the treatment for Karen's itch?
2. Would you expect a permanent cure?
3. Are there any associated conditions?
4. How would you use the opportunity to discuss the real problem?

R. M. Meyer, Johannesburg

468 AILEEN Z.   AGED 10   SCHOOLGIRL

Aileen Z. had an inflammatory disorder of her skin starting, her mother states, in infancy. She is sensitive to milk and at times develops bronchospasm and hay fever. The skin is slightly oedematous with areas of crusting, hyperplasia and keratosis mainly distributed on the flexural areas of the limbs. The condition relapses frequently when eating certain foods and on exposure to central heating in her school.

1. What is the diagnosis?
2. What is the treatment of this disease?
3. What is the management of this disease?

B. M. Fehler, Johannesburg

469 MR. P.B.   AGED 24   PUBLIC SERVANT

Mr. P.B., unmarried, has a life-long history of atopy: asthma, eczema, hay fever from early childhood. At the age of 10 he was desensitized against grass and house dust and subsequently there was a diminution in the frequency of asthma, with none for the past 4 years. The eczema flared 18 months ago and has become chronic. There are no social or family problems, no recent hay fever and no contact with obvious allergens.

On examination he has generalized eczema, worse on exposed areas, that is, face and hands. This responds to treatment with local steroid ointments and nocturnal sedation but as soon as these are ceased it returns. His IgE is greater than 1000 units per ml and RAST testing showed moderate to marked sensitivity to grasses, weeds, house dust and cat epithelia. This test showed no sensitivity to common food allergens.

1. How would you manage this man?
2. Why has his eczema returned?
3. Should he be desensitized again despite lack of respiratory symptoms?

P. F. Gill, Hobart

MR. C.A.   AGED 34   LABOURER   470

This 34-year-old labourer appeared in the office with a rash in both groins that had begun a month previously during warm summer weather. Extra bathing with the use of talcum powder had not helped. Past history revealed that his wife has had some vaginal discharge and perineal itching. The review of systems was negative except for some fatigue, possibly related to excessive weight gain over the past year, and more marked post-prandial.

Physical examination revealed mild to moderate obesity in addition to a symmetrical, semi-moist, slightly scaly, dull-red skin eruption in both groin areas, including the lateral scrotal skin.

1. What are the essential problems in development of a problem list?
2. What differential diagnostic possibilities exist in the male in the development of a groin rash?
3. What factors in patient education would be important in this case?

L. H. Amundson, Sioux Falls, SD, USA

MR. J.B.   AGED 23   INFANT SCHOOL TEACHER   471

Mr. J.B. has complained of an itchy rash on hands, forearms, groin and lower legs for approximately 6 weeks. There is quite intense itching which is often worse at night and not relieved by calamine lotion. He is not aware of any allergies. He admits to a lot of tension at work and doesn't get on with his senior. He is aware that some children have had a similar rash.

1. Where would you look to ensure the proper diagnosis?
2. What would make you think it was not psychological?

   3.   What investigations are necessary to prove the diagnosis?
   4.   What is the appropriate treatment?

D. S. Muecke, Adelaide

472   BRETT A.   AGED 13   SCHOOLBOY

Brett is brought in by his mother writhing in pain, crying, restless and
distressed. He is wearing a muddied track suit. After playing football at
school he became aware of smarting on his arms, thighs and around his
waist. He had a shower and the smarting turned to acute burning pain.
   The only striking physical finding is a patchy erythema of both arms
from shoulder to wrist, the middle and lower third of thighs and knees.
There are scattered vesicles and the general appearance is of a recent
burn.

   1.   What is your immediate management?
   2.   What is your working diagnosis?
   3.   What further steps would you take to establish the cause and plan
        further treatment?

J. A. Stevens, Ulverstone, Australia

473   RITA W.   AGED 47   FARMER'S WIFE

Rita is a farmer's wife, large, placid but energetic. Even as she sits in the
waiting room she is busily knitting.
   She has recently developed an itchy, scaling, eczematous patch,
roughly oval, around the dorsal surface of the right first metacarpophalangeal joint and a similar smaller area on the ulnar border of the left
wrist. Both are quite sharply defined and are almost certainly patches of
contact dermatitis.

   1.   To what is she allergic?
   2.   How would you confirm the diagnosis?
   3.   What is the management?

J. A. Stevens, Ulverstone, Australia

Other skin problems

JACOB H.   AGED 29   ACCOUNTANT

474

J.H., unmarried, has recently moved to the area and is attending for the first time.

He complains of sore red patches on both ankles, occasional back stiffness and also feels that he is slightly more breathless than usual after playing squash or running.

On each ankle there is a raised erythematous area about 4 cm diameter. Otherwise there are no abnormal physical findings.

1. What is your provisional diagnosis?
2. What are the possible causes of this condition?
3. What would be your management?

J. A. Stevens, Ulverstone, Australia

MRS. BARBARA F.   AGED 60   HOUSEWIFE

475

Mrs. F. presented 5 months previously with a 1 cm diameter ulcer on the lower ⅓ of her right shin. She had had it for the previous 6 months and although not painful, it would not heal and gave the suspicion of being a basal cell carcinoma. She was referred to a plastic surgeon for excision biopsy which he declined to do because of the patient's poor general health and poor peripheral circulation. He in turn referred her for X-ray therapy to the lesion after a conventional biopsy had confirmed Bowen's tumour. She next required medical attention from her general practitioner when he was called in an emergency one night for a haemorrhage from the wound. On examination he was horrified to see a 5 cm diameter ulcer on the skin approximately ½ cm deep with a floor of sloughing tissue from which there was a steady venous ooze. The haemorrhage was controlled by pressure and limb elevation and treatment of the ulcer was undertaken.

1. What treatment would be suitable for such an ulcer?
2. The patient is thinking of litigation – what would your attitude be?

R. M. Meyer, Johannesburg

MRS. B.Z.   AGED 52   HOUSEWIFE

476

A 52-year-old housewife came into the office with a 6 month history of blue discoloration of the heels and several toes of both feet. She suffered no coldness, pain, or numbness. The blue discoloration was not affected by exposure to cold and was fairly constant except for its disappearance with pressure. She denied pain in the calves on walking, or symptoms in the fingers or arms.

After an injury 4 months previously, an ulcer developed over the right lateral ankle which is not yet fully healed.

Review of systems was negative except for a history of moderate cigarette smoking.

Physical examination revealed that the right first and third toes and the left first and fourth toes were cyanotic. Irregular areas of cyanosis also appeared on the medial side of the left foot, with another on the left lateral heel. These areas blanched with pressure or with elevation. Blanching time was normal and venous filling times were prompt. A dry, crusted tender ulcer was present over the right lateral malleolus. Hair growth was present on the toes. Pulses in the legs revealed 2 + pulses in both femoral and popliteal arteries, a 1 + in the right dorsalis pedis, and 0 in the posterior tibial. On the left the dorsalis pedis pulse was missing with a 1 + pulse in the posterior tibial.

1. What are the possible aetiological factors in this lady's presenting complaint of blue toes?
2. What intrinsic problems might have an aetiological bearing, or serve as aggravating factors, in this lady's medical problem?
3. What therapeutic measures constitute good foot care irrespective of the diagnosis?

L. H. Amundson, Sioux Falls, SD, USA

CHAPTER 21

Lumps

This short chapter is a companion to the previous one. It presents lumps in the breast, neck and axilla. Breast lumps are amongst the most feared complaints presented by women and need careful and sympathetic handling by the family physician.

Breast lumps
---

477   **MRS. MARILYN B.**   **AGED 33**   **SINGLE PARENT**

This single parent, deserted by her husband, is upset after finding a lump in her breast 3 days ago. Her mother died of cancer of the breast. She is an hourly employee in a new job and has no relatives able to look after her three small children.

    1.   How would you manage the physical aspects of this problem?
    2.   How would you manage the social aspects?
    3.   What emotional supports can you offer this patient?

D. H. Johnson, Toronto

478   **MRS. J.D.**   **AGED 35**   **HOUSEWIFE**

Mrs. J.D. presented with her husband, a bank manager, because of her continued concern about her 'lumpy breasts'. She had very large 'fibrous' breasts and had regular breast examinations over the past 10 years. Her doctor examined her 3 months ago and said that the lumps (and one in particular) were no cause for concern. At this presentation there was skin tethering adjacent to a hard mass in the left breast.

    1.   What is the likely diagnosis?
    2.   How could you prevent this situation?
    3.   How would you manage this problem?
    4.   How would you conduct a management interview?

J. E. Murtagh, Melbourne

479   **MRS. LINDA A.**   **AGED 39**   **SALESLADY**

Mrs. Linda A. is the mother of two daughters aged 12 and 16 years. She works as a saleslady to supplement her husband's income. 'I first noticed this lump in my breast 4 months ago, doctor', she says. Examination reveals a mass, the size of a cherry, firm and immobile, with ill-defined edges, in the lower outer quadrant of her left breast. There are no palpable axillary glands. 'Is it serious', she asks.

    1.   What is your presumptive diagnosis?
    2.   How would you answer Linda's question?

3. Discuss your management of Linda after the performance of radical mastectomy.
4. Could the diagnosis have been established earlier?

Z. Cramer, Tel-Aviv, Israel

RACHEL S.   AGED 57

480

Rachel S. had had a mastectomy 18 months before, for a carcinoma of the left breast. She presented with what appeared to be skin secondaries around the operation scar. The doctor could find no other signs of the disease having spread and she felt extremely well.

He referred her back to the local hospital where the radiotherapy specialist suggested radiotherapy and chemotherapy. The patient, not keen to have treatment which would make her feel ill, returned to consult her own doctor.

1. How serious a problem is carcinoma of the breast?
2. What treatment is available for carcinoma of the breast?
3. How might the doctor react to Rachel's reluctance to undergo treatment?

J. C. Hasler, Oxford

Lymphadenopathy

---

481 | **MISS G.Y.** **AGED 22** **UNIVERSITY STUDENT**

Miss G.Y., a young single woman attending university, presented with a lump in the left side of her neck that had been present for 2 months. She felt generally well, had not experienced weight loss or other constitutional symptoms and specifically had not had night sweats.

On examination she had multiple, firm, rubbery, nodes, 1–2 cm in diameter in both supraclavicular regions of her neck, more prominent on the left side. The nodes were discreet, matted together, and non-tender. There were no nodes elsewhere and no hepatosplenomegaly. ENT examination including the thyroid gland was normal. General physical examination was also normal. Chest X-ray showed slight widening of the superior mediastinum. A full investigation was otherwise negative.

Following a cervical node biopsy, the patient was given a course of radiation therapy. Two years later she is clinically well without any recurrent disease.

1. How do you decide if a neck lump is significant?
2. How would you proceed to investigate this patient?
3. What determines the prognosis in a patient with lymphoma?

R. L. Perkin, Toronto

482 | **MR. J.B.W.** **AGED 84** **RETIRED SAILOR**

An old navy man, fair skinned, rugged and tattooed, comes for his usual check-up, with a warm smile and handshake. He has a past history of cardiac failure following atrial fibrillation 4 years previously, now well controlled.

He lives on his own since the death of his second wife. He is a little forgetful. Today he has a non-tender, hard, irregularly shaped lump in the right side of his neck behind the angle of his jaw. 'It's nothing to worry about, is it, Doc?'

1. How serious is this problem?
2. What treatment do you recommend?

G. M. Dick, Hobart

MR. B.P.   AGED 49   UPHOLSTERER

483

Mr. B.P. presents with a lump in his left axilla which is painful. He gives a history of mild diabetes and of several operations on his neck for nerve pressure. One of these operations resulted in osteomyelitis of the cervical spine. He is suspicious of physicians because they once tried to amputate his leg during the Korean War. He refused and his leg is now fine. The lump in his axilla has been expanding over the last several weeks. A biopsy of the node is performed.

1. What do you think is the nature of the lesion in this man's axilla?
2. How do you think this man's past contact with the medical profession might affect his attitude to his present illness?
3. How would you treat the pain this man is suffering from?

J. K. Shearman, Hamilton, Canada

CHAPTER 22

Musculoskeletal Problems

This chapter begins with spinal problems in the neck and the lumbar region. The ubiquitous low back pain is illustrated by a number of cases which demonstrate that there are traps for the unwary in diagnosing the cause. Then follow problems affecting the hip, thigh, knee, leg and ankle, after which problems affecting the shoulder, arm, elbow and hands are presented. The chapter concludes with several cases of rheumatoid arthritis.

Musculoskeletal problems are commonly presented to the family physician. The diagnosis can sometimes be most difficult and the management, particularly in the case of low back pain and rheumatoid arthritis, can test the skills of the doctor to the utmost.

Neck pain

484 **MISS SHEILA B.   AGED 23   TYPIST**

Sheila B. has long blonde hair. As she was washing it this morning, she jerked her head back to flick her hair, which was hanging over her face, over the top of her head. As she did so, she felt acute pain in her neck and has been unable to move it much since because of the pain.

She holds her neck stiffly, with her head bent to the right and her jaw slightly rotated to the left. She looks to be in considerable pain.

1. What is the nature of her condition?
2. What would you do about it?

W. E. Fabb, Melbourne

485 **MS. H.Z.   AGED 35   AIRLINE HOSTESS**

This patient complained of having a cold with a dry cough over the last 4 to 5 days together with pain and discomfort in the region of the left ear for 24 hours. She localizes the area of discomfort to just below the left mastoid. On examination hearing appears normal, temperature normal, there is a mild rhinitis, throat normal, ears – both drums appear normal and move with Valsalva's manoeuvre. Rinne and Weber tests normal. There is some tenderness over the upper sternomastoid muscle and pain which is aggravated on turning the head to the left and flexing the head to the left.

1. Is this likely to be a pathological or functional problem?
2. What is the natural history of this condition?
3. What advice would you give the patient?

T. D. Manthorpe, Port Lincoln, Australia

486 **MRS. E.C.   AGED 59   HOUSEWIFE**

Mrs. E.C. has been complaining of neck pain for over a year since a motor vehicle accident. Her lawyer has not settled the case because the doctor has not been definite about the prognosis. There are no neurological or radiological findings. An orthopaedic consultation was not helpful. There was minimal response to medications and physiotherapy.

1. To what extent can legal proceedings complicate the management of an accident-related medical problem?
2. How does a prolonged disability affect the patient's self-image, relationships with family and friends, and finances?

E. Domovitch, Toronto

Low back pain

---

487   **MR. B.B.   AGED 23   STOREMAN**

Mr. B.B. is brought to your office in pain. He slipped at work when moving a crate, and has had severe lower back pain since. He is normally fit and well, and consulted you for the 'flu' 3 years ago.

1.   What is the most likely diagnosis here?
2.   What would you expect to find on examination?
3.   What immediate investigations could you arrange?
4.   What is the immediate management?
5.   After the immediate episode, what then?

D. U. Shepherd, Melbourne

488   **MR. NATHAN S.   AGED 42   BUTCHER**

'My back's bad again doctor, I'd like a week off work please.'
'What started it this time Nathan, lifting carcasses again?'
'No, nothing, just leaning over the counter and bang it went on me.'
'Well you had better let me examine your back again; lie down.'
'Last time it was sore you said you couldn't find anything wrong.'

Last time I gave Mr. S. a week off he was seen at the races and there is a race meeting this week. He had an initial severe strain 10 years ago lifting a heavy carcass and had marked muscle spasm when seen then; 2 years later another lifting strain with classical neurological signs of sciatica. He's had at least one attack of low back pain a year since, occasionally with sciatica. X-rays of the spine last year reported slight narrowing of the fourth lumbar intervertebral disc space.

1.   Where are the possible sites of Mr. S.'s back pathology?
2.   What investigations are appropriate in chronic lumbar backache?
3.   How can recurrent backache and sciatica be treated?
4.   When is functional overlay or malingering diagnosed?

D. G. Chambers, Clare, Australia

489   **MR. J.D.   AGED 48**

The visit is to see Mr. J.D. at home. The last two entries in his notes read: *Four weeks previously* – 'Smelling strongly of cigarette smoke and alcohol. Minor backache. Nil O.E. ?What's going on here. ℞ Paracetamol. See 2 weeks.' *Two weeks previously* – 'Did not attend'.

Mr. D. has developed severe pain in the left lumbo-sacral region, while moving a washing machine 24 hours ago. He gives an impression of making the most of his symptoms, with hyper-reactive tenderness and somewhat inconsistent restriction in back movements.

After treatment has been prescribed, the doctor has a word with Mrs. D. downstairs, saying that Mr. D. appears to have 'lumbago'. 'Thank you, doctor,' says Mrs. D. 'To let you understand, we are separated – he doesn't live here now, but he turned up with this back trouble.'

1. What is the nature and pathogenesis of the relatively common 'lumbago' seen in general practice?
2. In Mr. D.'s case psychological and social elements are intertwined with the 'medical' condition. List as many (stated and implied) as you can.

J. D. E. Knox, Dundee

MRS. V.S.   AGED 48   HOUSEWIFE   490

Mrs. V.S. had symptoms of low back pain intermittently for many years. She reached into the trunk of her car to lift out some groceries when she suddenly experienced midline low back pain and had difficulty straightening up. Over the next few hours the pain became more intense with radiation to both buttocks but not down the leg. She had no sensory or motor symptoms in her legs or feet.

On examination her lumbar spine was flattened and she moved with difficulty. There was midline tenderness at L5–S1 with bilateral muscle spasm. Flexion of her back was not limited or painful, but hyperextension caused acute pain and was limited to 25% of normal. Straight leg raising was restricted to 60° bilaterally due to spasm in her back. There were no neurological changes.

The patient was treated with bed rest and analgesics and was better in 1 week.

1. What is the mechanism of this type of low back pain?
2. What is the natural history of such an episode of low back pain?
3. How would you treat the patient?

R. L. Perkin, Toronto

MR. R.   AGED 40   TRADESMAN   491

Mr. R., a Mediterranean by birth, is a company employed tradesman with a good work record. He presents initially with lumbosacral pain which developed after lifting a small box. He was seen by a doctor who had considerable experience assessing back injuries occurring at work. This examination revealed nothing more than minor muscle tenderness in the region of the 3rd and 4th lumbar vertebrae. Despite the patient's protests he was not X-rayed but was sent home to rest for 2 days and offered analgesics.

To the doctor's surprise he returned 2 days later complaining that his back was no better. Examination yet again revealed nothing of significance. He was reassured that he would certainly be fit for work after the coming weekend's rest but returned again on the Monday morning complaining once again of pain in his back and inability to work because of it.

1. Does 'Mediterranean back' exist?
2. Should the doctor have departed from his usual practice of treating back injuries with rest and analgesics and immediately embarked on a course of injections and manipulation which would appear to be closer to the treatment regime offered in the country of origin of this workman?
3. How would you treat the injury?

P. F. Gill, Hobart

492   MR. P.M.   AGED 38   SHIP'S CAPTAIN

Mr. M. was an energetic ship's captain and single-handed sailor, well-known to his doctor. He presented with back pain radiating down the right leg following lifting a moderately heavy box at work. X-rays were normal apart from a defective pars interarticularis on the left side of L5.

His simple sciatica did not respond to bed rest. Traction in hospital produced severe generalized back and neck pain, loss of sensation in his right foot and intractable headache.

A poor-quality myelogram showed some disc protrusion at the L4–5 level. Laminectomy was performed and the mildly damaged disc removed. Pain continued mainly in the left leg, with severe headache.

After a CT scan, further surgery on the 4th and 5th discs and fusion was carried out. Post-operative progress was satisfactory and the headache disappeared.

1. Is it possible to pick which cases of backache will do well?
2. How much does one's knowledge of the patient's personality influence management?
3. Do unusual pain features rule out organic disease?

A. L. A. Reid, Newcastle, Australia

493   MR. A.B.   AGED 38   LABOURER

Mr. A.B. has been unemployed for 2 years following an accident at work. He is receiving insurance benefits. He complains of lower back pain which is aggravated by bending and lifting. He has no radiological or neurological signs. He is not improved despite anti-inflammatory medication, physiotherapy and weight loss. An orthopaedic consultation agreed with the diagnosis of mechanical back pain with psychogenic overlay and agreed with the management. Most recently he has been to see a chiropractor at the suggestion of his friend. He was told his X-ray revealed subluxations and a curvature. After 2 weeks of vitamin and mineral therapy in addition to daily manipulations, he estimates he has improved 70%.

1. Why has this patient returned to the physician?
2. How can motivation be accurately assessed in problems with compensation, insurance and medicolegal complications?

E. Domovitch, Toronto

MR. D.F.   AGED 65   SEMI-RETIRED   494

The chief complaint is low back pain for 3 months. The patient states that the pain began as a 'sore back' but gradually over a 3 month period has worsened to the point where he refused to get out of bed. Coughing, straining at stool, and any motion of his back increased the pain. Two soft masses appeared on the scalp during the weeks before hospitalization, and he had lost 15 pounds since the onset of his illness.

Past medical history and review of systems were negative. He denied having any joint pain of any kind until the present illness.

Physical examination revealed that the patient appeared to have lost weight and looked ill. He would not move about in bed or attempt to get up because of back pain associated with motion of the spine. Examination of the skin revealed two subcutaneous nodules on the scalp. One nodule on the crown of the head measured 3 cm in diameter, and the other one, on the occiput, was 2.5 cm in diameter. Both were soft, nontender, and seemed slightly moveable. The liver, spleen, and kidneys were not palpable. The stool was negative for blood. Examination of the extremities revealed back pain on attempted straight leg raising. There was no oedema of the extremities. A blood count revealed a haemoglobin of 10.3 g, the indices showing a normochromic, normocytic anaemia, and white cells and differential within normal limits. The sedimentation rate was 48 mm in 1 hour. Urine revealed 2+ protein.

1. What are the essential problems in his problem list?
2. If in the clinical management of this patient, an intravenous pyelogram is considered, what factors should be kept in mind?
3. What are the main diseases to be considered in the differential diagnosis in a patient with this degree of back pain?

L. H. Amundson, Sioux Falls, SD, USA

95   MR. J.T.   AGED 50

Mr. J.T. has been coming to the doctor monthly for blood pressure checks since the diagnosis of essential hypertension was made 1½ years ago. Although it was initially controlled with a diuretic, his blood pressure remains at 160/110 despite treatment with increasing doses of diuretics, beta-blockers and hydralazine. He has not worked because of back pain for several months. The cause of his back pain is uncertain. A diagnosis of musculoskeletal lumbo-sacral back pain without neurological signs was made after examination and further tests by an orthopaedic consultant. He has not responded to medication and physiotherapy. He lives alone and has no family. He denies depression and has no somatic manifestations thereof. His financial situation has deteriorated but is not desperate. He develops a coin lesion on his chest X-ray.

1. Why might the BP have become difficult to control?
2. How can a doctor establish whether or not the patient is compliant?
3. Are there any underlying emotional factors?
4. What should be done about the coin lesion?

E. Domovitch, Toronto

496   MR. M.S.   AGED 68   RETIRED STEELWORKER

A 68 year old retired steelworker, an avid gardener, visited his family physician, having just returned from a winter spent with his wife in the warm climate of Florida. While in Florida, he had been having severe backache and in spite of several visits to a physician there, during which he had X-rays of his spine and several blood tests done, no diagnosis had been made. He reported that his pain was located in the mid-thoracic region and was worsened by either lifting or straining, and that little relief was obtained from analgesics.

His family physician performed a rectal examination as part of his attempt to determine the cause of the pain. He ordered an X-ray of the thoracic region and a bone scan and additional blood tests, because of the findings of his rectal examination.

1. What disease do you think the family physician is looking for?
2. If the diagnosis is made, is there any treatment?
3. What discussions might take place between the physician and the patient and his wife?

C. A. Moore, Hamilton, Canada

97   MRS. R.S.   AGED 24   HOUSEWIFE

Mrs. R.S. wanted a referral to a physiotherapist for her backache. She had attended a VD clinic because of concern with a vaginal discharge and irritation. She had not had intercourse for 4 weeks. Clinical examination disclosed no infection. She had a 4½ month child, her first, and her husband was an unemployed gambler 10 years older who had been divorced after his first wife left him.

The patient had not had any trouble with backache during her pregnancy or in labour. The husband often absented himself for a night or two at a time.

1. What are the possible causes of backache?
2. How could you diagnose this case?
3. How would a VD clinic manage this case?
4. What would be your management approach?

E. J. H. North, Melbourne

Lower limb problems

498 **MR. S.P.Y.   AGED 24**

Mr. S.P.Y. is single and a new patient. He complains of pain radiating down the back of the right leg from buttock to ankle of gradual onset 4 weeks ago. It is very bad on getting out of bed in the morning until he limbers up, but it aches at work. He has recently undergone special training to work on a saw bench at which he sits in a special swivel chair. There are no gross signs on physical examination. His physique is good. Straight leg raising is possible to 90° on both sides (but causing pain on the right). X-ray of the lumbosacral spine shows 'minor changes of old Scheuermann's disease with some Schmorl's nodes'.

1. What is your assessment of this situation?
2. What are your treatment plans for this man?
3. What additional patient education plans are indicated at this stage?

D. Levet, Hobart

499 **MR. A.S.   AGED 18   LABOURER**

Mr. A.S. presented with pain in the left thigh, aggravated by standing and walking. Examination revealed limited spinal flexion at the lumbar level and limited straight leg raising, more marked on the left.

After a period of bed rest the pain settled and he was able to resume work. However, 4 weeks later he presented again, this time with swelling of the ankles and lower legs and, on examination, was found to have distended veins over the abdomen.

1. What were the likely diagnoses at the initial presentation?
2. How do you cope with a situation in which you or one of your colleagues may have missed an important diagnosis?
3. What pathological process might account for the findings at the later consultation?

E. C. Gambrill, Crawley, UK

500 **ROBERT P.   AGED 4**

Robert's mother said he had been limping for 3 or 4 days. At first he had been reluctant to put his right foot to the ground at all. Now he could walk, but with obvious discomfort. He did not admit to pain anywhere.

On examination he was a healthy child with a limp but no generalized illness, fever or malaise. There was no weakness or wasting of the limbs. Movement of the right hip joint was restricted in all directions.

The doctor made a provisional diagnosis of 'irritable hip'. He advised the mother that the child should rest and not bear weight and arranged to see him again in 4 days time.

Four days later the child was symptom-free and walked without a limp.

1. What is 'irritable hip'?
2. Why did Robert limp?
3. Is rest an important part of the treatment?
4. What are the dangers of making a diagnosis of irritable hip?
5. What would you have done about Robert?

G. Strube, Crawley, UK

MR. FRANCIS M.   AGED 50   INVALID PENSIONER   501

Mr. M. is an invalid pensioner with cerebral palsy due to Rh incompatability. He lives with his wife, also afflicted with cerebral palsy; formerly a school teacher despite her handicap, now retired and an invalid pensioner like her husband.

Three months ago Mr. M. fell and fractured his left hip. A pin and plate were inserted and he made an excellent recovery. But 1 month after discharge from hospital he became ill with severe malaise, fevers and rigors and pain in and about the left hip.

1. Both general practitioner and orthopaedic surgeon suspected osteomyelitis. What steps were taken as a result of this provisional diagnosis?
2. After exhaustive tests the orthopaedic surgeon is unable to explain Mr. M.'s symptoms and signs and has referred him back to his GP. Meanwhile Mr. M. has lost 26 lb in weight, his pains continue in his left leg and his fever and sweats persist. What possibilities must the GP now consider?
3. In view of the fact that Mr. and Mrs. M. are very dependent upon each other and that she is confined to a wheel chair, what special considerations should govern the GP's management of the situation?

W. L. Ogborne, Sydney

JOHN Q.   AGED 15   SCHOOLBOY   502

John Q.'s father is a bricklayer. John has a mediocre academic record but is a fine athlete. His father brings John to the doctor complaining of pain in his left knee for a few weeks. His left tibial tuberosity seems swollen and is tender.

1. What is the likely diagnosis and what diagnoses must be excluded?
2. What are likely to be John's major worries when he presents?
3. Do you have any views concerning teenagers who are brought to you for treatment?

P. Freeling, London

503 MR. W.K. AGED 82 RETIRED SCHOOLMASTER

Mr. W.K.'s medical record is very scanty, as he seldom attends doctors. The last entry was nearly 30 years before. He comes now complaining of pain in his left knee and walks with a limp, though not using a stick. Movements of his hip are limited and rather painful; the knee is slightly swollen and crepitus is present but it is not severely affected.

His general health is satisfactory; he is not obese, does not smoke, and takes no medication. His main concern is that he cannot participate in his game of bowls. He asks for some pills to put him right.

1. What common joint diseases are likely to be causes of his symptoms?
2. Is a surgical opinion required now?

J. Grabinar, Bromley, UK

504 MRS. E.B. AGED 71

This elderly lady came to stay with her daughter but forgot to bring her pills for arthritis with her. Her daughter came to the office for a prescription for her mother and showed the doctor the name 'Butazolidin' written on a scrap of paper. The doctor was reluctant to prescribe a powerful and potentially dangerous drug for a patient he had never seen and asked if she was well enough to come to the office. The next day she came, walking with great difficulty, supported by her daughter. She told the doctor about the pains in her legs which were continuous even at rest. She indicated her thighs and shin bones. There was no swelling of the knee or ankle joints, or any restriction of movement. However, the tibiae were both tender on pressure. She was generally wasted and frail. On further enquiry it appeared that she had had a perforated stomach ulcer when she was younger and an operation had been necessary. She knew no further details.

1. What was the diagnosis given by her own doctor?
2. What is the true diagnosis?
3. How could this condition have been prevented?

A. G. Strube, Crawley, UK

MR. DONALD V.   AGED 48

505

Mr. Donald V., always previously healthy, worked as a farmer and part-time bartender, and lived with his wife in a rural area. All of his three daughters were married but living within a 60 mile radius of his home. He described his family as warm and close. He consulted his physician with complaints of skin rash, aching in his chest, and joint swelling and stiffness in the left knee. His appetite was poor and fever was present at 39.5 °C. Mr. Donald V. was convinced that some serious illness was occurring. He had never previously been hospitalized.

Physical examination revealed a new heart murmur never heard before and suggestive of endocarditis. Also present were a left knee joint effusion and a violet-coloured skin rash over the back and on the flexor surfaces of the wrist. The knee effusion was tapped and found to be sterile with only polynuclear cells present. Other laboratory analysis revealed a sedimentation rate of 45 mm in one hour, a complete blood count which was normal except for a white count of 11,500, and the anti-nuclear antibody test was negative. Cardiac echo revealed a mild peri-cardial effusion. Nine blood cultures were performed and found to be negative. Work up was otherwise unremarkable for positive findings.

After 19 days in a hospital located 35 miles from his home, and following a ten day course of IV antibiotic therapy for presumptive bacterial endocarditis, the true diagnosis was finally uncovered. A skin biopsy on the violet skin rash done to rule out systemic lupus erythematosus was reported to be positive for SLE. There had been no improvement with the antibiotic therapy, but after the diagnosis was made oral steroid therapy was instituted and Mr. Donald V.'s health began to improve.

1. What problems for Mr. Donald V., apart from the obvious medical illness, should have been considered by his physicians during his hospital care?
2. What are the unusual features of this illness?
3. Considering Mr. Donald V.'s inexperience with serious illness or hospitals, what further questions, apart from a medical history, should have been asked by his physicians?
4. What effects could the illness have had on Mr. D.V.'s psychological coping skills?

C. Driscoll, Iowa City

MRS. B.   AGED 75   WIDOW

506

Mrs. B., a 75 year old, very vigorous widow was pressured by her family to come to the doctor for a check-up. She had not seen a doctor for approximately 10 years. She was extremely active, working 5 or 6 days weekly assisting her sister in running a clothing business and had outside interests in various church and charitable organizations. Careful questioning revealed no physical complaints other than some occasional leg cramps at night. The cramps had increased in frequency in the previous few months so that virtually every night she was awakened by cramps. The pain was usually relieved by either rubbing her legs or using stretching exercises. There were no other significant complaints in the past or family history, or on functional enquiry.

A complete physical examination was normal. Her blood pressure was noted on two occasions to be 140/80. Investigations carried out included a full blood examination and urinalysis which were normal. Serum potassium, calcium and phosphorus were obtained to investigate the leg cramps. The calcium and phosphorus were normal but the potassium was 6.2 mmol/l on the first reading and on a repeat test it was 6.4 mmol/l. Further investigations, including serum creatinine and the blood glucose, were normal.

1. What are the most common causes of nocturnal leg cramps in a 75 year old lady?
2. What are the most common causes of an elevated serum potassium in an otherwise physically and biochemically healthy individual?
3. If the elevated serum potassium was persistent, what steps could be taken to prevent potentially serious consequences.

W. W. Rosser, Ottawa

507   MR. BRUNO G.   AGED 54   SHOP ASSISTANT

Mr. G. complains of shooting pains around the ankles for 3 weeks and pins and needles in the toes and fingers. His records showed coronary thrombosis 4 years ago; intermittent claudication in the calves diagnosed at last visit – advised to give up his heavy cigarette smoking. Reported still smoking – had unsuccessfully tried to stop many times.

Examination – clubbed fingers; very weak peripheral pulses in the legs; slight non-pitting oedema in both feet; hilar rales in both lungs.

1. What organs can be damaged by cigarette smoking?
2. What is the significance of Mr. G.'s symptoms and signs?
3. How can the morbidity from cigarette smoking be reduced?

D. G. Chambers, Clare, Australia

Upper limb problems

MRS. A.J. AGED 43 HOUSEWIFE   **508**

Mrs. A.J. presented with a 6 week history of pain in the right shoulder. Initially this caused trouble only when hanging washing on the line and on lifting weights. Gradually the pain became more persistent and she had pain on opening a jar top and turning off a tap. Subsequently the pain kept her awake at night and had also transferred along the outside of the upper arm to the elbow. There was no history of direct trauma.

She had not previously had this trouble. There is no significant past or family history of rheumatism or arthritis.

1. What is the most likely diagnosis?
2. Would any investigations help you?
3. How would you manage this problem?

D. S. Muecke, Adelaide

SYLVIA BLACK AGED 26 APPLE PACKER   **509**

Sylvia presents to you for the first time complaining of severe pain in her right forearm which has become worse gradually over the last 3 days. Any twisting or grasping movement with the right hand triggers the pain which causes her to drop whatever she is holding. The pain is stopping her from doing her job. She says it took her 3 months to find this job which she started 4 days ago. If she can't use her hand, she loses the job.

On further questioning you discover that Sylvia was married 5 years ago, has two children and has been separated from her husband for 6 months. She has moved in with her parents who are being 'very good' but she desperately wants to earn some money so she can look after herself and her children.

Examination findings confirm your suspicions from the history.

1. What is the diagnosis?
2. How would you treat her forearm?
3. What are the other aspects of managing this patient?

R. P. Strasser, Melbourne

MRS. P.R. AGED 51 HOUSEWIFE   **510**

Mrs. P.R. presented with a painful right arm that worried her from the shoulder to the hand for the past 7 months. She also had some pain in her back and left ankle. Her mother had rheumatism.

It hurt her to move her arm and when she lay on it. Washing and writing were becoming very difficult.

Examination disclosed localized tenderness in an area adjacent to the lateral epicondyle. Pronation and supination of the forearm produced discomfort. Movements of the shoulder and wrist revealed a full range of movement.

1. What process is at work?
2. How can it be treated?
3. What is the prognosis?

E. J. H. North, Melbourne

511   MOLLY A.   AGED 63

Molly A. has developed occasional lumbar pain and stiffness over the past 18 months. X-ray, blood count, RA latex screening, antinuclear factor and serum for LE cells are all normal and periodic courses of paracetamol and Naprosyn (naproxen) are rapidly effective.

She now complains of aching, weakness and stiffness in both arms, of her heart thumping particularly in bed, and of fitful and restless sleep. She thinks too that she has lost a little weight.

Examination shows general tenderness in the deltoids, some weakness in all arm movements but no objective neurological deficit. BP is 160/110, urine normal, chest X-ray normal. Full blood examination is normal but the ESR is 72 mm in one hour.

1. What is your provisional diagnosis?
2. What treatment would you prescribe?
3. How would you monitor the course of the disease?

J. A. Stevens, Ulverstone, Australia

512   MR. B.Z.   AGED 26   DENTIST

Mr. B.Z. complains of pain, stiffness, and swelling of the small joints of his right hand present for 1 week. On further questioning he gives a history of dysentery after returning from a holiday abroad 6 weeks previously. He is a known psoriatic with only minimal lesions on the elbows easily controlled with topical medication.

1. What is the differential diagnosis?
2. What further aspects of his history might be important?
3. What investigations would help in making your diagnosis?
4. What particular problems will be posed for this patient?

T. A. I. Bouchier Hayes, Camberley, UK

JULIE FREDRICKSON   AGED 28   TYPIST

513

Over the last 12 months, Julie has had intermittent episodes of soreness and stiffness in her right index finger and thumb and her left middle finger. With the cold weather of this last week, she had found all her fingers stiff and sore in the morning and that it takes ½ hour to 'work her fingers in' at the typewriter. She has been otherwise well in herself. Physical examination is unremarkable.

Julie says her mother and older sister have rheumatism and that her mother's hands are now badly deformed. She asks you if this will happen to her and whether she could do something to stop it happening.

1. What are the possible diagnoses?
2. What investigations are indicated?
3. How would you manage this problem?

R. P. Strasser, Melbourne

MR. G.C.   AGED 49   MANUFACTURER

514

This patient had started his own manufacturing company which at first was very successful and it had enlarged rapidly. Recently however, the recession had affected him badly as the market for his products diminished and he was forced to lay off workers, many of whom had become personal friends.

He developed pain in his hands which became increasingly severe. He was forced to seek medical advice when they became so stiff and weak in the mornings that he could hardly shave. The doctor noticed a puffiness surrounding the 2nd and 3rd metacarpophalangeal joints in both hands. His grip was weak and there was pain on gently squeezing the hands. The epitrochlear lymph node on the right was enlarged and tender. No other joints were involved. In spite of his easy manner, the doctor thought Mr. C. looked tired and drawn. He made a diagnosis of rheumatoid arthritis and this was confirmed by a positive test for rheumatoid factor with an ESR of 68 mm in the first hour, and a haemoglobin of 10.7 g with normochromic indices. The antinuclear factor test was negative.

In view of the evidence of activity, the doctor advised the patient to rest at home for at least 2 weeks, spending most of the time in bed. He also persuaded the patient to delegate more work to other members of his staff so that the stress of responsibility for the company was removed as far as possible. The doctor also felt that the activity of the rheumatoid process should be reduced as rapidly as possible before permanent damage to the joints could occur. He therefore prescribed a course of prednisolone and started him on a course of gold injections.

On this regime, the activity of the disease rapidly reduced and the ESR fell to normal. He was gradually mobilized and the prednisolone tailed off. He experienced a brief recurrence involving the metatarsophalangeal joints of the left foot. This followed an overseas visit on business but responded to a further period of rest and a brief course of steroids. The gold injections were continued until he had received a total of 2 g. He is currently in remission with haemoglobin 15.1 g and ESR 2 mm in 1 hour.

1. What factors may influence the activity of rheumatoid disease?
2. Discuss the treatment of rheumatoid arthritis.

A. G. Strube, Crawley, UK

515   MISS E.W.   AGED 52   UNEMPLOYED CLERK

This lady is unmarried and lives with her two elderly parents in a small house with three upstairs bedrooms. The parents are both over 80 years old but very sprightly.

Miss E.W. has had rheumatoid arthritis for the past 20 years. In the past she had a wide range of anti-rheumatic drugs but the disease is now quiescent, although she has considerable deformity of the ankles, knees, elbows, wrists and hands and is able to walk only short distances with the aid of two elbow crutches. She is prone to episodes of agitated depression occurring every 2 to 3 years and lasting for several months, which respond quite well to tranquillizers and anti-depressants.

1. What are the major causes of severe disability in middle-aged people?
2. What major problems are likely to arise for this family in the future?
3. What do you understand by the terms 'reactive' and 'endogenous' depression?

E. C. Gambrill, Crawley, UK

516   MR. P.   AGED 68   SELF-EMPLOYED ENGINEER

Mr. P. requests a home visit because of severe abdominal pain. On examination he has a left sided pleural rub and a tender enlarged spleen. He has not had to see a doctor in the last 5 years but does admit to increasing stiffness in his joints which he attributes to rheumatism. Examination of his hands indicate a mild active rheumatoid process. Further investigation reveals a high anti-nuclear and a high rheumatoid factor level plus an iron deficiency anaemia and a severe neutropenia. His ESR is normal.

1. What are the major management problems here?
2. How should his arthritis be treated?
3. What is the natural history of rheumatoid arthritis?

P. F. Gill, Hobart

CHAPTER 23

Injuries

This chapter is linked with the previous one. It begins with a number of cases of head and neck injury, followed by skeletal injuries to the shoulder, elbow, wrist and hand. Then follow knee, ankle and foot injuries. The chapter concludes with soft tissue injuries, which include a case of burns. Many of these cases are sports injuries. The family physician needs to be able to manage these conditions and be able to assess and manage where appropriate the more serious head, spinal and soft tissue injuries.

Head and neck injuries

517

S.C.   AGED 6 MONTHS

Mrs. C., an 18 year old married woman brought an apparently perfectly well 6 month old child to see the family doctor, as she had noticed swelling on one side of the child's head. An X-ray confirmed the suspicion that the child had a fractured skull.

The young mother appeared distraught when told of this and revealed the following history. She, the mother, had been in hospital for 5 days for a late postpartum haemorrhage. During that time, the child had been cared for by the father, by a next door neighbour who appeared to love the child as much as her own two children and by the child's grandmother and step-grandfather, who had kept her for one 24 hour period. When questioned carefully about any history of injury, or if she thought any of the caretakers were capable of inflicting harm on a child, the mother had no logical explanation.

1. What aetiology should the doctor be thinking about in this case?
2. Are there any features which might lead the family physician towards the causation of the fracture?
3. If the doctor's concerns are confirmed, what course of action should he take?

C. A. Moore, Hamilton, Canada

518

BILL D.   AGED 12   SCHOOLBOY

Bill has been brought to you early in the evening, 2 hours after falling from his bicycle and striking his head on a concrete path. No one saw the accident, so whether or not he lost consciousness is unknown. His parents are concerned because he 'looks so terrible'.

He is conscious, but pale and quiet. He responds appropriately to verbal stimuli. His BP is 100/60, pulse 70, his pupil signs are normal, and no neurological abnormality is detectable on examination. He has a small scalp haematoma in the right parietal area.

1. What diagnostic hypotheses would you have in mind?
2. What actions would you take?
3. What follow up would you order if it is decided to send Bill home?

W. E. Fabb, Melbourne

MR. DAVID D.   AGED 28   SCHOOLTEACHER

519

David D. is brought to you on a Saturday afternoon, following a blow on the temple with a cricket ball. His team mates say he was 'out to it' for perhaps ½ minute, left the field in a dazed state, but returned ½ hour later and resumed fielding. They have brought him in because he has a headache and they felt he should be 'checked over' and have a skull X-ray. The accident occurred 4 hours ago.

He is conscious and alert. He can't remember the accident or leaving and returning to the field afterwards. He can remember the last couple of hours of play. He complains about a severe generalized headache, which is worse over his left temple where he was struck.

His blood pressure is 130/85, his pulse 74, his pupil reactions are normal, he responds normally to verbal stimuli, and no neurological abnormality can be detected on examination.

1.   What diagnostic hypotheses would you entertain?
2.   What would you do for this patient?
3.   What follow up would you order?

W. E. Fabb, Melbourne

MR. GEORGE K.   AGED 48   UNEMPLOYED

520

This 48 year old male alcoholic is brought to the local hospital in a country town by the police following a fall in the street. He is conscious but confused. His speech is slurred and he can't remember the accident. His breath smells strongly of port. There is a 2 cm deep laceration over his occiput, which is bleeding freely.

1.   What actions would you take immediately?
2.   What actions would you take next?
3.   What condition(s) would you be watching for?
4.   What follow up care would you order when the patient is ready for discharge to his home?

W. E. Fabb, Melbourne

MASTER P.H.   AGED 8   SCHOOLBOY

521

This young man was taking a hayride during the fall in a small Canadian town. During the ride, he fell head first off the wagon and sustained injuries to his abdomen and chest. He did not obviously bang his head very hard and did not lose consciousness. Examination showed no obvious breaks in his chest apart from a broken clavicle. He is tender in his abdomen and has a few red cells in the urine. You admit him to hospital for observation. Later that day, you notice that he is holding his head very rigidly, not moving his neck. You X-ray the neck, this not having been done before because it was not a major symptom. X-rays show a fracture through the body of the first cervical vertebra.

1. What are the implications of this injury?
2. What will you do immediately?
3. What will you do next? (You are a long way, 120 miles, from the nearest orthopaedic surgeon).

J. K. Shearman, Hamilton, Canada

522 MRS. CARLA de P. AGED 36 HOUSEWIFE

Mrs. de P. is brought to your office following a motor accident in which she was hit from behind whilst stationary at traffic lights. Her head was thrown forward against the steering wheel and she has bruising of her forehead. She complains of a headache and pain in the upper part of her neck.

When you see her, she is lying quietly on the couch, and although she can move her neck, she is reluctant to do so.

1. What conditions would you suspect?
2. What would you do for her?

W. E. Fabb, Melbourne

Upper limb musculoskeletal injuries

G.H. AGED 9 SCHOOLBOY **523**

G.H. was brought to see the family doctor by his mother. He had hurt his shoulder playing football 2 to 3 weeks previously. It had seemed a relatively trivial collision, and the symptoms themselves not very alarming, but she remarked that she was a somewhat fussy mother of her only son. The doctor agreed that the symptoms and signs were not very notable, but a 'sixth sense' made him order an X-ray. The report came back that the condition was almost certainly osteogenic sarcoma of the humeral head with metastases locally.

1. How does a doctor gain a 'sixth sense' about clinical matters? In such a case as this, it was a valuable positive influence.
2. What is the morbid condition involved?
3. Clearly the technical treatment of this patient will be outside the province of the family doctor, but how does he go about supporting the rest of the family?

P. L. Gibson, Auckland

MR. KERRY McC. AGED 39 SCHOOLTEACHER **524**

Mr. McC. presents with a story of pain in his left mid upper arm, which began 3 to 4 days after lifting heavy tables and lockers at school 10 days ago. The pain has become worse over the last week, he is finding it difficult to move his arm, he cannot lie on it, and is finding it difficult to sleep.

Examination reveals limitation of all movements of the shoulder joint, especially internal and external rotation and abduction, the latter being limited to 20°. He is acutely tender under the acromion.

1. What is the probable diagnosis?
2. What would you do for this man?
3. What preventive measures would you advise?

W. E. Fabb, Melbourne

MR. B.F. AGED 42 BUSINESSMAN **525**

The patient is a sports enthusiast, plays squash regularly and tennis enthusiastically on weekends. For the past few months he has had increasing pain and discomfort in the region of his right elbow, especially with backhand strokes. The pain was aggravated 2 days prior to his consultation after participating in a tennis tournament. On examination there was tenderness over the right lateral epicondyle. Resisting wrist extension exacerbates his discomfort.

1. How do you make your diagnosis?
2. What is the treatment plan?
3. Future management problems?

B. M. Fehler, Johannesburg

526 PETER N.   AGED 3½

Whilst walking with his mother and brother, Peter wanted to be swung over driveways. He suddenly screamed and then had difficulty bending or straightening his left arm. The hand and lower arm were painful to any movement and were held in a pronated position. The situation was not relieved by support or analgesics. He was sent for an X-ray.

1. What are likely causes?
2. How would you treat it?

E. J. H. North, Melbourne

527 MRS. H.   AGED 55

Mrs. H. came to the office as an emergency with an injured right wrist. She was well known to her general practitioner. Several years previously she had had a right radical mastectomy for carcinoma of the breast. As a result of this she had some permanent oedema of the right upper extremity possibly more marked in the arm than in the forearm.

She was employed as a shop assistant, and whilst exercising her employer's dog in the park opposite the shop she fell and injured her right wrist. She presented with pain in the right wrist and gross swelling of the hand, wrist, and forearm. This swelling had appeared immediately following the injury. Clinically, she had a fracture, and this was confirmed radiologically.

It was apparent that for ideal results her fracture required manipulation and immobilization in a plaster cast. This undoubtedly would have added some reactionary swelling to the already present severe swelling, and it was felt that this could well jeopardize the subsequent viability of the hand and the forearm. The situation was discussed fully with Mrs. H. who agreed to accept a less than perfect outcome for the treatment of the fracture rather than take the anticipated risk of manipulation and immobilization. Her fracture therefore was treated with supportive splinting and bandaging.

Union of the fracture occurred readily but, as anticipated, she was left with a slightly deformed but an almost fully functional wrist. However, the gross oedema has persisted despite expert and specialized physiotherapy treatment.

Her injury was accepted as a Worker's Compensation liability and the employer's insurance company referred her to a surgical specialist for assessment of damages. The specialist in his report fully endorsed the action taken by the general practitioner.

1. What is the most likely diagnosis?
2. Was the general practitioner justified in making the initial decision on his own behalf?
3. What is the basis to support or otherwise a claim for liability under Worker's Compensation legislation for an injury sustained while taking the employer's dog for a walk?

D. A. Game, Adelaide

MR. DONALD G.   AGED 24   CLERK   528

Donald G. has been struck on the end of his right thumb with a fast moving cricket ball. His thumb is swollen and painful as far proximally as the wrist, and he has a small laceration at the tip of his thumb.

1. What possible injuries may result from this trauma?
2. How would you establish the diagnosis?
3. How would you manage each of the possible diagnoses?

W. E. Fabb, Melbourne

Lower limb musculoskeletal injuries

---

529 | **MISS DEBORAH C.   AGED 16   SCHOOLGIRL**

This 16 year old girl is brought in with a 'twisted knee' sustained at basketball 1 hour previously.

The right knee is grossly swollen and she cannot walk. It is so painful that she resists examination.

1. What specific enquiries would you make?
2. What conditions can result from knee injuries at sport?
3. What examination would you carry out?
4. What are the indications for X-ray in knee injuries?
5. How would you manage this situation?

W. E. Fabb, Melbourne

530 | **MRS. R.   AGED 36   HOUSEWIFE**

Mrs. R. limped into the consulting room and opened the consultation with 'my knee has gone again'. Examination of her history showed that 5 years ago she suffered an acute knee injury playing basketball, which failed to respond to rest and physiotherapy. A consultant orthopaedic surgeon confirmed a diagnosis of torn lateral meniscus. He advised arthroscopy and possible meniscectomy. The patient refused to take this advice.

In the intervening 5 years she has had five further attacks of a painful, swollen knee and has usually managed to see a different partner each time. She is convinced physiotherapy and a compression bandage will cure this attack as it has done in the past.

Mrs. R. admitted to increasing weight and increasing pain in her knee joint. She was worried about 'arthritis setting in'.

1. Is it justifiable to continue episodic treatment when surgery will probably remove the need for treatment?
2. Why has this patient avoided surgery?

P. F. Gill, Hobart

531 | **J.F.   AGED 17   STUDENT**

J.F. is planning to join the Army and has taken to running to get himself fit. He complains of pain in his left shin after running about a mile. The pain resolves after 10 minutes' rest. There is no abnormality on examination.

1. What conditions have to be considered?
2. What investigations would you do?
3. What advice would you give this patient?
4. What is the role of the general practitioner in the management of minor sporting injuries?

T. A. I. Bouchier-Hayes, Camberley, UK

MR. DOMINIC F.   AGED 32   ACCOUNTANT   532

Mr. F. is brought in by his fellow tennis players, unable to walk on his right leg. He reports that, whilst stretching for a volley, he felt a sudden sharp pain in the mid-calf as if he had been hit by a stone. Immediately afterwards, he found he could not walk because of very localized pain in the mid-calf.

1. What is the likely cause of this man's injury?
2. What would you do for him?

W. E. Fabb, Melbourne

MR. PETER M.   AGED 18   CIGARETTE SALESMAN   533

This 18 year old man is brought in from a local football match. He states he has 'sprained his right ankle' 2 hours previously.
His ankle is swollen and so painful that he is unable to walk on it.

1. What specific enquiries would you make?
2. What examination would you carry out?
3. What conditions can result from ankle injuries at sport?
4. What are the indications for X-ray in such injuries?
5. How would you manage this situation?

W. E. Fabb, Melbourne

MISS A.M.   AGED 17   SHOP ASSISTANT   534

Miss A.M. presents immediately following a basketball injury. She fell and twisted her ankle and had to leave the court. There is pain, swelling and tenderness over the lateral aspect of the ankle-joint.

1. What are the possible diagnoses?
2. Describe your management.

R. W. Roberts, Ravensthorpe, Australia

535 MR. DEREK J. AGED 29 SPORTS GOODS SALESMAN

Mr. J., who is a long distance runner, comes in because he can't walk on his left leg. He reports that he felt sudden severe pain in his heel while he was running this afternoon and now can't raise his heel from the ground.

1. What is the likely cause of this man's injury?
2. What would you do for him?

W. E. Fabb, Melbourne

536 MISS R.B. AGED 14 SCHOOLGIRL

This lass presented with her mother with a painful big toe which she injured at softball 3 weeks ago when someone trod on it. Since then it had become swollen and very painful. She had thought her nail was too long and had cut it. She was now limping and had a painful area under the ball of the foot. When examined she had an ingrowing toe nail and a small plantar wart.

R.B. asked what she could do for the pimples on her face which were bad at the moment and her mother asked what could be done for the painful heavy period R.B. had had over the past day.

1. Why are these conditions seen more commonly in the adolescent?
2. How would you go about treating this girl?

E. J. H. North, Melbourne

537 MRS. S.W. AGED 38 LIBRARIAN

Mrs. S.W. sustained a fracture of the proximal phalanx of her 4th right toe 24 days ago at work. She was seen by your partner, X-rayed, treated by strapping the 4th toe to the 3rd and put off work. She was reviewed by him a week ago and the period off work was extended by a further week because of pain on weight bearing. She was told to remove the strapping and return to work today, which she did. It is still painful. On examination the 4th toe is slightly swollen and slightly tender to deep pressure over the fracture site.

The patient has come with a request for another X-ray to 'confirm that progress is satisfactory in view of the fact that it is a Worker's Compensation case'.

1. What is the natural history of a fractured proximal phalanx of a minor toe?
2. What are the indications for re X-ray?
3. Assuming the re X-ray report reads 'fracture line remains evident', what will your further management be?

D. Levet, Hobart

Soft tissue injuries

MISS HELEN C.   AGED 18   TYPIST   **538**

Helen C., who has been working back late at work, is brought in at 11 p.m. following an accident at work in which she accidentally plunged her hand through a plate glass window. She has sustained a deep laceration across her right wrist, 3 cm above the distal wrist crease. It is 8 cm long and is almost transverse.

    1.   What structures might have been damaged?
    2.   How would you assess the damage?
    3.   What would you do immediately?

W. E. Fabb, Melbourne

MR. HARRY L.   AGED 42   SHEETMETAL WORKER   **539**

Mr. L. is a metal press operator. He is brought in by ambulance because he has crushed his right hand between the jaws of a heavy metal press. The hand is flail, with a number of lacerations, and is very swollen.

    1.   How would you assess this injury?
    2.   What would you do immediately?
    3.   What might be done for this man by the hand surgeon?
    4.   What factors other than the physical injury will be important in managing this man?

W. E. Fabb, Melbourne

WAYNE K.   AGED 3   **540**

This 3 year old boy has been rushed in to you by a frantic mother because he has burnt his right hand on a stove. The child was on a stool helping his mother cook when he slipped forward and placed his hand on the red-hot coil. The mother quickly removed him, but the palm and fingers of the child's hand look badly burnt.

    1.   How would you assess this situation?
    2.   What would your management be?

W. E. Fabb, Melbourne

CHAPTER 24

Tiredness

Tiredness is a ubiquitous symptom which leads the doctor to think of depression, metabolic disturbances such as thyroid disease or diabetes, electrolyte disturbances, infections, anaemia and malignant disease. All of these conditions are illustrated in this chapter. The family physician needs to be alert to detect serious disease, both physical and psychological, when the patient presents with tiredness, and to be able to take effective action.

541 MR. F.M.   AGED 50   PHARMACIST

Mr. F.A. is seen in the office complaining of tiredness, increasing in recent weeks. He gives a 3 to 4 month history of loss of energy with gradual onset of chest pains, abdominal cramping and backache. There has been some recent numbness of the fingers and toes and occasional weakness. He gives a history of 15 pounds of weight loss.

Past history reveals that he was quite 'run down' 15 years ago which was diagnosed on an office workup as exhaustion from overwork. A 'tonic' and vacation were prescribed following which he gradually improved and felt great until the recent symptoms began. His only medications had been proprietary drugs tried recently for sleep, but of little help.

Physical examination is essentially normal. The abdomen is slightly distended, but reveals no tenderness and no masses. There is mild to moderate prostatic enlargement. Mental status is clear and the patient is reasonably alert, but somewhat lethargic.

1. How should you approach the patient with multiple somatic complaints?
2. What classifications of drugs are available for use in the therapy of depression?
3. How can the family physician ensure a continuation of the primary care role before, during, and after diagnosis and therapy?

L. H. Amundson, Sioux Falls, SD, USA

542 MRS. D.H.   AGED 37   HOUSEWIFE

Mrs. D.H. whom you have known for some years complains of fatigue and insomnia, and weeps during the interview, especially when discussing the recent death of her dog. Her 20 year old daughter is married and her 19 year old son lives and works many miles away. Her husband, an executive, has recently been promoted to a demanding and responsible position. They own their own home. Her husband's parents are dead, her own parents live overseas. She has one sister living many miles away. Her husband has no close relatives. There is no family history of depression. She says she has no real thoughts of suicide. Sexual intercourse has recently left her unsatisfied and tense. She has few friends – her life revolves around her husband, children and housework.

1. What is the likely diagnosis?
2. Why does the recent death of her dog appear to have precipitated this problem?
3. Should the sexual problem be followed up? How?
4. Who else should be involved in this problem with her permission?

D. U. Shepherd, Melbourne

MR. CLEMENT K.   AGED 82   RETIRED FARMER

543

Mr. K. presented with a request for a 'check-up' because of increasing lack of energy and tiredness. Direct questioning led to an admission of disturbed sleep pattern with early morning waking. He also admitted that although happily married for 60 years, recently his wife had been nagging him a lot. After much gentle probing as to possible reasons he finally admitted that a sexual problem was the cause. Both partners still enjoyed active sexual relations, but his wife of the same age now had a stronger libido than he. Because he was unable to satisfy her sexual needs as often as she wanted she was convinced he must be having a sexual relationship with a young woman boarder.

1. What was the chain of events leading to the consultation?
2. What sexual problems can arise in old age?
3. How should this man and his wife be treated?

D. G. Chambers, Clare, Australia

MRS. E.N.   AGED 78

544

Mrs. E.N. had lived alone since the death of her husband 6 months earlier. She said she felt awful. She felt tired all the time, had no interest in anything and was losing weight. She slept badly, having difficulty getting off to sleep, waking frequently during the night, and would finally wake very early, feeling very depressed. She sometimes felt hungry and ate because she felt she should, but mostly had no interest in food. She complained of headaches, palpitations and of feeling 'swimmy' when she stood up. Her blood pressure, pulse rate and general examination were all normal but she was tearful, with a flat affect and depressed appearance. Urine test and full blood count revealed no abnormality. The doctor diagnosed depression, referred her to the community psychiatric nurse and gave her a prescription for imipramime 25 mg to be taken at night.

A few days later she telephoned asking for an urgent call about 7 p.m. She was breathless and complained of palpitations. She had taken only one dose of imipramime because it made her feel wheezy. Her pulse rate was 140 per minute, irregular and she had ankle oedema and raised JVP. The doctor diagnosed atrial fibrillation with congestive heart failure and sent her into hospital.

1. What are the causes of atrial fibrillation in an elderly person?
2. What is the connection between a life crisis such as bereavement, and physical disease?

G. Strube, Crawley, UK

545 MRS. JOAN W.   AGED 70   HOUSEWIFE

Mrs. W. walked slowly into the consulting room and sat down. After a short while she responded in a rather hoarse voice to the locum's greeting and questioning. It transpired that she was very tired and extremely depressed, but had come for a check-up and a repeat prescription. A search through the notes showed that she was taking digoxin, propranolol, a diuretic, potassium capsules, tranquillizers, hypnotics at night and various vitamins, costing her a sizeable portion of her income.

A limited examination showed a dry skin, coarse sparse hair, pulse 56 per minute, blood pressure 170/80 and slowly responding knee reflexes.

1. What primary hypothesis might the locum make?
2. What action might he take, regarding her drugs and the further elucidation of her problems?
3. How often may slowly developing changes in a patient escape the notice of a family doctor?

R. T. Mossop, Harare, Zimbabwe

546 MR. H. McG.   AGED 68   BREWERY WORKER

Mr. McG. stated that 5 months ago he was knocked over at work. Struck head and was briefly unconscious. A few days later awoke with shortness of breath, chest tightness, tingling fingers. Later noticed eyes persistently running, increasing disability with grip, increasing tiredness, falling hair. No previous illness. Non-smoker and virtually a non-drinker.

His wife offered the following observations. 'His skin has changed and is now rough and cracking. His hair is falling out, his eyes are running, his voice has changed, his face has swollen, he seems very cold, he drops things, seems a bit deaf. He walks much slower as if his legs are too heavy, his skin smells strange, he is short of breath. He's been like a clock slowly running down.'

1. What aspects of history taking are highlighted?
2. What features would you expect to find to clinch your diagnosis?
3. Does treatment pose a problem?

W. D. Jackson, Launceston, Australia

547 MRS. E.M.   AGED 50

This mother of three healthy girls came to the doctor with swelling of the ankles. She was also tired and exhausted and a blood count showed a haemoglobin of only 10 g. Her periods were rather heavy and it seemed likely that this was the cause of the anaemia and the ankle oedema. The doctor prescribed a course of iron injections but after a further month there was still no improvement and she had been forced to give up her work as a secretary as she felt so tired. The next time she came to the office her own doctor was on leave and so she saw one of the other partners who had not seen her for a year or so. He noticed a great change in her: she was fat and sluggish with a pale face but high colour in the cheeks. Her voice was husky and her speech slurred. When he took her hand she felt cold and her pulse slow.

He felt she had developed hypothyroidism and started replacement therapy. She made a complete recovery.

1. Why did her own doctor miss the diagnosis of hypothyroidism?
2. How would you treat Mrs. E.M.?

A. G. Strube, Crawley, UK

MRS. D.J.   AGED 47   HOUSEWIFE   548

You receive a letter from a local solicitor asking you for an opinion on this lady whom you have never previously met, although she is registered with you. She has been charged with obtaining goods on mail order by deception and he feels that a medical report may help her case.

You decide to visit this lady at home. It is a cold day. You find her only half dressed crouched over a small electric fire with a 'cotton bud' in each ear. She communicates quite rationally with you and complains of feeling cold and tired. On examination she is thin and pale. Her personal hygiene is poor and she has severe erythema ab igne on her shins. She denies all knowledge of the charges against her.

1. How would you define 'mental illness'?
2. On what grounds should society admit a person to hospital against their will?
3. How might you manage this particular problem?

E. C. Gambrill, Crawley, UK

SCOTT D.   AGED 13   SCHOOLBOY   549

Scott is the eldest of a family of three. You know his parents as solid and dependable and slightly over-anxious about their children. His paternal grandfather has recently died from Hodgkin's disease after the usual hopes and fears of chemotherapy.

Scott is 'just tired'. He comes home from school exhausted, often falls asleep at the evening meal, goes early to bed and rises reluctantly each morning. He is by turns surly and tearful.

He looks pale but has no physical evidence of disease. It transpires that he is heavily involved with football training, has recently been having daily swimming sessions, in which he is expected to cover some 24 laps and has expressed groundless fears of being overweight.

1. Is his condition mental, physical or both?
2. What would you see as the most pressing emotional elements?
3. Would you approach his teachers and coaches?

J. A. Stevens, Ulverstone, Australia

550 MISS F.T.　　AGED 19　　STUDENT

Miss F.T. consults you because she 'feels tired'. She is worried about her course, is not sleeping well, and feels her studies are not progressing. She has a room in a boarding house, but goes home for vacations. She has recently had a sore throat, and noticed she was feverish. Examination of the throat reveals pus on the tonsils, and some slightly tender cervical glands. She is febrile.

1. What other parts of the body would you specifically examine?
2. To determine if this is a physical illness, or an emotional problem or both, what questions would you ask?
3. What special investigations would you perform?
4. What other important questions should be asked?
5. If the diagnosis is confirmed as infectious mononucleosis, what advice would you give?

D. U. Shepherd, Melbourne

551 ANDREW M.　　AGED 15　　SCHOOLBOY

Andrew was brought along by his mother who offered the following history. He had been sick for 1 week feeling tired, listless, not eating and complaining of nausea. In the past 24 hours he had developed a temperature, headache and neck discomfort. Andrew is 15 and anxious to do well in his imminent examinations.

Last week his elder brother, a first year university student in the midst of examinations, was diagnosed as having glandular fever on clinical grounds and mono-spot test.

No abnormalities were found when Andrew was examined: in particular there were no glands, no spleen, no rash, only a slightly raised temperature.

1. What is 'glandular fever'?
2. Should the doctor have performed any further investigations before making the provisional but confident diagnosis of glandular fever in Andrew?
3. Should Andrew be allowed to sit for the examinations?

P. F. Gill, Hobart

MRS. VENERSTIA D.   AGED 30   PEASANT HOUSEWIFE

552

Mrs. D. presented to her district hospital in Africa complaining of tiredness, breathlessness on exertion and aching, slightly swollen legs. She believed she had been bewitched. She held up her pale palms. On the basis of local knowledge of faecal disposal habits and probability, together with rapid questioning concerning other possible causes of anaemia, a provisional diagnosis of hookworm anaemia was made. She was given a vermifuge and a course of iron tablets to take. Three weeks later she returned smiling, carrying a chicken as a present to the clever and kind clinician.

1. What is the life cycle of the hookworm?
2. Do you agree with Venerstia that the clinician had done a good job?
3. How may attempts to promote health be hindered by a firm belief in witchcraft (or even a belief that all illness arises from the will of God)?

R. T. Mossop, Harare, Zimbabwe

MRS. C.A.   AGED 75   PENSIONER

553

This woman presents with mild aches and pains, general malaise, tiredness and wants a tonic. Examination revealed only minor degenerative joint disease and a slight pallor.

Blood examination
Hb 9.5 g/dl
MCV 95 cμ
MCHC 31%
WCC 5000/cmm
Platelets 190,000/cmm
Film – some hypochromic red cells

1. What is her problem?
2. Are any other laboratory investigations necessary?
3. How would you manage this problem?

T. D. Manthorpe, Port Lincoln, Australia

MRS. V.G.   AGED 32   DOMESTIC

554

Mrs. V.G. has been treated for wheezing episodes, with a diagnosis of asthma, relieved in part by oral theophylline preparations for several years. At the end of today's interview, which had been directed at regulating her theophylline treatment, she complains of feeling more tired than usual, of night sweats and poor appetite. Her record demonstrates a 10 lb weight loss in the past 4 months. As she was about to leave, she also mentioned off-handedly that she had noticed a firm lump in her neck for the past few months.

1. What diagnoses would you consider at this time?
2. What tests would you order?
3. What would you tell the patient about her problem?

K. F. Weyrauch, Charleston, SC, USA

555 MR. W.P.   AGED 24   BANK TELLER

Mr. W.P. aged 24 presented to his family physician complaining of fatigue and a tendency to develop bruises after even minor trauma. A blood test revealed that he was suffering from acute myeloblastic leukaemia.

He was admitted to hospital and after two courses of chemotherapy, his disease went into remission. His hospital course was a stormy one, in that the patient exhibited great fear of injections and venepuncture, which were so much a part of his treatment. After the first few days he refused to eat hospital food, and henceforth his wife and other family members brought him his food from home. On the surface he was very nonchalant about his disease and did not share his feelings with his physicians. When discharged home in remission, he not only resumed his hobby of golfing several times per week, but also joined a baseball team. Although he was on maintenance therapy, he often had excuses to miss appointments and on one infrequent visit, revealed to his doctor that he had stopped all treatment several months previously. Later he was informed that the peripheral blood smears suggested that his disease was recurring and more definitive therapy was in order. The following day the family physician was advised by the patient's wife that she was now 3 months pregnant and that her husband had decided that he would not undergo further treatment.

1. What are the implications of the diagnosis of acute myeloblastic leukaemia?
2. What are the apparent dynamics in this case?
3. What are the issues related to the pregnancy?

C. A. Moore, Hamilton, Canada

556 MRS. M.R.   AGED 70   WIDOW

Mrs M.R. has been a widow for 35 years and lives with two spinster sisters in a middle class district. She has been known to her present family physician for the past 20 years, during which time her only health problem has been repeated bouts of bronchitis. She has tried diligently, but unsuccessfully, to stop smoking. On this occasion M.R. consults her family physician because of weight loss and fatigue of at least 3 months' duration. On functional enquiry, she admits to a blood stained vaginal discharge. Pelvic examination reveals a large fungating mass which appears to be replacing her cervix.

1. What is the relationship between smoking and bronchitis?
2. Why has the patient waited so long to consult her physician?
3. What is the significance of a patient presenting with fatigue?
4. Is it unusual to have this lesion in a patient of 70 years of age?

C. A. Moore, Hamilton, Canada

MR. I.J.   AGED 45   ENTERTAINER   **557**

Mr. I.J. consults his family doctor because he does not feel too well, has lacked energy, and has had trouble with boils. His career as an entertainer has resided in the fact that he is obese, happy-go-lucky, and a great socializer. The doctor quickly establishes that he has significant hypertension, and finds that he has glycosuria.

Subsequent testing confirms that he has frank diabetes and significant hypertension (160/115). His socializing involves him in regular beer drinking and he smokes about 30 cigarettes a day. A chest X-ray is clear. His act as an entertainer depends substantially on his obesity and joviality.

1. How would one manage the physical illnesses?
2. What other elements are there in the 'total diagnosis' of this patient?
3. What are the likely effects of his illness on himself and his life, his family and his employers?
4. What are the likely psychological and social effects of his illness?

P. L. Gibson, Auckland

MR. B.   AGED 55   CIVIL SERVANT   **558**

Mr. B. had presented on four previous occasions with a non-productive cough, recurrent low-grade fevers and general fatigue. He had received two previous courses of antibiotics. Several previous physical examinations had revealed occasional rales over both lung fields but no rhonchi. No sputum test had ever been conducted because he had not raised any sputum. Tuberculosis tests and skin tests for histoplasmosis and coccidioidomycosis were all negative. The patient was becoming somewhat depressed. He lived in a suburban area of the city, married at the age of 34 and had five daughters aged between 11 and 21. They were very active and he had a very busy life at home. He was finding great difficulty in maintaining the pace. His married life had been stable and solid and his wife was very concerned about his health.

A physical examination at this time revealed some rales over both lung fields but no other abnormal findings. Enquiry about his activities of daily living revealed that his five daughters were all involved in a nearby riding school and although he was not himself a rider he frequently visited the barn and helped them care for two horses they owned.

1. What further investigations would be indicated in arriving at a differential diagnosis?
2. Should this man be admitted to hospital for further investigations?
3. What role does organic illness play in the development of depression?

W. W. Rosser, Ottawa

559   **MISS K.   AGED 21   AU PAIR GIRL**

Miss K. who recently arrived from Switzerland and was working for a Canadian family for the previous 6 months presented to the office complaining of weakness. Her past history was completely negative. Her history indicated some vague renal problems in her father and one brother. On further questioning she admitted that she was lonely although she had other friends from Switzerland in the city who were doing the same type of work. She complained that her work was rather boring and the family that she was working with was not particularly supportive or warm. She did not appear depressed. The physical examination was completely normal. The weakness was described as varying in degree from day to day but sometimes becoming so severe that she was forced to sit down. A complete blood count and serum electrolytes were ordered. The blood count was normal, but the serum potassium was found to be 2.4 mmol/l.

A serum potassium was repeated and again was found to be 2.2 mmol/l. Further investigations of renal function were negative.

1. What are the most likely causes of hypokalaemia in an otherwise healthy 21 year old female?
2. What simple investigations would help you to decide whether this was a psychologically or organically based problem?
3. How would you manage this problem if it were psychologically based?

W. W. Rosser, Ottawa

CHAPTER 25

Weight Loss

Weight loss is always a worrying symptom which leads the doctor to think about serious disease, such as malignancy, thyrotoxicosis, diabetes and severe infection. All of these are illustrated in this chapter. The family physician also recognizes that anxiety and depression can result in weight loss. The diagnostic skill of the family physician is often taxed to the utmost in elucidating the cause of weight loss.

560 PAUL S. AGED 6 SCHOOLBOY

Paul developed an upper respiratory tract infection with associated con-junctivitis, followed by a rash typical of measles on the fourth day.

Symptomatic treatment only was advised and he avoided any of the common complications of the disease. However, his mother, always an anxious person, complained that he did not seem to be recovering properly and ten days later he became lethargic and was obviously losing weight rapidly.

1. What other conditions may present in a similar fashion to measles?
2. What factors may influence the degree of anxiety which parents feel about a sick child?
3. What conditions may account for the deterioration in Paul's condition?

E. C. Gambrill, Crawley, UK

561 MR. B. AGED 59 BRICKLAYER, MRS. B. HOUSEWIFE

Mr. B. aged 59, a bricklayer, had been under treatment for hypertension for a number of years. He required a lot of medication but was well controlled. He presented with a very sore throat for which an assistant had prescribed an antibiotic one week previously. It was noted now that he had a very dry mouth, and further questioning and examination revealed the typical symptoms and signs of a well defined clinical entity. The diagnosis was confirmed by simple but appropriate biochemical testing.

He responded well to treatment but Mrs. B., normally a very placid person, whilst attending for a knee injury, expressed her extreme anxiety and fears about the future management of her husband's illness. He apparently refused to take any interest in organizing the appropriate changes in his life style or his ongoing therapy. He left all this to her, and she was extremely concerned particularly as Mr. B. did most of his work away in the country when he would live by himself.

Four months later Mrs. B. again presented herself with the story that her anxiety and concern had become much worse. She was now very shaky and generally upset. She had lost nearly 6 kg in weight since the onset of her husband's illness. She felt she could not manage any longer and would have to give up her part-time secretarial job. She wanted to know why she was not now coping.

1. What are the possible diagnoses of Mr. B.'s condition?
2. What are the possible diagnoses of Mrs. B.'s condition?
3. Could the general practitioner have anticipated Mrs. B.'s condition?
4. What is the management of this family?

5. Was the general practitioner justified in accepting his own diagnosis and instituting treatment for these disease processes?

D. A. Game, Adelaide

MRS. R.H.   AGED 23   HOUSEWIFE

562

Mrs. R.H., happily married and the mother of a healthy 3 year old boy, is a very anxious but pleasant and cheerful individual who consults with her physician indicating that for several months she has noticed a painless swelling in her lower central neck, has become increasingly fatigued and irritable, has lost 6 to 8 pounds and has been more nervous than ever before in her life.

1. What is the most likely cause of Mrs. H.'s symptoms?
2. What advice would you offer this lady regarding treatment?
3. If Mrs. H. suggested that she was about 6 weeks pregnant and you were able to confirm this, how might your recommendations for investigation or treatment be modified?

G. G. Beazley, Winnipeg

JOHN P.   AGED 48   LABOURER

563

In mid-April 1978, Mr. P. complained of muscular weakness for 2–3 weeks. He had a heavy labouring job digging holes in roads and was unable to do his share. He had no other symptoms except that of tiring quickly. He felt well, had a good appetite and all bodily functions were normal. He was lean and had recently lost about 10 lb in weight. He was a non-smoker and had no previous history of illness. His first wife had died some years before aged 32 from a cerebral tumour, leaving him with two small sons, now aged 8 and 12 years. He had recently married again.

On examination, the most striking feature was exophthalmos with lid lag. He was very thin, had a fine tremor, pulse 98, regular, BP 120/80. He had no palpable goitre. The doctor made a diagnosis of hyperthyroidism. Relevant investigations were as follows:

Serum thyroxine	181 nmol/l
	(normal range 60–138 nmol/l)
Serum T$_3$ uptake	73.7% retention
	(normal range male 43–60% retention)
Free thyroxine index	1334
	(normal range male 258–828)
Chest X-ray normal	

He was treated with carbimazole 30 mg and propranolol 60 mg both daily in divided doses. Within 1 week he was feeling much better but 3 weeks after the start of treatment he had severe urticaria, covering his whole body, accompanied by painful joints. He felt very poorly. His WBC was 12,200/cm with 80% neutrophils. The carbimazole was stopped, the propranolol continued and 5 days later the rash and arthralgia had disappeared.

On the 6th June he had a dose of I^{131} as an outpatient. This was his only hospital visit. He started to reduce the dose of propranolol a month later and by mid-July he felt completely well, had gained 7 lb in weight and returned to work. Early in August, he still felt fit and was coping well with the job, he gained a further 7 lb and his pulse rate was 60 per minute. Arrangements were made for him to have routine thyroid function tests at the end of September before seeing his GP for a check-up in October. The thyroid function tests were as follows:

Serum thyroxine	< 10 nmol/l
Serum T_3 uptake	32.9% retention
	(for normals see previous report)
TSH	> 50 mU/l
(thyroid stimulating hormone)	(normal range < 1.5–6.0 mU/l)

When he attended for routine check-up, he admitted to feeling tired and lethargic and had gained a further 12 lb in weight. His face looked bloated and he talked and moved slowly. He was treated with thyroxine 0.1 mg daily, increasing after 2 weeks to 0.2 mg daily. He was completely his normal self within a month and continued well. He was seen every 6 months and a year later had lost a little weight and had a resting pulse rate of 72 per minute. The dose of thyroxine was reduced to 0.1 mg daily and he has continued extremely well. He is now seen annually by his general practitioner.

1. What are the most likely causes of muscular weakness and weight loss in a man of this age?
2. What other methods are used in treating hyperthyroidism?
3. What was the rash and arthralgia due to?
4. What is the value of routine follow up in thyroid disease?
5. How would you have managed this problem?

G. Strube, Crawley, UK

564   MR. MARK L.   AGED 56   WARDSMAN

Mr. L. came to the office complaining of rectal bleeding for 3 years. It had been getting worse for 6 months. It occurred after each bowel motion and was more than just spotting. It was bright red blood. He had a sensation of fullness in his abdomen and had been passing a lot of flatus for the past 6 months. He had a weight loss of 3 kg in the past 2 months.

1. What other symptoms would you enquire about?
2. What would your physical examination include?

3. What would you say to the patient before any other investigations are carried out?

M. D. Mahoney, Brisbane

MR. M.N.　　AGED 63　　INSURANCE AGENT

565

Mr. M.N. comes to your office because his friends have told him he looks pale. He has had a 12 kg weight loss over the past year. In addition, he has been constipated for 4 months and has had rectal bleeding for 2 months. On rectal examination you feel no masses. His haemoglobin is 9.0 g/dl.

1. What investigation would you conduct?
2. While you are investigating him how would you explain to him what you are doing?
3. What might be the therapy?
4. What would you do if he refuses investigation?

E. V. Dunn, Toronto

MRS. G.S.　　AGED 76

566

Mrs. G.S. came during December complaining of a dry, tickly cough which she had had for a month. She was generally well. There were no abnormal physical signs. She was a non-smoker. A chest X-ray was reported as follows: '. . . the left hilar shadow is a little prominent. I think this is probably within normal limits. I suggest a further film in 3 weeks' time.' A further film was reported as showing no change but the cough had improved and the chest remained clear. In the meantime she developed nausea on Christmas night, which persisted. When next seen, in February, she had lost her appetite, her weight had dropped from 76 kg to 70 kg, the tickly cough had returned and she complained of nausea and of solid food sticking at the lower end of the sternum. There were no abnormal physical signs except slight epigastric tenderness. She was obese despite the loss of weight. A barium swallow and meal was reported as normal.

1. What do you think is wrong with Mrs. G.S.?
2. What would you do next?
3. What are the risks of delay in investigating this problem?

G. Strube, Crawley, UK

MR. W.　　AGED 67

567

You are called to the Ws' house because Mr. W. is weak and has lost his appetite.

He suffers from mild deafness and maturity onset diabetes treated with a small dose of glibenclamide. He has the heart murmur of mitral incompetence following rheumatic fever and takes digoxin 0.25 mg daily, frusemide 40 mg each morning and slow release potassium tablets. This controls his mild congestive failure.

He tells you that he was quite well until he went on holiday 3 weeks ago. He caught diarrhoea from friends, but this settled quickly though he had not regained his appetite. He had lost 2½ kg in weight.

Other history and physical examination were non-contributory, his urine was sugar free. All investigations which seemed appropriate were normal except that the ESR was 80 mm in 1 hour. His condition slowly deteriorated and he became confused. Hospital admission was refused by the medical registrar who examined him in outpatients and said he was 'getting old'. His IgA was found to be very raised.

Finally, 6 weeks after he was first seen, his diagnosis became manifest, he responded rapidly to treatment in hospital and is now well (although markedly deaf) on the same treatment as when you first saw him.

1. What investigations would seem to be appropriate?
2. Could all this have been caused by 'getting old'?
3. What are the diagnostic possibilities in this case?
4. The general practitioner is frequently concerned with undifferentiated illness. How does he manage this?

A. L. A. Reid, Newcastle, Australia

CHAPTER 26

Iatrogenic Illness

The incidence of iatrogenic illness is alarming. Much of it is the result of the use or misuse of medications. This chapter illustrates this, beginning with cases of polypharmacy, after which a number of cases demonstrating adverse reactions to cardiac drugs, anti-hypertensives, anti-inflammatory drugs, the contraceptive pill, tranquillizers and steroids is presented. The chapter includes some of those tragic cases where the doctor's words or actions have inflicted psychological wounds on the patient, leading to the development of cardiac neurosis.

The family physician has a wide range of therapeutic tools at his disposal. He needs to be aware of their risks as well as their benefits, and alert to the adverse reactions which may occur. He needs too, to be aware of the effect of his own words and actions on the patient's psyche. The problem of iatrogenic illness is probably much bigger than it seems at first sight.

568 MISS L.   AGED 66

Miss L. comes to you as a new patient without a letter from her former doctor. She presents the following shopping list:

Lanoxin PG 2 mane for heart and ankle swelling.
Isoptin 40 mg 2 t.d.s. for palpitations.
Nicotinic acid 100 mg 2 t.d.s. for brain circulation.
Stemetil 5 mg t.d.s. for giddiness.
Indocid cap. 1 t.d.s. for arthritis.
Span-K 1 t.d.s.
Lasix 1 midday.
Vit. C., Ferrous sulphate tabs., Vit. B$_{12}$ 1000 units weekly.
Serepax ½ nocte.
Isordil 1 q.i.d. for angina.
Zyloprim 1 daily.
Colchicine 1 daily.
Anginine p.r.n.

1. What illnesses does this patient probably have?
2. What difficulties might one encounter in reducing therapy?
3. What do we know about the patient's doctor?

A. L. A. Reid, Newcastle, Australia.

569 MRS. D.   AGED 55

Mrs. D. had a thyroidectomy 30 years ago for thyrotoxicosis and, because of the changes in the employment of her husband, has had numerous residences necessitating attending different doctors. Lately, she had been attending the out-patient department of a public hospital and she rarely sees the same doctor more that once.

She presents requesting a repeat of tablets. She is taking a diuretic and a beta blocker, 300 mcg of thyroxine, calcium and vitamin D, in addition to sleeping tablets and two lots of tranquillizers. Further history reveals that she was getting attacks of chest pain suggestive of angina, was agitated, had a tachycardia at times and despite tranquillizers and sleeping tablets was not sleeping well.

After some argument, the patient agreed to the general practitioner's suggestion to stop all treatment and remain in contact with one doctor. Over a period of weeks medication was gradually withdrawn and the patient's symptoms appeared to be well controlled with a diuretic only for hypertension and glyceryl trinitrate for angina. Two months after the cessation of medication her thyroid function tests were normal. Three months after cessation of medication the patient was obviously myxoedematous with confirmatory thyroid function tests.

1. List this patient's problems.
2. List the doctor's problems.

3. What responsibility does a hospital outpatient department have in such cases?

P. F. Gill, Hobart

MRS. ANNIE W.   AGE 86

570

This patient has long standing congestive heart failure, hypertension, and anxiety state. She is becoming frail, lethargic and forgetful, but still lives by herself. Her present medications are digoxin 0.25 mg daily, hydrochlorothiazide 50 mg daily, diazepam 2 mg tid.

1. Are you worried about continuing these drugs and these doses?
2. What adverse drug reactions might occur in this patient?
3. Do the risks of treating hypertension in the elderly outweigh the benefits?

D. H. Johnson, Toronto

MRS. MARGARET S.   AGED 78

571

Mrs. S. is an elderly female patient who has congestive heart failure and renal failure. Over a short period of 6 weeks this formerly alert individual became moderately demented. Except for the change in mental status, the neurological and remaining physical examination remained unchanged. Your records show that her medications are digoxin 0.125 mg daily, and frusemide 40 mg daily.

1. What further history do you want from the patient or her husband?
2. What is your plan of investigation?
3. What community help can be offered to help maintain this person in optimum health at home?

D. H. Johnson, Toronto

ERNEST W.   AGED 78

572

Mrs. W. asked the doctor to call because Ernie was having another one of his tummy upsets. 'Very queer he is' she said on the telephone. He had had a previous attack 5 months before when he was visited and found to be weak and feeble and vomiting but with no abnormal physical signs. A diagnosis of viral gastritis was made. He recovered in 24 hours. He gave a history of similar less severe attacks of vomiting lasting about 20 minutes every 2 weeks or so for 6 months. He had been well between attacks. When seen he felt awful and was vomiting. On examination he was fully conscious, alert, a good colour and could move all his limbs normally. He was not giddy and had no nystagmus or any abnormal physical signs except minimal ankle oedema and some epigastric tenderness. His pulse rate was 78, regular, and of normal volume.

He had moved to the area 10 years before with a history of paroxysmal tachycardia 5 years before that. This had caused angina and mild congestive heart failure and led to his early retirement from work as a bus driver. He had been admitted to hospital initially and when he registered with this practice he was taking: frusemide 40 mg daily, digoxin, 0.25 mg daily, Slow K two daily, amitriptyline 75 mg daily and propranolol 50 mg daily in divided doses. These were all continued unchanged except the amitriptyline which was stopped and the digoxin which was reduced to 0.125 mg daily. He had been well on this regime until 6 months before this episode.

1. Can you make a provisional diagnosis?
2. Are there any tests which could be useful?
3. What would you do next?

G. Strube, Crawley, UK

573   MRS. A.D.   AGED 83

Mrs. A.D. was a house-bound, obese, blind woman, with osteoarthrosis of most joints and ischaemic heart disease, causing atrial fibrillation and chronic congestive heart failure. This was fairly well controlled with digoxin 0.125 mg daily and Navidrex K, 2 daily. She had been constipated all her life and took laxatives from time to time. She was seen frequently by the doctor with numerous different complaints.

The doctor was asked to visit her because she felt weak and faint and had vague pains across her chest and abdomen. The constipation was worse than usual. She looked more than usually frail but there were no new physical signs. Her abdomen was very obese but bowel sounds were present. Rectal examination revealed soft faeces only. Over the next 2 weeks she became weaker and developed abdominal distension. She was admitted to hospital with a diagnosis of intestinal obstruction. Her serum potassium was found to be 2.8 mmol/l. Her blood urea was normal. She recovered with conservative treatment.

1. What is the significance of the serum potassium?
2. What are the symptoms of potassium depletion?
3. What are the dangers of potassium depletion?
4. How can a doctor guard against missing a new diagnosis in an old patient with multiple pathology whom he sees frequently?

G. Strube, Crawley, UK

MR. J.F.   AGED 80

574

Mr. J.F., whose wife had just recently died, came for his routine blood pressure check. He complained of tired legs, and was found to have a normocytic, normochromic anaemia. ESR was not raised. Cold agglutinins were present and his Hb was 11.2 g/dl. Physical examination, apart from the anaemia, was normal. He was taken off methyldopa, and his BP remained at 150/90. After several months when his Hb was 8.8 g/dl he was given a transfusion and regained his former vigor, able to walk into town and back, and resume his gardening.

1. Are any other investigations worth pursuing?
2. How long will symptomatic treatment give relief?

G. M. Dick, Hobart

MR. A.B.   AGED 79   PENSIONER

575

Mr. A.B. presents because he is vomiting coffee-grounds material. There has been a delay in his examination because of confusion over names at the group general practice. His usual doctor is on leave. By the time he is seen, Mr. B. is pale and mentions incidentally that he has a painful lump in the groin.

On examination, he appears to have bilateral inguinal herniae – one of these is quite tender on palpation. A barium meal examination 3 months previously revealed a scarred duodenum but no evidence of active ulcer. The patient's only medication is indomethacin prescribed for joint pain by another doctor in the practice.

1. Who defines an emergency? Should it be the patient, the receptionist, the relatives or the doctor?
2. Who is responsible in a group medical practice for each patient's care?
3. In this case, how much care should be provided by the primary care doctor?

B. H. Connor, Armidale, Australia

JAN WILLIAMSON   AGED 21   PRIMARY TEACHER

576

Jan is seeing you for the first time, although she has seen other doctors in the practice several times before. Each time over the last 18 months, when she has presented for a six monthly check-up and repeat pill prescription, her blood pressure has been slightly elevated. Twelve months ago she saw the cardiologist who manages her father's hypertension and, on that occasion, her blood pressure was normal.

Today, Jan rushes in late for her appointment and starts telling you how busy she is with preparations for her forthcoming wedding. She says she can hardly find time for her regular netball and squash together with her school activities and time spent watching her fiancee (Tom) play football and basketball. Although she says she 'never felt better', you find her blood pressure remains 135/95 after two quiet 5 minute intervals on your examination couch.

You arrange to see her again first thing Saturday morning when her blood pressure is 125/85.

1. Will you treat Jan's hypertension?
2. Will you continue her on the pill?
3. What non-drug treatment is appropriate?

R. P. Strasser, Melbourne

577 GILLIAN A. AGED 24 SCHOOLTEACHER

Gillian has been attending the Family Planning Clinic for advice on contraception. She is unmarried and has no history of previous serious illness. On several recent visits to the Clinic her blood pressure has been consistently elevated at 160/100 and, for this reason, she has been referred to her general practitioner.

1. What is the significance of a blood pressure of 160/100 in a 24 year old female taking oral contraceptives?
2. What factors would influence the doctor's decision to advise Gillian for or against continuing to take her oral contraceptive?
3. What alternatives are available to Gillian if a decision is taken to stop her oral contraceptive?

W. L. Ogborne, Sydney

578 MISS C.T. AGED 33

Miss C.T. comes to a new doctor having recently moved requesting a repeat prescription for diazepam 5 mg q.i.d. which she has been taking for the past 4 years. She describes a free floating anxiety partially alleviated by the medication. Withdrawal results in unbearable tension. She had two previous psychiatric consultations in which gradual withdrawal accompanied by temporary substitution with phenothiazines was suggested. Both resulted in half-hearted attempts and full-blown failures. At present she has no desire to discontinue the drug.

1. To what extent should an attempt be made to persuade her to alter the use of her medication?
2. Is the medical profession in any way culpable for this patient's addiction?
3. If the doctor feels that he cannot in all good conscience fulfil her request, how should he manage the case?

E. Domovitch, Toronto

MR. O.P. AGED 27 UNEMPLOYED

579

Dr. Z. is consulted on a Sunday morning, when he is seeing patients on an emergency basis for a group of five partners. Mr. P. seems an unusual sort of person. His approach is diffident; he appears ill at ease. He states that he was discharged from prison 10 days ago, that his nerves feel terrible, he cannot eat and is sleeping poorly. He states that, while in prison, he was seen by a doctor and was treated with Valium (diazepam) and/or anti-depressants. He feels in desperate need of something to settle his nerves immediately. He agrees that he attracts doubt and suspicion in making such a request at such a time.

1. Should the doctor carry out a full clinical examination?
2. Should he make out the prescription or refuse to do so?
3. Should he try to communicate with the prison doctor concerned to see if the patient's story is correct?

P. L. Gibson, Auckland

MR. K. AGED 66 PAINTER

580

Mr. K. first presented 5 years ago. He stated that 6 months previously he had had a sudden attack of pain in the left side of his chest and left arm. He was seen by a doctor and told that he had had a 'small heart attack'. He had come because he was still having some bouts of chest pain.

Full assessment suggested a normal cardiovascular system. ECG showed no abnormality or evidence of previous myocardial infarction.

Further discussion revealed the fact that his wife had Parkinson's disease and had had a myocardial infarction 3 years previously. Also, his brother had died recently of myocardial infarction.

Over the ensuing months he maintained he was having continuing attacks of pain and was unable to work. He required sickness certificates. Assessment by a cardiologist failed to convince him that he did not have significant cardiovascular disease.

After 12 months he was told he would be given no further sickness certificates. He applied for a job but, on the day of the interview by the prospective employer, he had 'one of my attacks'. Following this he made several attempts to obtain a permanent invalid pension.

Protracted discussion between the general practitioner and the medical officer of the Social Security Department finally resulted in his being granted an invalid pension.

He is now living in active retirement. He travels around the country pursuing his photography hobby, and does the odd painting job. He has had no therapy or medical attention, except for a minor injury, since he obtained the pension 3 years ago.

1. What are the disease processes, if any, in this man?
2. How should this case be managed?
3. Were sickness certificates and later the Invalid Pension justified?

D. A. Game, Adelaide

581   MR. G.   AGED 45   WORKSHOP MANAGER

Mr. G. was taken in an emergency from his place of employment to the emergency department of a teaching hospital. He was a very conscientious man working under great pressure with reduced staff. It appears that, following a disagreement with the general manager of the company, he had become acutely short of breath and tight in the chest. Both Mr. G. and the other employees were greatly alarmed so he was taken to the hospital.

After a rather cursory assessment and without any investigations, the very busy intern at the hospital told Mr. G. what he considered his problem was and sent him home with a bottle of tablets to take if and when the condition returned.

Mr. G. reported to his general practitioner the next day. After careful assessment of the history it was apparent that he had suffered from a minor disability without any of the implications of the diagnosis made by the intern. However, from that day it was impossible to eradicate from his mind the positive diagnosis made in the emergency department, even despite thorough assessment by appropriate specialists.

He had several further similar episodes precipitated by disagreements with his employer. Finally he was dismissed from his employment. Subsequently, over a long period of counselling, Mr. G. was able to take on employment in a less stressful situation, but deep down he was obviously still anxious about his physical condition.

The company for which he originally worked subsequently went out of business because of unsatisfactory trading results. Mr. G. continues to attribute his 'illness' to the stresses of work. The failure of the company he feels is proof of the strain under which he was working. He has sought advice from his general practitioner on the advisability of seeking disability allowance under Worker's Compensation legislation for his illness.

1. What is or are the disease process/es exemplified here?
2. How does the general practitioner cope with the ongoing 'medical' problems created by others?
3. Are there any grounds for compensation for Mr. G. under the provisions of Worker's Compensation legislation?

D. A. Game, Adelaide

582   MRS. A.W.   AGED 74

Mrs. A.W. has been an insulin dependent diabetic for many years increasingly disabled by CCF, osteoarthritis and angina pectoris. Circulation in legs increasingly compromised with obvious evidence of occlusive vascular disease and neuropathy. Web space infection of foot difficult to clear. Admitted to hospital and left sympathectomy done with improvement in perfusion of leg but came home with pressure sore of heel. Mental and physical condition deteriorated rapidly and could no longer be nursed at home. Readmitted to hospital, septicaemia diagnosed. Deterioration of leg necessitated amputation. Post-operative myocardial infarct and despite all efforts died after some 2 weeks.

1. What complications of diabetes threaten life?
2. Does sympathectomy or bypass surgery have much place in treating vascular complications?

W. D. Jackson, Launceston, Australia

MASTER M.C.C.   AGED 6

583

This Chinese boy is taken to see the doctor because he has been 'falling all over the place' and is suffering from 'weakness of the knees'. According to Mrs. C., M.C. has been 'eating like a horse' and gaining a lot of weight. He also appears to be losing a lot of hair, and bruises easily.

After examining the boy, the doctor concluded that M.C. must be either suffering from Cushing's syndrome, or taking corticosteroids over a long period of time. On questioning the mother, she admitted that M.C. has been suffering from asthma for many years, and though he has been treated by private specialists and at government special clinics, his asthma has not been satisfactorily controlled.

Six months ago, a herbalist using his 'Magic Powder' 'cured' M.C.'s asthma. Mrs. C. informed the doctor that he was not to worry about M.C.'s asthma any more but that M.C. now required treatment for the 'weakness of his knees'.

1. What are the problems?
2. What is the role of the GP as a health educator?

N. C. L. Yuen, Hong Kong

Questions
and Sub-questions

MRS. T.　　AGED 30　　HOUSEWIFE　　　　　**1**

1. Why had Mrs. T. consulted the general practitioner six times in the past 3 weeks with her baby?
   a. What is the meaning and significance of the term 'high user'?
   b. What is meant by the child being 'the presenting symptom of the mother's illness' (Balint)?
   c. Why did the mother find it necessary to present her baby each time if she really wanted help with her own problems?
   d. Was Mrs. T. necessarily **aware** that she was wanting help for **herself** rather than her baby?
   e. What causes mothers to be over-concerned about their children's health?
   f. What is meant by the 'door-handle sign'?

2. What were the reasons for the baby's and the mother's insomnia?
   a. Can maternal depression affect a baby?
   b. What role do feelings of inadequacy as a mother play in causing post-partum depression?
   c. What role do marital and psycho-sexual problems play in causing post-partum depression?
   d. What feelings can a mother who is having difficulty relating to her baby be expected to experience?

3. How should the general practitioner manage this situation?
   a. Of what value is reassuring the mother that all is well with her baby?
   b. Should the GP refer the baby to a paediatrician in an effort to 'convince' the mother that her baby is healthy?
   c. Should the GP prescribe hypnotics or other psychotropics for the baby and/or the mother?
   d. How should the GP go about eliciting the patient's feelings about her situation?
   e. How should the GP respond if the patient expresses negative feelings towards her baby e.g. resentment, aggression, rejection?
   f. Is there any place for involving the patient's husband in the management?

S. Levenstein, Cape Town

MRS. E.S.　　AGED 30　　HOUSEWIFE　　　　　**2**

1. What disorder is she suffering from?
   a. How often do patients present with a minor problem which is not their main reason for coming? Why?
   b. What other information would you wish to obtain?

2. What is the prognosis of this condition and what are its risks?
   a. What are the risks to the mother?
   b. What are the risks to the infant?

3. How would you manage this condition?
   a. When is hospitalization indicated?
   b. Does chemotherapy help? Is it safe in a lactating woman?
   c. How would you counsel the mother? When would you see her again?
   d. Would you arrange to see her husband? What would you discuss with him?
   e. Would joint consultations be considered?

4. Why might she have dyspareunia?
   a. Is it likely to be due purely to psychological causes?
   b. What physical factors might she have after childbirth to cause this?
   c. Do hormonal factors play a part?

5. Does the baby have a sleep disorder? If so, how would you manage it?
   a. Should the baby sleep in the same room as the parents?
   b. Are sedatives indicated? If so, which one?
   c. When is hospitalization indicated?

H. C. Watts, Perth, Australia

3 JOHN McALISTER   AGED 9 MONTHS

1. Who is the 'patient' in this case?
   a. Is the 'patient' always the one presented to you?
   b. Would you describe John as 'sick'?
   c. Can there be more than one 'patient'?
   d. Is Mary exhibiting 'illness behaviour'?

2. How would you describe 'the problem(s)' in this case?
   a. What is a 'problem'?
   b. What is a 'diagnosis'?
   c. Is there a 'disease' involved?
   d. Can the problem(s) be labelled in one or two words?

3. Outline your management of this case.
   a. Is a stronger sedative for John indicated?
   b. Would referral to a paediatrician help?
   c. Would you give Mary a sedative?
   d. How would you involve Bill in your management?
   e. Who else in the community might you involve?

R. P. Strasser, Melbourne

MRS. A.B.   AGED 34   HOUSEWIFE

4

1. What sort of examination would you undertake?
   a. What are the indications for a routine physical examination in the first year of life?
   b. What are the indications for a psychomotor assessment? How many should be undertaken during the first five years of life and when?
   c. Does undergraduate or postgraduate training provide one with the knowledge and skills to do such assessments? If not, why not?
   d. What would you expect to find in such an examination of a 4 month old child?

2. Following a normal examination, what sort of questions would be a reasonable follow up?

3. Who is the patient?
   a. Do mothers usually present an apparently normal child to a doctor for a check at 4 months? Especially when the examination confirms the normal appearance of the child.
   b. What worries either about this child or another person might make a mother request such an examination?
   c. Should further questioning include – Is the child's immunization status appropriate?

4. Closer observation reveals that mother is very tired and anxious. How might you go about further questioning?
   'Mrs. A.B., she's really quite normal (assuming she is) for her age. Was there some special reason for bringing her?' (You might have asked this at the outset).

   OR

   'Mrs. A.B., you look very tired and a little worried. Is there something else with which I might be able to help?'.

5. The mother had had no sleep for almost 2 weeks, awakening at each movement or cough of the child at night for fear of another SIDS which occurred with her first child 9 years ago. Her marriage is becoming strained. What can you offer?
   a. What would you do about the marriage situation?
   b. Why might she not have been in contact with the local SIDS support group?
   c. How might you inquire and arrange help with this? Even if you don't feel it is your kettle of fish, it is clearly important to the health of this family.

A. J. Radford, Adelaide

5 MRS. M.L.   AGED 26   HOUSEWIFE

1. What do you understand by 'organization of disease'?
   a. Do you think any 'harm' could be done by the doctor ignoring this patient's shoulder?
   b. Does the fact that she never mentioned her shoulder again surprise you?
   c. Should the doctor make mention of this?
   d. What would the doctor's motivations and/or needs be for re-discussing the patient's shoulder?

2. What are the possible organic causes for a painful shoulder?
   a. How do you diagnose these?
   b. What diagnosis did the surgeon have in mind here?
   c. Do you think that the surgeon could have been 'pressured' by doctors and the patient?

3. Does depression often present through organic symptoms in family practice?
   a. What do you understand by the term 'masked depression'?
   b. What somatic symptoms are found in depression?
   c. Do you think there may be problems in Mrs. L.'s second marriage?
   d. Are the children at any special risk?
   e. Which child, if any, would be at greater risk?

4. What are the advantages and disadvantages of putting this (a young) patient on anti-depressants?
   a. What type of anti-depressants are available in your country?
   b. In which situation would you use one group instead of another?
   c. What are the side effects of anti-depressants?
   d. Is dosage standard in the administration of anti-depressants?
   e. What information would you provide to this patient about her being put on anti-depressants?

J. H. Levenstein, Cape Town

6 MRS. K.   AGED 18   SECRETARY

1. What was the patient's actual reason for coming to see the doctor?
   a. Why did the patient complain about her breasts?
   b. What are the possible problems facing this patient?

2. How should the GP manage this situation?
   a. What is the value of reassuring the patient that her breasts are normal?

b. What approach should the GP adopt to the patient's contraceptive status?

c. What approach should the GP adopt to the patient's sexual dysfunction?

d. Should the GP ask to see the patient's husband?

e. To what extent does this situation demonstrate the potential for preventive work in general practice?

f. What can the GP anticipate in respect of future consultations from this patient and/or her husband?

S. Levenstein, Cape Town

MARK B.   AGED 23   7

1. Why has Mark come to see you?
   a. Is Mark genuinely concerned about an infection?
   b. Could he be concerned about some other physical problem?
   c. Could he have some emotional problem?

2. With the story and findings what could be your attitude to this patient?
   a. Do you find yourself being angry or judgmental if
      - the patient thinks he has a physical problem and hasn't
      - a fit young man comes with a story you can't substantiate.

F. Mansfield, Perth, Australia

MRS. G.H.   AGED 26   HOUSEWIFE   8

1. Is it likely that the need for an annual check-up is the real reason for the visit?
   a. Would it be useful to suggest a follow-up visit?
   b. Would you consider speaking with the husband?
   c. Are there others who might be contacted who might shed some light on the reason for this patient's severe distress?

2. What sort of treatment, if any, would you offer?
   a. Would tranquillizers shorten the course of this 'illness'?
   b. Would anti-depressants shorten the course of this 'illness'?
   c. When would you consider referral to a psychiatrist in a situation like this?
   d. Is it possible that marital counselling might be useful?

3. Would you make use of the laboratory in managing this total situation?
   a. How often should women using IUCDs have a Pap. smear?
   b. Would a haemoglobin estimation and urinalysis be indicated?

    c.   With negative history and physical findings is it likely that thyroid function studies would be abnormal?

4.   Is it likely that this patient's distress is related to a normal grief reaction?
    a.   Might this patient have been having an affair with the deceased?
    b.   Might Mr. H. have been having an affair with the wife of the deceased?
    c.   Would you think the death might have been suicidal?
    d.   Would you think the death might have been homicidal?

G. G. Beazley, Winnipeg

9   MRS. V.   AGED 40   *AND*   GLORIA   AGED 18

1.   What significance (if any) may be attached to consultations when more than two people (patient and doctor) are present?
    a.   If you wanted to talk to Gloria on her own, how might this be accomplished without making her mother feel excluded?
    b.   What ethical and medico-legal issues are inherent in the situation described?

2.   What might prompt Gloria and Mrs. V. to consult at this time?
    a.   How does the family doctor cope with his own feelings when faced by continuing failure to relieve symptoms?
    b.   If Mrs. V. is using Gloria's continuing symptomatology as a 'cover story' to present problems of her own, you may need access to her record – how do family doctors organize and use records?

3.   What are common causes of nasal complaints such as Gloria's?
    a.   What features distinguish the various types of rhinitis from one another?
    b.   Could self medication be involved?

J. D. E. Knox, Dundee

10   MASTER C.M.   AGED 14   SCHOOLBOY

1.   What was Cecil's **actual** reason for consulting the GP?
    a.   Why did he find it necessary to complain about the scar when his real concern was elsewhere?
    b.   Why had he not asked the surgeon the questions he had asked the GP?
    c.   Why did he ask about the prosthesis?
    d.   What feelings might an adolescent undergoing this operation be expected to experience?

e.   Why did the surgeon make no attempt to anticipate Cecil's anxieties?

2.   How did the GP facilitate the expression of the patient's fantasies?
a.   What is the importance of confidentiality in relating to adolescents?
b.   What is the importance of 'permission' in enabling adolescents to express their feelings?
c.   To what extent do adolescents ordinarily divulge their feelings to a GP and why?

3.   How should the GP have responded when asked 'Will I ever be able to have children'?
a.   What was the patient's prognosis for fertility?
b.   What were the psychological implications for the patient of the question he had asked?

4.   What lasting psychological effects could the operation be expected to have on Cecil, if any?
a.   Has the surgeon failed in his treatment?
b.   Would the boy's mental state have any bearing on his reaction to the operation?
c.   Would parental attitudes have any bearing on his psychological adjustment to the operation?
d.   What role would the GP have in preventing psychological ill-effects from the operation?

S. Levenstein, Cape Town

MR. D.C.   AGED 46   BOOKKEEPER   11

1.   Do you agree with the doctor's use of home management for acute myocardial infarction (AMI) in this instance?
a.   What is the natural history of AMI?
b.   Would you have treated this patient's blood pressure?
c.   What do you think the doctor's medications could have been?
d.   When, where, and how often would you like to see this patient again?
e.   What are the electrocardiographic changes of acute myocardial infarction?

2.   What type of personality did this patient have?
a.   What alerted the doctor that something serious may be wrong?
b.   Does the long break between consultations have any significance?
c.   What defence mechanisms was the patient using in relation to his pain?
d.   Now that this condition has been diagnosed, do you think this patient will change his 'approach to life' unassisted?

   e.   How do you think he generally copes with his emotions and
        conflicts?

3.   Could anything have been done to prevent this attack?
   a.   What steps could you take to avoid this happening in your
        practice?
   b.   How would you recognize patients at risk?
   c.   What strategies would you use to screen and counsel them?

J. H. Levenstein, Cape Town

12   MS. J.R.   AGED 23   OFFICE SECRETARY

1.   What do you feel could be the problem/s in this consultation?
   a.   Do you feel the doctor was justified in not believing this was due
        to the pill?
   b.   What made him feel that it was not due to the pill?
   c.   Should he have conducted any further examinations or tests to
        rule out the possibility of the pill being the causative factor of
        this woman's presenting problems?
   d.   What is your approach when the signs and symptoms do not fit
        into a logical pattern?
   e.   What are the side effects of the contraceptive pill?

2.   Why do you think the patient burst out crying?
   a.   What is the significance of the patient crying?
   b.   What attitudes do you think the doctor used to catch the
        patient's mood?
   c.   Should you start something you can't finish or are not 'con-
        tracted' to undertake?
   d.   Do you think the doctor probed too deeply?

3.   What do you understand by the 'termination of a consultation'?
   a.   Do you feel that the doctor terminated this consultation appro-
        priately? too early? too late?
   b.   If too early, what should the doctor have done?
   c.   Should you ever leave a patient in this state at the end of a
        consultation?
   d.   What do you understand by 'offers'?
   e.   How would you generally terminate a consultation?

J. H. Levenstein, Cape Town

13   MRS. M.S.   AGED 26   SINGLE MOTHER

1.   What are the aetiological factors in this situation?
   a.   What do you understand by the term 'cycle of deprivation'?

b. What influence does poverty play in situations like this?

2. How would you handle this situation?
   a. How would you go about weaning her off medication?
   b. Would you give her sleeping tablets?
   c. How much time can you afford in counselling this family?
   d. Are social situations such as this really a family doctor's responsibility?

3. What social agencies would you use?
   a. What help can you get from social/welfare workers?
   b. Do 'self-help' groups assist such people?

R. W. Roberts, Ravensthorpe, Australia

MISS C.   AGED 12   SCHOLAR   14

1. What are the likely causes of C's refusal to attend school?
   a. What should be the basis of excluding organic disease?
   b. Are any investigations justified, and if so, which?
   c. What is the mechanism of psychosomatic illness in a child?

2. What would be your approach to elucidating this problem?
   a. What skills does the general practitioner require to persuade C. to talk to him?
   b. How can the general practitioner involve the father in elucidating the problem?
   c. Is the general practitioner justified in delving deeply into this family's dynamics?
   d. Should he directly discuss the problem with C.'s school teacher?
   e. Are there others who could assist?

3. What would be your approach to the management of this problem?
   a. What do you understand by family therapy?
   b. Who is the patient?
   c. Are there any other persons whose assistance you could enlist. Who are they, and in what way could they help?
   d. In plain practical terms, how do you get C. to go back to school?

D. A. Game, Adelaide

ROSEMARY C.   AGED 8   SCHOOLGIRL   15

1. What are the causes of bedwetting in an 8 year old girl?
   a. How does one distinguish on history between psychological and organic causes?
   b. Although this sounds psychological, should one do investigations, and if so which ones?

   c.   If the causes are psychological, which lines should be pursued?

   d.   Sexual interference could cause this, but incest is very rare: true or false?

2. Why should a bright and intelligent child like Rosemary be labelled as dull and stupid?

   a.   Are her home problems interfering with her school work?

   b.   Could she be suffering from a specific learning difficulty (dyslexia)?

3. What is Rosemary's real problem and how may it best be helped?

   a.   What are the early hallmarks of specific learning difficulty?

   b.   How is specific learning difficulty best managed?

   c.   What are the probable outcomes?

   d.   Which professionals can help a child whom one suspects has a special learning problem?

A. L. A. Reid, Newcastle, Australia

16 MASTER M.P.   AGED 2 YEARS

1. Is Mark retarded?

   a.   What is the most likely diagnosis?

   b.   How do you differentiate between autism and retardation.

   c.   Can a child be both autistic and retarded?

   d.   What other conditions must be excluded?

2. What is the single most important method of reaching a diagnosis?

   a.   What particular aspects of the history are important?

   b.   What characteristic features would you look for in Mark's behaviour?

   c.   How do autistic children react to changes and to other children?

3. What is the treatment of the condition?

   a.   Do psychotropic drugs help?

   b.   Is there a place for psychotherapy?

   c.   What is the long term prognosis for Mark?

   d.   Is this condition hereditary?

   e.   What agencies are available for help?

W. F. Glastonbury, Adelaide

17 MRS. A.B.   AGED 71   PENSIONER

1. What evidence is there for asthma being a psychosomatic disease?

   a.   Do you think the sex problem in Mrs. B.'s case could be the triggering factor in her late onset asthma?

b. If you made the above diagnosis, would you gradually withdraw her medications?

c. What additional stress had been placed on Mrs. B.?

2. What assessment tools are available to measure lung function in primary care?
   a. Is listening to the chest and taking a history a good enough assessment of lung function?
   b. Do you think Mrs. B. is on the 'right' treatment for her intractable asthma?
   c. What are the dangers and advantages of steroids in the treatment of asthma?
   d. What dosage schedule would you aim for in steroid management and why?
   e. Do more people die from under or over treatment of asthma?
   f. What is the advantage of beta 2 stimulant inhalants over oral therapy and vice versa?

3. Would you agree with the clinical assessment of Mrs. B.'s sexual status?
   a. If you were to initiate sex therapy in this patient, how would you go about it?
   b. What are common problems in sexual activity in elderly people and their possible management?

4. How do you feel the doctor should have responded to the fact that he was reputed to be 'wonderful'?
   a. What could this tell you about Mrs. B.'s personality?
   b. What are the dangers in inappropriate responses to Mrs. B.'s statement?

J. H. Levenstein, Cape Town

MISS L.T.   AGED 22   BALLET STUDENT   18

1. Is a consultation indicated?
   a. What are the implications of a referral to a psychiatrist to the patient, to the doctor, and to society?
   b. What are the risks and benefits of such a referral?
   c. Are there any non-psychiatric consultants in your area who might be appropriate?
   d. Are the implications of a referral to someone other than a psychiatrist any different?
   e. How should one prepare a patient for such a referral to ensure optimal results?

2. What are the therapeutic goals?

    a.   How much does the cost of treatment enter into your decision on management?

    b.   Is this a potentially life-threatening situation?

    c.   If a consultation is felt to be indicated how does one deal with the patient's refusal to be referred?

3.   When a family physician undertakes extensive psychotherapy with a patient, how does it affect the doctor–patient relationship?

    a.   Does it alter in any way his ability to deal with general medical problems?

E. Domovitch, Toronto

19   HILDA M.   AGED 58   HOUSEWIFE

1.   What explanation can be made of the processes going on in this relationship?

    a.   How much of the behaviour pattern could be due to the patient's medical and social history?

    b.   How much could be due to her husband's personality?

2.   How far should the general practitioner proceed in trying to unravel the possible psychological disturbances underlying the situation?

    a.   Does failure to proceed any further constitute the 'collusion' described by Balint?

    b.   Is acceptance of 'collusion' as a solution necessarily undesirable in all situations?

3.   What are the possible causes of dysuria and frequency in a patient of this age?

    a.   What examination should be made?

    b.   What investigations may be necessary?

    c.   Which drugs are most frequently used in the treatment of infections of the bladder?

J. G. P. Ryan, Brisbane

20   GRAHAM B.   AGED 50   BANK MANAGER

1.   How do you establish a therapeutic relationship with such a personality?

    a.   How can you weld the group of doctors involved into an effective and co-operative treatment team and who should lead it?

    b.   How much effort should you make to reach him and what priority should you give him in the many other claims on your time?

2. What are the likely psychodynamics?
   a. What factors in personality, upbringing, life pattern, work, home and social milieu would you consider significant?
   b. Should you explore them or leave it to the psychiatrist?
   c. How would you manage the anal problem that brought him to you?

3. What is the best approach to managing the total situation?
   a. At what point, if at all, should you raise personal issues as outlined above?
   b. Should you discuss the problem with his wife or seek further information from the other sources available in a small country town?

J. A. Stevens, Ulverstone, Australia

GWENDOLINE W.   AGED 69   HOUSEWIFE   21

1. Is she sick?
   a. Are further physical investigations necessary or wise?
   b. How far should you accept your specialist colleagues' conclusions and impressions?
   c. How do you define 'disease' in this context?

2. What is the diagnosis?
   a. Is a label useful to you or does it prejudice further management?
   b. Is a label useful to her? Does it give her symptoms 'respectability' or simply delay analysis and perhaps resolution.

3. How can you help?
   a. Is symptom relief (of pain, of anxiety) by medication justifiable?
   b. How far should you go in probing her personality, life history and situation in search of causes?
   c. Should you involve her husband and how?
   d. Does she require the psychiatrist to help?

J. A. Stevens, Ulverstone, Australia

MASTER B.   AGED 8   SCHOOLBOY   22

1. What was the cause of Michael's abdominal pain?
   a. How would you distinguish between organic and non-organic causes of abdominal pain?

    b.   Is psychogenic abdominal pain diagnosed only by excluding organic causes?

    c.   If the GP can find no organic cause for Michael's pain, would extensive investigations be indicated or justified?

    d.   Could Michael have been 'the presenting symptom of his mother's illness'?

    e.   Can children develop psychosomatic symptoms as a result of emotional stress in one or both parents or as a result of marital discord between the parents?

    f.   Will the child be likely to develop psychosomatic symptoms if the parents claim that there is no open quarrelling in front of him?

    g.   Can psychosomatic symptoms or illness in a child serve to divert attention away from the parents' marital conflicts?

2.   Why did Mrs. B. present with tension headaches?

    a.   Why do patients often present with somatic manifestations of underlying stress?

    b.   What feelings might Mrs. B. have been experiencing during her extra-marital affair, and could these have contributed to her tension headaches?

    c.   Why did the headaches persist after the extra-marital affair had terminated?

    d.   How can tension headaches be distinguished from organic causes of headache?

    e.   What hypotheses can be generated about the relationship between Mrs. B. and her husband?

    f.   Is there any connection between Mrs. B.'s symptoms and those of her son?

3.   How should the GP manage this situation?

    a.   How should the GP have reacted to being told about Mrs. B.'s extra-marital affair?

    b.   Is it appropriate for the GP to express his personal views about marital fidelity in this situation?

    c.   Is it appropriate to give advice in this situation?

    d.   Is it possible that the GP's ability to manage this situation could be affected if he is not in touch with his own feelings about sexual behaviour?

    e.   How can the GP stop the child from being the 'patient' in the family?

    f.   Should the GP attempt to involve Mrs. B.'s husband in the management?

    g.   How might any previous contact with Mr. B. affect his chances of involving him in this situation?

S. Levenstein, Cape Town

KARL Z.   AGED 2   **23**

1. What is the likely cause of the child's condition?
    a. What role does maternal anxiety and obsessiveness play in toilet training problems?
    b. How does the condition become established?
    c. What psychological problems can this condition create?

2. How can the situation be managed?
    a. What measures can be instituted immediately?
    b. What advice would you give mother?
    c. What opportunities for health promotion and preventive care does this situation present?

W. E. Fabb, Melbourne

MISS V.   AGED 18   TYPIST   **24**

1. Who was the patient, the 18 year old woman or her mother?
    a. Is the patient with the presenting complaint necessarily the one most in need of help?
    b. Why should a patient wanting help with her psychological problems come to see the GP with her daughter who has a physical complaint?
    c. What deductions can be made about the relationship between the mother and her daughter?

2. What is the diagnosis?
    a. Is the infective process (possibly precipitated by contact dermatitis from the deodorant) an adequate diagnosis?
    b. Does the mother's psychological state form part of the diagnosis?
    c. Is the mother–daughter relationship part of the diagnosis?
    d. Is the presence of the mother at her 18 year old daughter's visit to the doctor part of the diagnosis?

3. How would you manage this situation?
    a. Should the use of under-arm deodorants be discouraged in the presenting patient?
    b. Should antibiotics have been prescribed at the first consultation?
    c. Should the GP have acceded to the mother's request for tranquillizers?
    d. What psychotherapeutic approach should be adopted with the mother, the daughter, and the mother–daughter relationship?
    e. Why did the mother make a point of thanking the GP for his help at the end of the second consultation?

    f.   How should the GP have responded to the mother's expression of gratitude?

    g.   What can the GP anticipate in respect of future consultations by the patient and/or her mother?

S. Levenstein, Cape Town

25 MRS. J.   AGED 23   *AND*   BABY AGED 20 WEEKS

1. What further history or clinical information would you like?
    a.   Do you need to examine the baby?
    b.   Do you need to examine the mother?
    c.   Do you know enough about the mother's home circumstances?

2. What is your response to the tears?
    a.   Do you ignore the tears?
    b.   If you don't ignore them how do you react to them?
    c.   Do you ever touch patients of either sex to console them?

3. What is your management?

F. Mansfield, Perth, Australia

26 MRS. L.   AGED 40   HOUSEWIFE

1. How do you begin to manage this problem?
    a.   What governs your ability to manage the problem?
    b.   Should you involve the husband, if so how and when?
    c.   What does her problem list tell you?

2. Might it be better left alone?
    a.   Is there a point at which you do not try to resolve such a complex problem?
    b.   How is this point recognized?
    c.   When patients hide real problems behind a facade of functional symptoms, are they at risk?

3. What does the final statement suggest to you about (a) the patient; (b) her gynaecologist?
    a.   Enumerate some of the risks of such a statement in the case under discussion.
    b.   When does it profit a patient to have the defensive facade systematically dismantled?
    c.   Are there dangers in doing this?

W. D. Jackson, Launceston, Australia

MRS. ANNA N.   AGED 27   RECEPTIONIST

27

1. Why did the doctor seek details of her home life?
   a. What sort of questions are appropriate for exploring this?
   b. How does the doctor know when to ask these questions?
   c. Are there clues which patients give which invite exploration? Give examples.
   d. What significance would one place on the words, 'I was divorced.'?

2. What are the problems faced by divorced women?
   a. How easy is it for divorced women to meet suitable male companions?
   b. What are the hazards of being a divorced woman?
   c. What reactions do divorced women evoke from married women, married men, single men and their friends now married?
   d. What are the emotional problems consequent to divorce?

3. What response should the doctor make to self-deprecating remarks?
   a. What is the meaning to the patient of the expression, 'blubbering female'?
   b. What other self-deprecating remarks have you heard females use?
   c. What actions could or should the clinician take when such remarks are made?
   d. Can such remarks be used for exploring self-image and self-esteem?

4. How could one manage this situation in a 10 minute consultation?
   a. How does one avoid completely missing the emotional component of an interview, especially when the presenting symptom is physical?
   b. How does one avoid a superficial exploration of emotional aspects in a short interview?
   c. Are there any key questions or techniques which facilitate rapid but meaningful exploration of emotional issues?
   d. What alternative strategies does the doctor have if time constraints are severe?

W. E. Fabb, Melbourne

MRS. FRANCINE S.   AGED 29   HOUSEWIFE

28

1. The consultation appears to have been very effective to the present time. What has made it so?
   a. What skills has this doctor demonstrated?

b. Would the use of these skills during all consultations enhance both your efficiency and diagnostic processes? If the answer is 'yes', why?

c. Are you competent in the skills demonstrated by this doctor? If not, where would you learn such skills?

d. What kinds of things do general practitioners commonly do during the consultation which delays, or prevents them from ascertaining the patient's 'real' concern?

2. What would you 'do' next?
    a. Do we always have to initiate some action during the consultation in order to be effective?
    b. How do we demonstrate empathy?
    c. How do you react to patients who cry during the consultation?

M. W. Heffernan, Melbourne

29 MRS. M.S.   AGED 71   HOUSEWIFE

1. How do you explain this patient's behaviour?
    a. Why has she waited so long to report this?
    b. Has she seriously tried to correct the glycosuria herself?
    c. Does she feel guilty, or that she has failed?
    d. How do you elicit a patient's fears?
    e. Is she afraid that she will have to have insulin injections?
    f. Is insulin indicated here, or another hypoglycaemic?

2. What are the possible causes of her loss of control?
    a. Has she strayed off her diet intentionally or unintentionally?
    b. Her husband is a 'difficult' man. Could the problem be related to stress?
    c. Could another latent disease or infection be the cause?
    d. Is she intentionally or unintentionally concealing symptoms of another disease for fear of the diagnosis?
    e. Has there been some change of life-style?

3. Are any further investigations indicated?
    a. What investigations would you perform?
    b. How extensive a physical examination is indicated?
    c. What short term complications can you expect if this poor control continues?

W. F. Glastonbury, Adelaide

30 MRS. C.B.   AGED 30   HOUSEWIFE

1. Who is the patient in this situation?
    a. What effect does the mother's state of mind have on the baby?

    b.   Which child-rearing practices are helpful and which are counter-productive in ensuring a happy, contented child who will develop normally?

2.   What are the causes of 'wind', 'colic' and irritability in babies under 7 months old.
    a.   What difference, if any, is there between breast-fed and bottle-fed babies in this regard?
    b.   What medicines might be helpful in this situation?
    c.   Which serious conditions should be excluded if these symptoms persist?

3.   What risks are inherent in this situation?
    a.   What are the characteristics and circumstances of parents who harm their children?
    b.   How would you assess the risk of non-accidental injury to a child?
    c.   How would you assess the risk of a suicide gesture in a patient under stress?

4.   What measures could you take to help this family?
    a.   What do you, as a doctor, have to offer?
    b.   What other agencies are available to help? How do you contact them?
    c.   What would you expect them to provide?

E. C. Gambrill, Crawley, UK

MR. E.S.   AGED 42   TRUCK DRIVER   **31**

1.   Why did the GP not test for glycosuria at the first consultation?
    a.   Should the urine be tested routinely at all first consultations?
    b.   Was there any indication for testing the patient's urine from the history?
    c.   Did the delay in testing the urine have any effect on the outcome of the patient's illness?

2.   Was a provisional diagnosis of myocardial ischaemia justified at the end of the first consultation?
    a.   What is the relative importance of history and physical examination in diagnosing myocardial ischaemia?
    b.   To what extent was this history suggestive of myocardial ischaemia?
    c.   Of what value is the ECG in assessing patients with chest pain?

3.   Of what importance was the patient's psycho-social background in the diagnosis and management of the patient's problems?

    a. Could the history of alcoholism have had any bearing on the onset of the illness?

    b. Could the patient's imminent marriage have played a part in the onset of the illness?

    c. Could the patient's work situation have contributed to his condition?

4. Why was the patient's compliance poor?

    a. What information about his personality and behaviour may have made non-compliance more likely in his case?

    b. What role could the side-effects of anti-diabetic drugs have in causing non-compliance?

    c. What is the importance of the doctor–patient relationship in determining patient compliance?

5. How would you manage this situation further?

    a. Under what circumstances is a switch to treatment by insulin injection indicated?

    b. How should the GP attempt to establish a relationship which would improve the chances of the patient's compliance being better?

    c. To what extent is patient compliance the responsibility of the GP?

    d. What attitude should the GP adopt to the patient's obesity?

    e. What approach should the GP adopt to the patient's relationship with his fiancé?

    f. What approach should the GP adopt to the patient's work situation?

    g. What assessment can the GP make of the patient's personality and how would this affect his overall management?

S. Levenstein, Cape Town

32 MR. A.O.S.   AGED 67   PENSIONER

1. How does a GP come to terms with an intense feeling of animosity towards his patient?

    a. Could the patient's manner be a facade for inadequacy?

    b. Is it reasonable to accept incompatibility and work towards a break?

    c. How aware are patients of our feelings towards them?

    d. What prospects are there of this patient establishing a mutually happy relationship with any doctor?

    e. If the answer is 'none' should one be prepared to take the rough with the smooth?

    f. Should his obvious physical incapacity affect the issue?

g. What effect do harmful attitudes have on the clinical quality of the consultation?

2. How does a GP distinguish between the wants and needs of his patient?
   a. Does topical addiction (with withdrawal rebound) to steroids exist as a clinical entity?
   b. How often is the vehicle in a topical medication the therapeutic agent?
   c. How often is response to topical medication merely a placebo effect?
   d. If two anti-inflammatory drugs (aspirin and ibuprofen) are being given simultaneously is it possible that one is unnecessary?
   e. In the doses used in this patient, could either or both be acting merely as a placebo?
   f. If a single morning dose of an anti-inflammatory agent appears to produce benefit, how is one certain that the reduction in symptoms later that day were not merely a feature of the illness?

3. How does a GP effectively apportion his time in this type of situation?
   a. What proportion of time should go into history taking, examination, prescription writing, patient education, and so on?
   b. When can a physical examination be omitted?
   c. Is it reasonable to ask one's staff to give longer appointments to 'difficult' patients?
   d. When is it reasonable to ask the patient to book another appointment for his less pressing problems?
   e. How much longer does it take not to write a prescription than to write one?

D. Levet, Hobart

BRIAN M.   AGED 55   33

1. How would you manage Brian in the rest of the consultation?
   a. Would a physical examination be helpful?
   b. Would you prescribe any medication? If so, what?

2. What is the most likely diagnosis?
   a. Is it likely to be physical, psychological, or both?

3. How would you manage Brian in the next few weeks?
   a. What would the likely effect be on his work?
   b. What would the likely effect be on his marriage?
   c. Might any other professionals be helpful in this case?

J. C. Hasler, Oxford

34 MRS. P.A. AGED 44 INVALID PENSIONER

1. What is the differential diagnosis?
   a. What features of depression would you look for?
   b. What endocrine disorder, if any, should be excluded?

2. What further information would you want?
   a. Is family history important?
   b. What, if any, special investigations would help elucidate the problem?

3. How would you manage this patient?
   a. Would referral to a psychiatrist help?
   b. What is the role of drug therapy?
   c. What social agencies would you use?

R. W. Roberts, Ravensthorpe, Australia

35 MRS. H. AGED 83 HOUSEWIFE

1. What do you consider to be the main problem?
   a. List the physical, psychological, family problems evident and implicit in this situation.
   b. What is the natural history of low backache in family practice?
   c. What blood tests, if any, would you have done in this patient?
   d. What are the risks of depression in a patient of this age?

2. What would your two priorities be in the management of this patient?
   a. What do you understand by counselling?
   b. What counselling techniques do you know of?
   c. Which one would you use in this situation?
   d. How do you see the role of anti-inflammatory drugs in this situation?
   e. Would you prescribe an anti-depressant?
   f. How would you cope with her anger 'at no one taking notice of her' and 'doctors not making her better'?

3. What do you understand by 'limit-setting'?
   a. What would you tell this patient about future visits from you and your clinic?

J. H. Levenstein, Cape Town

36 MRS. D.B. AGED 48 MEDICAL PRACTITIONER'S WIFE

1. What other information would you wish to obtain from her?

2. What is the nature of the problem?

    a.   Who is the patient – the wife, the doctor or the relationship?
    b.   What disorders could Dr. A.B. be suffering from?
    c.   How much credence can be put on the views of one partner in an inharmonious marriage?

3.   How would you manage the problem?
    a.   How does the fact that he is a doctor influence your management?
    b.   How would you counsel the wife?
    c.   Should you be directive in circumstances like these?
    d.   Should you approach Dr. A.B. – if so, when and how?

4.   What problems do doctors and their families have in obtaining medical care?
    a.   Does the medical background influence the way other doctors treat a doctor and his family? Should it?
    b.   To what extent should doctors treat their own families?
    c.   Do doctors have problems adopting the 'patient' role?

5.   How should doctors reconcile the immediate demands of their work with the needs of their families?

H. C. Watts, Perth, Australia

K.L.   AGED 17   STUDENT   **37**

1.   How high a suicidal risk is this patient?
    a.   Is the rate of teenage suicide higher or lower than average?
    b.   How would you assess his suicide potential?

2.   What types of pressure contribute to stress at this age?
    a.   Do teenagers need to conform?
    b.   How do parents pressure their children?
    c.   What other expectations are placed on teenagers?

3.   What other sources are available to assess the situation?
    a.   Would you talk to his parents?
    b.   Would you call the school?
    c.   Can his peers help him?

4.   How would you proceed to manage his depression?
    a.   Do anti-depressants help these cases?
    b.   What criteria would you use to decide on a referral or hospital admission?

E. V. Dunn, Toronto

38 MALCOLM R.   AGED 16   STUDENT

1. The increasing pressure of senior school examinations during the
    past six months has seen Malcolm requiring more and more frequent
    injections, usually of dihydroergotamine, Maxolon and pethidine.
    What should be the GP's major concerns for this boy?
    a. What factors should be explored by the family doctor in
        thoroughly reappraising Malcolm's problem?
    b. Are there any appropriate investigations that should be
        considered?
    c. What matters should be discussed with Malcolm's mother?

2. Malcolm is an intelligent lad and has good insight into the relation-
    ship between the emergence of his migraine and the family break up.
    He has tried all the known drug regimes and is very much aware of
    the risks he runs if the current situation continues. What therapeutic
    strategies are available to his family doctor?
    a. Malcolm has disclosed that his mother has made several suicide
        attempts since her divorce and that he has lived in fear as a
        result. In what way should the doctor respond to this revelation?
    b. Malcolm is deeply religious but is a 'loner' in his fellowship
        group at church. He needs friends but has difficulty relating in
        a meaningful way with his peers. What, if anything, can
        Malcolm's general practitioner do to help him develop the
        relationships he clearly recognizes as important?
    c. Malcolm's religious convictions are presently narrow and rigid.
        He is suspicious of psychotherapists and distrusts such alter-
        natives as hypnotherapy. Given that these may be important
        therapeutic alternatives, what could be done to encourage
        Malcolm's interest in them and to gain his acceptance of them as
        meaningful treatments?

W. L. Ogborne, Sydney

39 MR. J.A.C.   AGED 18   STUDENT

1. How might a GP feel when confronted by such a referral request?
    a. What factors govern medical referrals from GP to specialist?
    b. What is the difference between a consultant and a specialist?
    c. Should the GP convey his feelings to the specialist?
    d. Should the GP convey his feelings to the patient?
    e. Should the GP attempt to define the problem prior to referral?
    f. What are the indications for psychiatric referral?
    g. Is psychological medicine too time consuming for general prac-
        titioner involvement?

2. What are the possible reasons to explain the 'depression'?

a. Is depression before final exams more likely to be caused by working too hard or not working hard enough?

b. What is the relationship between intellect and motivation?

c. How common is endogenous depression at this age?

d. Is being told that one is a failure likely to bring out the best or the worst in an adolescent?

e. Would the assessment be altered by the patient having a smiling face rather than a sad one? If so, in what way?

3. What aspects of health promotion/preventive medicine apply to this situation?

a. Does smoking have any special significance in a person with ankylosing spondylitis?

b. Do adolescents from broken homes have any particular predisposition to alcoholism?

c. Does sexual awakening have any bearing on educational failure at the end of secondary schooling?

d. What part do secondary schoolboys play in the epidemiology of unplanned pregnancy and sexually transmitted disease?

e. Does counselling reduce the incidence of future marital breakdown in adolescents from broken homes?

f. Can anything be done to slow down the progress of ankylosing spondylitis?

g. What genetic counselling could be applied to this family in respect of ankylosing spondylitis?

D. Levet, Hobart

JOHN P.   AGED 48   SCHOOLMASTER   40

1. What is your immediate action (a) on receipt of the first call? (b) on receipt of the second call?

a. What are your criteria for estimating the possibility of suicide?

b. Is admission for observation appropriate on his return given that the son's police training has accustomed him to dealing with the drunk?

c. Is sedation appropriate, and if so, what?

2. What is your further plan of management?

a. Of the three problems mentioned (money, health and work) which would you give priority in exploration?

b. How would you deal with the distress of both family and patient over this wholly uncharacteristic behaviour?

c. What sort of answer would you give to enquiries from the school authorities about his suitability for, and likely continuance of, his present job?

3. What prognosis can you give?
  a. What factors would you consider in giving a prognosis?

J. A. Stevens, Ulverstone, Australia

41 MR. J.L. AGED 55 STORE PROPRIETOR

1. What is the cause of this patient's headaches?
  a. Is headache a common feature of hypertension?
  b. What are the characteristics of headaches due to hypertension?
  c. Are there any other possible causes of this patient's headaches?
  d. What additional questions might help to clarify the cause?

2. What is the effect of medical treatment on the natural history of hypertension?
  a. What are the possible complications of untreated hypertension?
  b. Which complications can be reduced by effective treatment?
  c. What are the criteria of effective treatment?
  d. What clinical or epidemiological surveys have been published which support your answers to these questions?

3. How would you plan your management of this patient?
  a. What factors would influence your utilization of further investigations and laboratory tests?
  b. What is the role of diet in his management?
  c. What factors would influence your choice of medications?
  d. How often would you follow-up this patient?
  e. What aspects would you clarify and examine at follow-up visits?

4. What are the possible implications of your treatment for the patient and his family?
  a. Physical activity?
  b. Work conditions?
  c. Social habits?
  d. Sexual behaviour?

M. R. Polliack, Tel-Aviv, Israel

42 MR. JOHN T. AGED 43 SMALL BUSINESS PROPRIETOR

1. How common is alcoholism?
  a. Discuss hidden ways alcoholism may present.
  b. What medical problems are associated?
  c. What psychological problems may precipitate it?
  d. Would you expect a background history of similar problems in the family?

2. How would you approach this situation?
   a. Discuss the pros and cons of direct confrontation.
   b. If he agrees to a 'drying out', describe how you would set about this.
   c. What advice should you give to his family?
   d. Would you involve a specialist in his treatment?
   e. If so – how and for what reason?

3. What agencies exist in the community to help?
   a. Discuss the role of AA – ALANON – ADA and how and when they can be involved.
   b. In long term follow up, have these agencies a particular value?

4. What tests would you do?
   a. Discuss the value of blood alcohol levels and liver function tests in diagnosis and treatment.

5. During withdrawal what additional therapies can be used?
   a. What is the role of Hemineurin (chlormethiazole) and diazepam?
   b. What is the role of vitamins?
   c. Discuss the pros and cons of Antabuse (disulfiram).

6. What long term prognosis would you offer?
   a. What factors affect long term prognosis?
   b. Do you feel the doctor's personal interest and support bear a relationship to relapse?

K. C. Nyman, Perth, Australia

MRS. D.F.   AGED 57   RETIRED TEACHER   **43**

1. What may have caused these psychiatric symptoms?
   a. Do psychological stresses cause this kind of problem?
   b. Is this bizarre thinking a form of schizophrenia; if it is, does that knowledge help?
   c. The 'lesion' seems to have been vascular rather than neoplastic. Is this relevant? How can we further clarify its nature?

2. What special difficulties arise from living with a passive dependent alcoholic?
   a. Do the spouses of alcoholics collude with them to ensure which one gets the abnormal label?

3. What approach should one take in talking to someone who can carry out an entirely rational discussion about a system of beliefs which seem totally irrational?

    a.   How can one tell that she is not describing real events?

    b.   Should one use diagnostic labels like 'schizophrenia'?

4.   What part do psychotropic drugs play in this kind of problem?

    a.   Why should *she* take drugs anyway – her husband has the problem?

    b.   Which class of drugs may be helpful?

    c.   If the 'lesion' were a slow growing tumour rather more anterior than this one, it just might cause the symptoms; would drugs be of any help in that case?

A. L. A. Reid, Newcastle, Australia

44   MRS. E.G.   AGED 82   AGED PENSIONER

1.   When do you suspect someone has an alcohol problem?

    a.   What is the definition of alcoholism?

    b.   What physical, mental and social effects of excessive alcohol consumption might she show?

    c.   Would you endeavour to get her to reduce her alcohol consumption? How?

2.   What could you do to help this couple to manage at home?

    a.   What community facilities do you have available?

    b.   What alterations to her home might help her?

    c.   What drug therapy might help her?

3.   Should doctors play a role in forming community attitudes towards social problems such as alcohol and tobacco? How?

4.   What is the value of home visits?

    a.   What information can you obtain which is not obtainable in a surgery consultation?

    b.   How often do you do home visits?

    c.   What type of patient do you most frequently visit?

H. C. Watts, Perth, Australia

45   MR. A.   AGED 62   CUSTOMS OFFICER

1.   What was the syndrome that Mr. A. was suffering from?

    a.   What is the incidence of alcoholism in your community?

    b.   What proportion of hospital admissions are alcohol related?

    c.   What are the common physical effects of alcoholism?

    d.   What occupations are at greatest risk of alcoholism?

    e.   What is the prognosis of Korsakow's syndrome?

    f.   If there was an external ocular muscle palsy what would the diagnosis be?

2. What principles would you observe in the management of alcoholism?
   a. What do you regard as the general practitioner's role in the management of alcoholism?
   b. What do you understand are the features of Wernicke's encephalopathy?
   c. How would you define alcoholism?
   d. What is the role of confrontation in the management of alcoholism?
   e. What agencies might be used to assist in the management of this man?
   f. Would he be eligible for any form of Worker's Compensation benefits?

J. G. Richards, Auckland

MRS. B.W.　AGED 55　　46

1. What do you think is the importance of the duration of the symptom?
   a. Does the absence of physical signs except excoriation exclude an organic diagnosis?
   b. Would you carry out any pathological investigations?
   c. Would you do any examination other than perineal or vulvo-vaginal?

2. Could this lady's social history be of importance?
   a. How do you manage itch of probable emotional origin?

F. Mansfield, Perth, Australia

MRS. E.I.　AGED 68　WIDOWED PENSIONER　　47

1. Under what circumstances should a doctor accept a request from another person to visit a patient?

2. How can you conduct an interview with this patient?
   a. Do you have access to an interpreter?
   b. Have you had training in the use of a medical interpreter?
   c. How will she follow instructions about any medication prescribed?

3. What other arrangements will you have to make concerning her welfare?
   a. How will she cope with shopping?
   b. How will she cope with meals/cooking?
   c. How will she cope with housekeeping?

    d. How will she cope with finances?

    e. Would you anticipate any problems related to medication?

4. Is her probable 'isolation' likely to cause any problems?
    a. Could lack of contact cause depression?
    b. Can visits from suitable people speaking her language be arranged?
    c. Can outings be arranged?

D. U. Shepherd, Melbourne

48 MRS. K.T.   AGED 49   HOUSEWIFE

1. What is the likely diagnosis?
    a. Could the problem be iatrogenic? i.e. What the doctor said and/or prescribed?
    b. Is hyperthyroidism a distinct possibility, even in the absence of eye signs?
    c. How do you clinically distinguish between an anxiety state and hyperthyroidism?

2. How would you manage this problem?
    a. Would it be appropriate to contact the previous doctor?
    b. Should you refer her for multi-phasic screening?
    c. Should you organize thyroid function tests?
    d. Should you comply with the previous doctor's opinion?

3. What are special problems faced by immigrants?
    a. Are migrants with genuine organic diseases disadvantaged when consulting 'foreign' doctors?
    b. Should ethnic doctors be freely available for these special groups?
    c. Is there a significant difference in disease patterns between national groups?

J. E. Murtagh, Melbourne

49 MRS. MARGARET C.   AGED 55   HOUSEWIFE

1. How would you cope with this immediate situation?
    a. Should you hand her some 'tissues', tell her to have a good cry and go on with the consultation when she is ready?
    b. Should you postpone the consultation and tell Margaret to come back when you have more time?
    c. Should you patiently take a full history there and then?

2. People commonly hold incorrect views about the role of vitamins in health. As doctors, should we always dissuade them?
   a. Discuss the placebo effect. Would you ever use vitamins to obtain this effect?
   b. Would thiamine in fact be likely to help this patient?
   c. Which groups in the population need vitamin supplements and why?
   d. Do doctors have a health education role to counter the massive propaganda for vitamins and tonics?

3. Your detailed history reveals Margaret as a recent migrant without relations in this city and living apart from her husband. In addition she is menopausal. Would these facts influence your probable diagnosis and treatment?
   a. Discuss depression in the menopause.
   b. What are common precipitating causes of 'reactive depression'?
   c. Would your attitude be optimistic in this case?

4. What avenues of therapy would you consider in this case?
   a. Is psychotherapy valuable?
   b. How would you use anti-depressants in such a case?
   c. Could oestrogen replacement therapy have a role?
   d. Since involvement could be the key to this lonely lady's life, what positive steps could you take to help her achieve this?

K. C. Nyman, Perth, Australia

MRS. K.L.   AGED 28   HOUSEWIFE   50

1. What is your response to this cry for help?
   a. What is your responsibility in a case like this?
   b. How can you best give help to the woman?
   c. What avenues are open to you to obtain protection for her?

2. How do you think the husband will respond to you if you intervene in this situation?
   a. Do you think that you are putting yourself in danger?
   b. You admit the patient to hospital as there is no other available route to protect her. The husband subsequently gets drunk and shoots himself through the chest with a rifle. He is in a small house in town and the police call you to go out with them to attend him. He still has the rifle. How will you handle this situation?

J. K. Shearman, Hamilton, Canada

51 MRS. V.C.   AGED 29   HOUSEWIFE

1. How much investigation does the present problem require?
   a. Should her sexual relations be discussed?
   b. What initial examination and tests would you perform?
   c. Should she be referred to a fertility clinic?
   d. When should her husband be brought into the discussion?

2. What questions does the diagnosis 'salpingitis' raise?
   a. Is venereal disease an important cause in general practice?
   b. Should salpingitis be treated at home?
   c. What investigations are needed?
   d. Should the patient have been referred to a VD clinic?

3. What does her history reveal of her personality?
   a. Can you predict anything about her relations with her parents and husband?
   b. Would simple psychoanalytic probing be helpful?
   c. Would she respond to simple reassurance?

J. Grabinar, Bromley, UK

52 MRS. C.A.   AGED 28

1. What is your initial response to this request?
   a. What ground rules do you set down for this decision-making process?
   b. How important to your assessment is the age of your patients?
   c. Would you be party to sterilization if you had talked with only one partner?

2. How would you follow this through?
   a. Do you feel the husband should be involved in discussion?
   b. What determines which partner is sterilized?

W. D. Jackson, Launceston, Australia

53 DAVID J.   AGED 27   COMPANY EXECUTIVE

1. What steps should the doctor take to define the cause of David's symptoms?
   a. What elements of history taking are critical to the definition of the problem?
   b. If after thorough history taking and physical examination the cause of the symptoms is thought to be emotional stress, what investigations, if any, are warranted?

    c.   If it is decided to proceed on the basis of the history and physical examination without recourse to further tests, what therapeutic strategies could be employed in order to promote David J's recovery?

2.   What is the doctor's responsibility to David's previous doctor?
    a.   Should he be informed that David has sought a second opinion?
    b.   If it is decided to notify the doctor previously consulted, how could this best be done? What would be the nature of that communication?
    c.   What ethical considerations govern the patient's request for a second opinion and the relationship between the patient and both doctors created by such circumstances?

3.   Should the doctor consulted for a second opinion learn that David has also sought the help of a hypnotherapist, what influence will this have on the consultation?
    a.   Should the doctor contact the hypnotherapist?
    b.   Is it appropriate to inform David's previous doctor of these facts?
    c.   Is it appropriate to pass on findings and clinical assessment to the hypnotherapist?
    d.   Is it appropriate to seek an opinion from the hypnotherapist as to the patient's problem and is it appropriate to ask the hypnotherapist for details of the strategies being employed?

W. L. Ogborne, Sydney

MRS. E.M.   AGED 43   HOUSEWIFE   **54**

1.   What is the value of psychotherapy in such cases?
    a.   Are there risks in probing this patient's unconscious thoughts?
    b.   Is psychotherapy helpful?
    c.   Does ordinary psychiatry help, and how?

2.   Why does she come every month?
    a.   Is a regular contact of therapeutic value or does it perpetuate the illness?
    b.   Should her treatment be continued indefinitely?
    c.   What feelings are aroused in doctors by such patients?

3.   What non-medical help can be offered?
    a.   Are there self-help groups for patients with obsessional neuroses?
    b.   How can her family and friends co-operate in her care?
    c.   Is she likely to recover?

J. Grabinar, Bromley, UK

55 MR. R.P.   AGED 38   MUNICIPAL WORKER/LAVATORY
                             ATTENDANT

1. What facts about the natural history of schizophrenia are illustrated
    by this story?
    a. To what degree are age, pre-morbid personality, and gender
        predictive of the outcome of a first diagnosis of schizophrenia?
        What is meant by the 'theory of social drift'?
    b. What are the risks and advantages of injected drugs in the
        management of schizophrenia?
    c. What are the side-effects of phenothiazines? Is flupenthixol
        decanoate a phenothiazine? Do you have any views about
        dependence and autonomy and the rights of schizophrenics?

2. What do you understand by 'the collusion of anonymity'?
    a. What can be done to avoid a patient being the subject of a
        collusion of anonymity? Does such a collusion indicate things
        about the patient, or about the doctor, or about both? Is social
        deviance illness?

P. Freeling, London

56 MS. H.S.   AGED 30

1. When do you first start to worry about this mother's potential
    parenting skills?
    a. Is it possible to predict which persons may have trouble with
        parenting?
    b. If you suspect there may be trouble, what can you do about it?
    c. What rights have the mother and the father in this case?
    d. What rights has society to take care of the child?

2. What factors are important in deciding to remove the child from its
    parents' care?
    a. What evidence has to be available in order to justify removal?
    b. Is there a better way of handling this?

3. Having removed this child from the parents, what can one do about
    subsequent children?
    a. Does your country have a network to follow such parents?
    b. Do we have the right to sterilize parents who have great diffi-
        culties with parenting?

Follow up note: This mother subsequently had a child which she took to
another province in Canada with another father and we heard she had
gouged the child's eyes out.

J. K. Shearman, Hamilton, Canada

MRS. J.R.   AGED 48   HOUSEWIFE   **57**

1. Mrs. J.R. presents with a somatic complaint for which no obvious pathology is found. Is this a common way for a life stress problem to present?
   a. Do patients find it difficult to present the doctor with problems of a personal nature?
   b. How can we make it easier for them?
   c. How should we deal with the somatic complaints?

2. When faced with marital complaints, is it your job as a physician to help them stay together or help them to part?
   a. What may be the role of the family physician in dealing with marital problems?
   b. Who else might he call upon for help?
   c. What should be the nature of that help?

3. What do you think Mrs. J.R. will feel on learning of her husband's death?
   a. She refused to talk to him last night when he called in a drunken state. How will this affect her feelings about his death?
   b. Do you have any predictions about her future course in life?

J. K. Shearman, Hamilton, Canada

MRS. I.M.   AGED 57   **58**

1. What do you think is the major problem that has to be dealt with in this lady?
   a. Is there any way you can put all these complaints together?
   b. What can we offer Mrs. I.M.?
   c. Do you think it possible to produce a change in her way of dealing with her life?

2. What do you think is the most efficient way for the health care system to handle the kind of problem this lady has?
   a. Who do you think should co-ordinate the multiple problems Mrs. I.M. has?
   b. Is this the kind of patient you would like to have in your practice?

3. How would you approach each of the medical problems she presents with?
   a. We found that over the last eight years Mrs. I.M. had had 10,000 millirems of radiological investigations. Is this acceptable?
   b. Is there a cumulative risk from repeated investigations?

J. K. Shearman, Hamilton, Canada

59 MRS. G.R.   AGED 47   HOME DUTIES

1. How may a busy GP properly manage this first interview?
   a. Is one option the refusal to prescribe further tablets?
   b. Should the existing tablets be increased in dose or changed to a different type?
   c. Is there any urgency to investigate the problem?

2. What is the predominant cause of insomnia seen in general practice in this age and sex group?
   a. Should organic conditions be excluded first or is this unnecessary at this stage?
   b. Are any investigations necessary other than a full history and brief physical examination?
   c. Is it necessary to offer a definitive treatment at this first consultation?

3. What strategies are available in the long term management of this problem?
   a. Is this a problem that can properly be managed by a GP?
   b. What group of allied health professionals may be of assistance in management?
   c. What alternative strategies to drug therapy are available?

T. D. Manthorpe, Port Lincoln, Australia

60 MR. D.N.   AGED 49   INVALID, LIVES AT HOME

1. What is the cause of his left-sided paralysis?
   a. What investigations might be needed to establish a diagnosis in this case?
   b. When should they be done?
   c. Where should they be done?

2. What physical problems could be responsible for the hemiplegia?
   a. What premonitory symptoms might have indicated that this man had a physical problem?
   b. Assuming that in this case the reason for the hemiplegia is physical, what long-term complications might be expected?
   c. What is the long-term outlook for the hemiplegia?

3. Who is responsible for this patient's care?
   a. What support services should be used to help him and his family?
   b. How will his accommodation need to be altered to help him?
   c. What is the role of the hospital in the care of this patient?
   d. How will the family's strong religious beliefs affect the overall management of the patient?

e. How can this man be made to feel more independent?
f. If he feels threatened by a member of the caring team, what should be done?

4. How often do family stresses contribute to physical illness?
   a. What should be done to help this man's wife?
   b. How will the two retarded boys be educated and employed?
   c. How will all the boys cope with an invalid father who requires that they help him rather than the usual expectation of him being there to help them?
   d. How available should the general practitioner be to help in the care of a family like this?

B. H. Connor, Armidale, Australia

MR. L.M.   AGED 29   BIRD FANCIER   61

1. When is an invalid not an invalid?
   a. What artificial aids are available for people with limb deficiencies?
   b. Who takes the overall responsibility for the care of a person with a chronic physical handicap?
   c. How often do medical practitioners cause chronic invalidism through unawareness of the total problem?
   d. How can assistance be arranged for someone who is physically handicapped but of normal intelligence?
   e. How can an invalid be trained to be a useful and satisfied member of the community?

2. How can the effects of long-term hospitalization be minimised in a young person with a chronic disability?
   a. What community facilities are available to circumvent hospitalization?
   b. What transport systems are required to take a disabled person to centres for treatment or entertainment?
   c. What can be done to help the family of a person with a chronic disability when it has been decided to continue treatment at home?

3. What is alcoholism?
   a. How punitive should society be as far as alcohol is concerned?
   b. How often is alcoholism a symptom of family stresses?
   c. What techniques can a primary care doctor use to help a person who appears to be developing a dependence on alcohol?
   d. How does a doctor confront a patient who consumes excessive amounts of alcohol?

B. H. Connor, Armidale, Australia

62 MRS. O. AGED 53 HOUSEWIFE

1. Why did the general practitioner supervisor say that physiotherapy would be as unsuccessful as the anti-inflammatory drugs?
   a. What are the possible problems leading to these symptoms?
   b. How would you approach the task of elucidating the possible basis of the symptoms?
   c. What is the relationship of the X-ray findings to the symptoms presented?

2. What would have been the correct management of Mrs. O's problems?
   a. What, if any, are the motives and the disadvantages of 'shopping around' for medical care?
   b. What was the basis of the general practitioner supervisor's 'hunch' that the management to date had been inappropriate?
   c. Would you have been surprised that adequate history revealed major domestic problems including the caring for an invalid husband?
   d. What are the indications (if any) for physiotherapy or drug therapy.

3. What is your definition of a general practitioner/family physician?
   a. What aspects of your definition are exemplified in this case?
   b. What are the implications of episodic care as opposed to 'total patient care'?

D. A. Game, Adelaide

63 MISS LINDA W. AGED 26

1. What further information do you want?
   a. What motivations and skills does the husband-to-be offer?
   b. If the proposed partner appears to have Klinefelter's syndrome, how does this change your problem list?
   c. If they have a child, will it likely be of subnormal or normal intelligence?

2. Identify the problems to be managed.
   a. Would you involve the parents of this couple?
   b. What form of birth control would you urge?
   c. Is epilepsy an absolute contraindication to birth control pills?
   d. If it is impossible to insert an IUD in this tense, nulliparous patient, how far would you go – insertion under general anaesthesia?
   e. What community help will be needed for this couple to be as independent as possible in the future?

f. What are the problems if a child of apparently normal intelligence is born to this couple? How would you help to safeguard and nurture the child?

3. Can/should society intervene?
    a. Should society recognize a legal contract (marriage) undertaken by such a couple?
    b. Are there circumstances when you feel forced sterilization, or forced giving up of a newborn should occur?

D. H. Johnson, Toronto

MRS. P.   AGED 32   **64**

1. Is the contraceptive pill prescribed too easily?
    a. What history should be taken?
    b. What examination should be performed?
    c. Can one doctor rely on the fact that a predecessor has initiated therapy and on that basis continuation is justifiable without a. and b. above?

2. Should the doctor, despite the patient's objection, try to treat social and medical problems together?
    a. Should the doctor try to involve the estranged parents of one or both adults?
    b. Should he give precedence to one or other problem?
    c. What should be the doctor's response when he learns a colleague has prescribed the pill on the patient's request?
    d. Why bother with non co-operative patients?

3. How far does a doctor's responsibility go?
    a. Should the doctor have arranged for a social worker to call?
    b. Should the doctor inform voluntary helping organizations that there is a family in the district in need of help?
    c. Has the fact that another doctor has provided a change of pill absolved the doctor from any further action?

P. F. Gill, Hobart

MR. S.   AGED 76   **65**

1. What is the most likely cause of this man's presenting signs and symptoms?
    a. How would you define a delayed grief reaction in this man?
    b. Could depression account for the physical findings?
    c. What would be the most likely malignancy to suspect in this man?

2. What other information about this man's lifestyle would be important to know between his first and subsequent visits?
   a. Would a detailed smoking history be of assistance?
   b. Would an alcohol intake history be of assistance?
   c. Would a history of his daily living be of assistance?

3. Why would this man deny the aetiology of his problem?
   a. How important is the social history in this problem?
   b. How important is the man's religion in this situation?
   c. How common are alcohol problems in the elderly?
   d. How important is the man's relationship with his family in this
      situation?
   e. What role may the doctor play in assisting normal grief re-
      actions after the death of a spouse?
   f. How may this situation have been prevented?

W. W. Rosser, Ottawa

66 MR. H.S.   AGED 82   RETIRED BUSINESSMAN

1. Why has an 82 year old man undergone an elective hernia repair?
   a. Do some hernias put the patient more at risk than others?
   b. What are the risks of surgery in this age group?
   c. What role should the family physician play in the decision
      making?
   d. What community services are available to assist with his wife
      during his absence?

2. What would be the normal expected length of stay for an uncomplicated hernia repair?
   a. Does the unusual pain suggest a complication, and if so, what?
   b. Do you think that the patient is using the pain for secondary
      gain?
   c. What is secondary gain?
   d. How does the physician confront that issue?

3. What is the likely explanation of this sudden appearance of a swollen
leg?
   a. Do you think it is related to surgery?
   b. Is he particularly susceptible to such a complication?
   c. What measures might have been taken to prevent such a
      complication?
   d. How should his leg problem be investigated?
   e. What possible therapy should be undertaken and for how long?

C. A. Moore, Hamilton, Canada

MR. J.B.   AGED 81   RETIRED PHARMACIST

67

1. How would you manage this man's congestive heart failure on an ambulatory basis?
   a. How frequently would you see him?
   b. Would you see him in your office or at home?
   c. What regimen do you use in your medical locale?

2. What advice do you give such a patient about his living conditions?
   a. How long can such a patient live at home and in what kind of a home?
   b. If he has to stay at home, what modifications can make life easier for him?

3. What advice would you give this patient in relation to the future?
   a. Will you talk to him about his prognosis?
   b. Will you help him deal with the idea of impending death?

4. How will you help his wife cope with his illness?
   a. His illness will put a heavy burden on his wife. Can you help to ease that burden?
   b. Does your community have facilities that will keep this man out of hospital?

J. K. Shearman, Hamilton, Canada

MRS. P.   AGED 84   WIDOW

68

1. What are the possible medical conditions from which Mrs. P. is suffering?
   a. What is senile dementia, and what are the pathological changes, if any?
   b. Is senile dementia different from confusion in the elderly, and if so how would you differentiate them?
   c. What investigations should the general practitioner perform in this case?
   d. What medication would be appropriate for Mrs. P.?

2. What is meant by family dynamics?
   a. What particular behavioural patterns are the three siblings portraying?
   b. What effects are these behaviours having on Mrs. P., and the management of her problem?
   c. Would the general practitioner be justified in attempting to modify their behaviours?
   d. How could he do this?

3. What can the general practitioner do (as demanded by the daughter)?
   a. How can he co-ordinate those assisting her?
   b. How can he involve the family in this process?
   c. What are the indications or criteria for admission of an elderly person to a nursing home?
   d. How far does the general practitioner's responsibility lie in the problems presented by Mrs. P.?

D. A. Game, Adelaide

69 MRS. S.W.   AGED 82   RETIRED

1. How would you assess her mental state?
   a. What is 'senile dementia'?
   b. What other disorders may present in this way?
   c. What treatment is available?

2. How would you advise her relatives?
   a. Is the family history of significance in dementia?
   b. Is drug therapy of any value?
   c. What is the prognosis for this old lady?

3. What resources do you have in the community to help in the care of this old lady?
   a. What help can social services provide?
   b. What are the functions of a psychogeriatric day hospital?

4. On what grounds should elderly people be encouraged to give up their independence and enter some form of sheltered accommodation?
   a. How would you assess whether she is capable of managing her own affairs?
   b. What is your role as a doctor in this situation?

E. C. Gambrill, Crawley, UK

70 MRS. F.F.   AGED 82   WIDOW

1. Is this likely to be an organic or psychological problem?
   a. What historical features help to distinguish an organic lesion?
   b. What would you look for on physical examination?
   c. Are there simple office psychological tests which might help you distinguish an organic lesion?

2. What are the common causes of rapid deterioration of mental status of an elderly person?
   a. What types of physical illness can precipitate such a change?

b. Do many medications do this?
c. Can masked depression present in this way?

3. What investigations would you do?
   a. Will any laboratory tests help?
   b. Would you ever consider X-rays or other tests?
   c. Can psychological tests help?

4. How would you manage this patient?
   a. Could she be managed at home?
   b. Would any medication help before a more definitive diagnosis is made?
   c. How would you mobilise others to help in her care?

E. V. Dunn, Toronto

MISS M.B.   AGED 82   RETIRED NURSE   **71**

1. Should she be persuaded to have more medical care?
   a. What community service might be available?
   b. What are the laws governing admission of patients against their will?
   c. What should be the goals of the doctor's intervention?

2. Is there any indication for the use of anti-depressants?
   a. What is the efficacy, tolerance, dosage, and risk/benefit ratio of drugs used to treat depression in the elderly?

3. How can family physicians assist patients requiring considerable care to remain at home and out of institutions?
   a. What conditions would make it impossible for this patient to remain at home?

E. Domovitch, Toronto

MRS. A.T.   AGED 83   WIDOW   **72**

1. Was the surgeon's recommendation of chemotherapy reasonable?
   a. What beneficial effects can be expected from treatment with 5FU?
   b. How long will the effects last?
   c. What other treatment can be offered if the chemotherapy is ineffective?

2. What do you think the doctor's reaction to the telephone requests would be?

    a.   Could the doctor have done anything to avoid the apparently sudden request by the niece's husband to institutionalize Mrs. A.T.?

    b.   What is the place of a family conference in such a situation?

    c.   What factors in the care of a sick elderly person do families find least tolerable?

3.   Which of his patients, Mrs. A.T., her niece, and the niece's husband, should the doctor consider most when making decisions about admitting Mrs. A.T. to a nursing home?

    a.   Was the niece's health at risk because she was working so hard for her aunt?

    b.   What could be done to ease the stress for each member of this family?

G. Williams, Iowa City

---

73   OLIVE N.   AGED 61   EXECUTIVE

1.   How do you propose to conduct this consultation?

    a.   What do you tell Mrs. O.N.?

    b.   How and what do you tell her daughter?

2.   What is the likely course of her disorder?

    a.   What plans do you make for her care?

    b.   What specific problems do you anticipate?

    c.   How will you deal with them?

    d.   How will her family cope?

J. Fry, Beckenham, UK

---

74   J.H.   AGED 7   SCHOLAR

1.   Could you list the possible causes of this boy's enuresis in order of probability?

    a.   Would you first eliminate an organic cause for the enuresis?

    b.   What investigations would you employ?

    c.   What positive results would influence your management?

2.   Do you think this is a dysfunctional family and if so, why?

    a.   If you diagnosed a dysfunctional family how would you set about managing the situation?

    b.   Would you make use of a marriage counsellor, family therapist, psychiatrist for individual therapy, child psychologist or try to initiate counselling yourself?

    c.   How would **you** set about it in this family?

3. What is/are the natural history/ies for asthma in children?
    a. What basis is there for believing asthma is a psychosomatic disease?
    b. What would your management plan be for a child with chronic asthma?
    c. Do you have any instruments to measure 'asthma' and its response to treatment in family practice?

4. What do you understand by a 'mother presenting through the child'?
    a. Is this a common occurrence in family practice?
    b. Why would a mother 'want' to present through her child?
    c. What would make you aware that the mother may be presenting through her child?

J. H. Levenstein, Cape Town

MRS. C.B.   AGED 35   HOUSEWIFE, PART-TIME JOB IN NURSING HOME   75

1. Who should you treat first – mother, father, child or the whole family unit?
    a. Will psychotropic drugs help this patient?
    b. If you feel they will, what will govern your choice?
    c. What are the risks to the child?
    d. Should the patient continue working at week-ends?

2. Does the fact that you don't often see father and son mean anything?
    a. How might a visit to the home assist you?

3. Given the common problem of multiple patients in a family but access limited to one, what might you achieve?

W. D. Jackson, Launceston, Australia

THE A. FAMILY   76

1. What functions does the family doctor discharge in the on-going care of families like the A.'s?
    a. What agencies might already be involved in supportive family case-work?

2. What should be done at this time of night?
    a. How might the family doctor resolve the apparent conflict between being a 'personal doctor' and a human being needing a night's sleep?
    b. What roles might the police have (if any) in the current crisis?
    c. Does drug therapy have a place in the immediate management of Mrs. A.?

3. What psychiatric diagnoses might be represented in this family?
   a.   What is a psychopath?
   b.   What are the benefits of attempting to treat the family as a unit, and how might this be achieved?

J. D. E. Knox, Dundee

77 MRS. D.H.   AGED 33   HOUSEWIFE

1. What is one definition of the 'family life cycle'?
   a.   At what stage is this family in their life cycle?
   b.   Is it possible for one family to be at different stages of the life cycle at one point in time?
   c.   What kinds of medical crises might be considered to be 'high risk' events in the family life cycle?
   d.   What kinds of non-medical crises might be considered to be 'high risk' events in the family life cycle?

2. Other than routine, what additional measures might be utilized regarding the investigation and management of this pregnancy?
   a.   Is there a need for amniocentesis at this time?
   b.   Is immediate termination of the pregnancy worthy of consideration?
   c.   Is there a need for ultra-sound in the next few weeks?
   d.   Should the question of post-partum tubal ligation be raised at this time?

3. What is meant by the concept of the 'family as the patient'?
   a.   What would your strategy be for the management of this 'patient'?
   b.   How would you use anticipatory guidance in dealing with this 'patient'?
   c.   How does the concept of tertiary prevention apply to the management of this 'patient'?

G. G. Beazley, Winnipeg

78 MRS. L.M.   AGED 28   PROFESSIONAL MODEL

1. What is the problem list for this patient?
   a.   Are all the problems a manifestation of her anxiety state?
   b.   Could the patient be the cause of the basic sexual problem?
   c.   Could the doctor be an 'obstacle' to this patient? Is depression likely to be a significant problem?
   d.   Is she likely to have a negative attitude towards her children?

2. Who is the real patient?

    a. Is the husband the basic cause of the pathos?
    b. Who is likely to be at fault with their sexual dilemma?
    c. Is it imperative to involve the husband in the management?

3. What has gone wrong with the management of this family?
    a. Is the gathering of a true psycho-sexual history an embarrassing problem for family doctors?
    b. Do VIP patients present special problems in eliciting sensitive information?
    c. Why has a communication problem developed?
    d. Should a proper vaginal/pelvic examination spot the problem?
    e. Should these patients be treated with tranquillizers?

4. How should the family doctor manage this problem?
    a. Is the problem solvable?
    b. How would you involve the husband in the counselling?
    c. Can the general practitioner cope with this type of problem?
    d. Should the responsibility be handed over to specialists and marriage guidance personnel?

J. E. Murtagh, Melbourne

MRS. M.   AGED 45   HOUSEWIFE   **79**

1. What is the likely disease process producing Mrs. M.'s painful joints?
    a. How could rheumatoid arthritis be diagnosed in general practice?
    b. What is the treatment of Mrs. M.'s rheumatoid arthritis?
    c. What is the prognosis?

2. What is meant by total patient care?
    a. How do Mrs. M.'s medical problems exemplify this?
    b. Would the particular medical treatment prescribed for Mrs. M. be influenced by her relationship with the whole family?

3. What is family medicine?
    a. Indicate how family dynamics influence the health of the M. family.
    b. Could the family have had any effect on the type or severity of Mrs. M.'s illness?
    c. How should the general practitioner handle this family's dynamics?
    d. Could and/or should the general practitioner assist in improving the relationships with Mrs. M. Snr?
    e. What are the implications of S.'s presentation to the general practitioner?

D. A. Game, Adelaide

80 MRS. P.B. AGED 23 HOUSEWIFE

1. What is the significance of a patient arriving in the office accompanied by a relative or friend?
   a. How would you deal with the problem of the patient's mother monopolizing the consultation?
   b. How do you react to a patient's suggestion that she might wish to change her doctor?
   c. Which member(s) of this family is/are the real patient(s)?

2. What conditions would you consider when a patient complains of tiredness?
   a. What are the possible causes of anaemia in a woman of childbearing age?
   b. What are the possible presenting features of hyper- and hypothyroidism?
   c. What advice would you give to a patient suffering from insomnia?
   d. How would you assess the risk of suicide in a depressed patient?

3. What might lead the family practitioner to suspect a disturbance of family dynamics?
   a. What agencies might be enlisted to help problem families?
   b. What are the possible reasons for this family failing to re-appear in the office?

T. A. I. Bouchier Hayes, Camberley, UK

81 SHELLEY AGED 14 MONTHS

1. Should this child and family be requested to stay with one doctor except in emergencies?
   a. Why did Shelley have a 'glue ear'?
   b. Are there dangers in casual management for episodic illness?
   c. How does one handle parents who are accustomed to episodic care only?

2. Does Shelley have a chronic ENT problem?
   a. Is teething a factor in otitis media?
   b. What is the place for prophylactic antibiotics?
   c. Should this child be referred to an ENT surgeon for adenoidectomy and/or the insertion of a grommet?

3. Does this family have a problem?
   a. Who is responsible for the child's health: the doctor; the family; or both?
   b. Should the practice insist on the family staying with one doctor?

c. How can one motivate the mother to accept the responsibility for deciding whether medical attention is necessary?

P. F. Gill, Hobart

MRS. I.C.   AGED 28   HOUSEWIFE   **82**

1. What advice would you give to the patient?
    a. How could you control her diarrhoea?
    b. What is your diagnosis?

2. How do you treat this family unit?
    a. Which member of the family requires your advice?
    b. Would you counsel the family as a unit or individually?
    c. What problem solving processes would you use?

3. Is medical treatment required?
    a. Would you hospitalize the patient?
    b. Do the son and the patient require therapy?
    c. Does the husband require advice?

4. What further advice may be required?
    a. Is a psychiatrist of help?
    b. Would a psychologist be of help?

B. M. Fehler, Johannesburg

MRS. T.   AGED 49   CHINESE MEATSTALL OWNER   **83**

1. What are the problems?
    a. Can congestive cardiac failure (CCF) be treated at home?
    b. How much rest can you expect with such a home environment?
    c. Can CCF be treated without proper rest?

2. How would you manage the husband as part of the overall problem?
    a. Will counselling help?

3. How do you manage this situation?
    a. Is this a family, social or medical problem or the combination of the three?
    b. As a doctor, which of the three problems is the easiest to manage; which is the most difficult?

N. C. L. Yuen, Hong Kong

84 MRS. D.G.   AGED 42   HOUSEWIFE

1. What were the inherent deficiencies in the management of this family?
   a. Did the arrival of the baby precipitate this crisis?
   b. Would you look for other reasons leading to the marital break-up?
   c. Should they have been advised to institutionalize the baby?
   d. Should amniocentesis have been performed antenatally with a view to termination if the syndrome was detected?
   e. Should the husband have been present at counselling sessions?

2. What preventive measures could have been adopted to help this family?
   a. Is it a mistake to counsel one parent only?
   b. Should the family doctor carry out impromptu social home calls when all the family are likely to be at home?
   c. Would attention to postnatal birth control and sexual counselling have prevented this crisis?
   d. Are there community support agencies that could help parents with handicapped children?

3. How would you manage the present situation?
   a. Would you look for possible underlying reasons apart from the stress of the child?
   b. Would you advise the patient to 'cool it' and leave the door open for her husband?
   c. Would you advise her to separate?
   d. Should you attempt to contact her husband?
   e. Would you advise institutionalization of the child?

J. E. Murtagh, Melbourne

85 PETER B.   AGED 18 MONTHS

1. What sequence of events could have led to the diagnosis of Down's syndrome either having been overlooked or not communicated to the parents?
   a. What are the stigmata that the baby would have presented in the early weeks of its life?
   b. How could the diagnosis have been confirmed?
   c. With what condition could Down's syndrome be confused in the first year of life and how could the distinction be made on clinical grounds and by investigation?
   d. What are the implications of an error in diagnosis between these two conditions?

2. How does the doctor deal with the problem presented by this 18 months old child?
   a. What treatment should be prescribed for the upper respiratory tract infection?
   b. Should antibiotics be prescribed?
   c. How should he go about explaining to the parents the fact that their child has Down's syndrome and its prognosis?
   d. What social and psychological problems in the parents and siblings may result from this knowledge?
   e. To what extent is it the general practitioner's responsibility to counsel the parents and manage these problems?

J. G. P. Ryan, Brisbane

MASTER ROBERT S.   AGED 2   86

1. What is wrong with the child?
   a. How accurately can motor and intellectual development predict the child's prognosis?
   b. What other diagnostic manoeuvres could be undertaken?

2. What should the parents be told?
   a. What community and hospital-based resources are available and when should they be brought to the attention of the parents?
   b. Is there any harm in deferring further action?

3. Who is the patient?
   a. How does a doctor assess the family's ability to cope with this situation?
   b. What can be done to assist them to cope?

E. Domovitch, Toronto

HANNA W.   AGED 6   SCHOOLGIRL   87

1. How should toilet training be done?
   a. At what stage of child development should toilet training begin?
   b. At what stage should a child be 'dry'?
   c. What factors in the parent–child relationship enhance or disturb training?
   d. Why should a 'trained' child begin bedwetting?

2. What is the diagnosis for Hanna's problems?
   a. What is onset enuresis?
   b. What factors in her family and environment could be contributing to her bedwetting?

c. Why is she reluctant to go to school?
d. Can you make any predictions regarding the interpersonal relationships between members of this family?

3. What additional investigations could help to clarify the problems?
   a. What further information would you try to elicit from the mother?
   b. How would you exclude an organic cause?
   c. What is the relevance of her initial toilet training?
   d. How could the school nurse or teacher be helpful?

4. How would you manage Hanna's problems?
   a. What are the roles of her parents in her treatment?
   b. Should the mother continue to lift and carry her, or to wake and escort her to the toilet at night?
   c. What possible modification in the home or school environment could you explore?
   d. Is drug therapy indicated?
   e. What other methods of treatment could be tried?

Z. Cramer, Tel-Aviv, Israel

88 MR. M.S.   AGED 18   PAINTER AND DECORATOR

1. What is the significance of a couple coming together to see the doctor?
   a. How do you feel about a joint consultation?
   b. What effect does it have on the doctor? Why?

2. What is the problem?
   a. What do you understand by the term 'minimal cerebral dysfunction'?
   b. What investigations may help to clarify the problem?

3. What is the likely prognosis?
   a. Is the condition likely to improve after adolescence?
   b. What is the likelihood of epilepsy as an associated condition?
   c. Is drug therapy likely to be of any value?

4. What can you do to help this family?
   a. What other agencies are available to help?
   b. What is the role of the GP in this type of situation?
   c. What is 'family therapy'? Could it be of value in this case?

E. C. Gambrill, Crawley, UK

STEVEN H.   AGED 13   SCHOOLBOY

89

1. What help was mother seeking?
   a. How would you deal with the request for wart treatment?
   b. Who in the family are the patients?
   c. How often do parents use a physical excuse to present a child with a psychological problem?

2. What problems can adoption cause?
   a. How and when should a child be told he is adopted?
   b. How would you counsel this family concerning the adopted child's wish to find his natural mother?

3. What problems relating to male puberty might present to the doctor?
   a. Do all boys face problems at puberty?
   b. What factors lead to the development of significant problems?

4. How should children be given sex education?
   a. What is the parents' responsibility in sex education?
   b. What health education should be in the school curriculum?
   c. What is the family doctor's role in sex education?

5. How would you handle the complaint of bestiality?
   a. Is bestiality a perversion or a variation of normal behaviour?
   b. How common is bestiality?
   c. What factors lead to bestiality occurring?
   d. How would you counsel this family on the subject?

D. G. Chambers, Clare, Australia

MRS. H.   AGED 35   HOUSEWIFE

90

1. What other clinical entities may be brought on by continuous psychological stress?

2. How would you manage her dilemma?
   a. 'In a divorce neither party wins.' Do you agree with the statement in this case?
   b. How would you approach the husband over her complaints?
   c. What are the early symptoms of a suicidal tendency?

3. Would you accede to her request for admission to a hospital? Give your reasons.
   a. What are the resources available in your community for her problem?
   b. How would you best utilize these resources for her needs?

F. E. H. Tan, Kuala Lumpur

91 MRS. S.   AGED 22   HOUSEWIFE

1. What are her problems?
   a. Are there particular problems associated with mixed marriages?
   b. How may cultural differences and marital disharmony present as psychosomatic illnesses?

2. How can the problems be solved?
   a. Does her husband need help?
   b. How best can the GP broach the subject with the husband?
   c. Would a marriage counsellor be of help?

N. C. L. Yuen, Hong Kong

92 MRS. Y.H.   AGED 42   NURSING SISTER

1. What are the main considerations to be discussed?
   a. What are the early symptoms of Huntington's chorea?
   b. May her symptoms be prodromal to the disease?
   c. What likelihood do the children have of inheriting the disease?
   d. Can Huntington's chorea be predicted?

2. What responsibilities does the doctor have?
   a. What kind of care will help this patient?
   b. Should the children be involved?
   c. Should the daughter be protected against pregnancy?
   d. Should the husband be informed?

G. M. Dick, Hobart

93 MR. I.   AGED 32   UNEMPLOYED LABOURER

1. How might initial contact be made with Mr. I.?
   a. What formalities are necessary to establish Mr. I. and Ian as your patients?

2. What diagnostic problems are inherent in this situation?
   a. What clinical features would confirm suspicions that Mr. I. had Huntington's chorea?
   b. How might you obtain objective information on Mr. I's past medical state?

3. What legal and ethical issues are raised by the problems inherent in this situation?
   a. How far can the doctor go in dealing with Mr. I. if there is evidence of an advanced state of the disease?

b. What considerations govern management decisions regarding Ian?
c. What legal issues are raised by the presence of the son, Ian?

J. D. E. Knox, Dundee

MR. W.G.   AGED 40   AIRLINE PILOT   94

1. What is the natural history of Huntington's chorea?
    a. What are the genetic factors?
    b. Can his chances of developing the illness be altered?
    c. What diagnostic tests are available?
    d. What are the early and late signs and symptoms?
    e. What are the principles of management of established cases?

2. Where do your professional responsibilities lie?
    a. Will a 'regular check-up' be of any value?
    b. Should he be sterilized?
    c. Can he fly safely now?
    d. Can you respect his request not to inform his employer?
    e. What responsibilities do doctors have to: (i) society; (ii) bureaucracies; (iii) patients; (iv) patients' families?

P. R. Grantham, Vancouver

MR. A.B.   AGED 45   MID-LEVEL EXECUTIVE   95

1. What is the minimal history and physical examination you would consider appropriate for this visit?
    a. Is a chest and cardiovascular examination necessary? If so, why?
    b. What are the common complications seen at this time?

2. What effect is this episode likely to have on his life style?
    a. How will it affect him, his wife, children and work situation?

3. When would you permit this patient to return to full activities?
    a. How soon can he return to work, engage in strenuous activities, drive a car, and resume sexual activity?

4. What opportunities present for patient education, health promotion and preventive care?

E. V. Dunn, Toronto

96 MR. E.L. AGED 47 PIPE FITTER

1. At what different stages of the development of a disease can prevention be applied?
   a. What is meant by primary prevention?
   b. What is meant by secondary prevention?
   c. What is meant by tertiary prevention?
   d. What kind(s) of prevention might be applied in this case?

2. What therapeutic measures might be useful in managing Mr. L.'s disease?
   a. Given the usual natural history of the disease from which Mr. L. suffers, is it likely that medication would be of use?
   b. What is the place of counselling in this situation?
   c. What is a risk factor?
   d. What personality trait does Mr. L. exhibit that might make counselling difficult?

3. What are lifestyle problems?
   a. What lifestyle problems does Mr. L. demonstrate?
   b. Could chronic anger be characterized as a lifestyle problem?
   c. Could marital separation be characterized as a lifestyle problem?

G. G. Beazley, Winnipeg

97 SUSAN M. AGED 3 MONTHS

1. What is the significance of the infantile spasms?
   a. What exactly are they and at what age do they normally present?
   b. What causes them?
   c. If a paediatrician had said they were caused by the pertussis vaccine, would you believe him?

2. What facts would you present to help the parents decide whether their baby should be vaccinated or not?
   a. Is whooping cough a serious disease?
   b. Is medical treatment for it satisfactory?
   c. Is vaccination effective?
   d. What minor reactions may the vaccine cause?
   e. Does the vaccine cause fits?
   f. What is the risk of brain damage from the vaccine?

3. What are contraindications to pertussis vaccine and why?
   a. The American Academy of Paediatrics states that a history of fits in the child is not a contraindication while the Department of Health and Social Security (UK) says it is. Which should we believe?

    b.   Do infections such as a cold increase the likelihood of a reaction to the vaccine?

    c.   Is there a distinction between brain damage and progressive degenerative disease of the nervous system or are both contraindications?

4. Should the childhood immunization programme be made compulsory for all children?

A. J. Moulds, Basildon, UK

MRS. A.B.   AGED 25   SOUTHERN EUROPEAN MOTHER   98

1. How would you react?
    a.   Do you feel threatened when your medical authority is questioned?
    b.   Is anger a likely response; if so, how do you handle anger?
    c.   How much should one bow to ethnic mores in this situation?

2. How will you explain the process of immunization?
    a.   Which immunization products are alive?
    b.   What is a toxoid?
    c.   At what age is a baby's immune system able to produce antibodies?
    d.   Can you immunize too early?
    e.   At what age is immunization carried out for
        – diphtheria?
        – pertussis?
        – tetanus?
        – poliomyelitis?
        – mumps?
        – rubella?
        – measles?

3. Are there any dangers to immunization?
    a.   What specific contraindications exist to any immunization regime?
    b.   Are there any dangers in rubella immunization?
    c.   Can side effects of rubella immunization cause permanent disease?
    d.   If an adult seeks immunization against rubella, what pathology tests do you carry out?
    e.   What level of antibody titre constitutes significant protection?
    f.   What precautions do you advise before immunizing an adult against rubella?
    g.   How soon can the patient become pregnant?
    h.   If she conceives before this date, what will you say to her?

4. Is immunization always effective?
    a. What percentage of non-immunized people do you need in a community to produce an epidemic?
    b. How often are booster doses needed for each immunization process?
    c. If you are a community physician, how could you ascertain that your community was safe against a disease epidemic of diphtheria or poliomyelitis?

A. Himmelhoch, Sydney

99 MR. J.R.   AGED 22   UNIVERSITY STUDENT

1. For which three groups of disease should immunization be considered for travellers?
    a. Why is there a case for adults who received a full Salk course of vaccination to receive at least one, if not a full course of Sabin before travelling abroad?
    b. Which three areas require yellow fever immunization and for how long is such vaccination valid?
    c. Would you offer to immunize this young man with gamma globulin? If not, why not?
    d. What advice would you give regarding protection from another sort of hepatitis? Which activities can be associated with its passage?

2. Can you give cholera and typhoid immunization in the same syringe?
    a. The protection is months with one component and years with the other. Which is which?
    b. What single umbrella medication will markedly reduce the length and intensity of local and systemic complications of these immunizations?
    c. Why is intradermal immunization for typhoid, at least after the primary dose, advised by many doctors?

3. What medicine kit would you advise this young man and his companions to take?
    a. Medical care can be very expensive abroad. How much insurance should each person carry? For what particular event should this coverage be taken out?
    b. What antimicrobials might reasonably be taken just in case?
    c. What essential information should always be sought from, and advice given to, travellers about current medications?

A. J. Radford, Adelaide

JILL B.   AGED 20   STUDENT

100

1. What range of topics should a pre-marital consultation cover? Should you plan for a long consultation to cover them?
   a. What community role can the family doctor play in pre-marital counselling, parenting?
   b. When did you last open the conversation about the issues of living as 'two' instead of 'one', of sexual knowledge and contraceptive processes in someone who was engaged but who didn't initiate an enquiry? Is it a routine in your practice?
   c. Who was more embarrassed? Who had more to lose?

2. Let us assume that you are really uncomfortable on finding out that she is both totally sexually ignorant and minimally experienced. How would you proceed?
   a. What would you tell her? No, not the topics, what would you actually tell her?
   b. Three months after the marriage she turns up again and says she 'feels nothing' when her husband makes love to/at her. What is your line of questioning?
   c. Would you call him in? If so, what would be your line of questioning?
   d. You find he 'fires' almost before he's started. What would be your line of questioning and probable suggestions?

A. J. Radford, Adelaide

MR. J.B.   AGED 30

101

1. How can the doctor motivate the patient?
   a. To what extent are diabetic complications related to the control of the disease?
   b. Is his lack of compliance related to his unwillingness to accept his illness?
   c. How can diet and insulin administration be made more flexible?

2. What can be determined from the fact that the patient continues to visit his regular family physician albeit irregularly?

3. What is the doctor's role in this patient's life?
   a. Of the many possible roles – dictator, parent, friend, advisor, teacher, helper, consultant – that a physician may adopt, which one is likely to be most advantageous to the patient? to the doctor? Is this always the case?

4. Should family physicians take the position that patients should be given appropriate advice and the extent to which they follow that advice is their own responsibility?

    a. Should we expect patients to comply unequivocally with the doctor's advice?

    b. Why do we react the way we do to 'non-compliance'?

    c. What physician's role would minimize expenditure of unproductive emotional energy?

E. Domovitch, Toronto

102   G.H.   AGED 11   STUDENT

1. What home factors might contribute to poor diabetic control?
   a. What are the problems of diet management in a child at home?
   b. Do children have consistent physical activity?

2. Do you expect the mother to comply with instructions in this case?

3. How can G.H. be taught to help herself?

4. What other people can be engaged to help?
   a. What about the father?
   b. Can the visiting or school nurse be helpful?
   c. Is it appropriate to ask the teacher to help?

5. What problems is G.H. likely to encounter during her adolescence?

E. V. Dunn, Toronto

103   L.W.   AGED 42   VOLUNTEER WORKER

1. How would you manage the problem of diabetes control in this patient?
   a. What oral hypoglycaemic agents are available and why would you choose one or another?
   b. Who is a candidate for these agents and who must be treated with insulin?
   c. What is the value of high fibre diets in managing insulin dependent diabetes mellitus?
   d. What variables offset this patient's compliance with medical treatment?

2. How do cultural and personality variables influence your management decision?

3. What do you think is a reasonable treatment goal for this patient?

K. F. Weyrauch, Charleston, SC, USA

MRS. RUTH S.   AGED 54   WIDOW

104

1. What model of doctor–patient relationship would you pursue?
   a. Describe three models of doctor–patient relationships, e.g. parent/child.

2. What further information would you wish?
   a. Is her depressed mood a relevant concern?
   b. How would you proceed if she was afraid of needles?
   c. How would you proceed if she told you that an insulin reaction caused her husband to crash his car and this led to his death?
   d. Describe the process of patient education you would carry out in this case.

D. H. Johnson, Toronto

MR. P.B.   AGED 68   NAVY - RETIRED

105

1. What techniques might increase Mr. B.'s compliance with diet and insulin?
   a. Would you consider switching from insulin to an oral hypoglycaemic?
   b. Which of the oral drugs are contraindicated especially in the elderly patient?

2. What degree of claudication would require angiography?
   a. What are the risks of arterial surgery in this patient?
   b. What nonsurgical techniques might improve symptoms?

3. Are there any effective techniques to help Mr. B. discontinue smoking?
   a. What effect does the physician's repeated exhortations to the patient to stop smoking have in the long term?
   b. Do behaviour modification techniques offer anything to the smoker who wishes to quit?

C. T. Lamont, Ottawa

MR. M.   AGED 72   RETIRED SCHOOLTEACHER

106

1. What is the problem?
   a. Organic?
   b. Psychological?

2. Is confrontation the answer?
   a. How often will this approach succeed?
   b. How curable is alcoholism?

3. What can the doctor do?
   a. What can he do himself?
   b. Is psychiatric help useful?
   c. What community resources could be helpful?

J. G. Richards, Auckland

107 MISS S.H. AGED 20 CLERK

1. How much preventive medicine can be carried out at this interview?
   a. What relationship has hypertension to overweight?
   b. What medical and surgical conditions are more likely in the obese?

2. What aetiological factors induce overweight?
   a. What endocrinological factors must be ruled out?
   b. What part does her emotional state play in the aetiology of her obesity?
   c. With other members of the family overweight, is the prognosis for cure altered?

3. What is the programme of treatment?
   a. What success rate have anorectic medications?
   b. Does exercise help?
   c. Should one be realistic in setting a target weight?
   d. Can one alter her body image?
   e. Can her aims be changed permanently?
   f. How important is appearance to her?
   g. What is the value of group therapy?

G. M. Dick, Hobart

108 DAVID J. AGED 29 FARMER

1. What pathological conditions might lead to this type of story?
   a. What vascular problems present like this?
   b. What is the relationship to lifestyle?

2. Is there any way in which such an outcome might be prevented?
   a. Will counselling help?
   b. If this were Buerger's disease at work would cessation of smoking have a beneficial effect?
   c. Would cessation have to be complete?
   d. Would the patient be likely to continue to smoke surreptitiously?
   e. If his wife reported that she knew he was continuing to smoke, despite vehement denials, what should the doctor do?
   f. How can his wife best be supported?

3. Where does responsibility lie?
    a. How far can a doctor go in the process of providing information, ensuring comprehension, changing of attitudes and finally providing the motivation for change of habits?

R. T. Mossop, Harare, Zimbabwe

MRS. JESSIE A.   AGED 78   **109**

1. How would you verify whether she is taking her drugs?
    a. What blood or urine tests would help?
    b. Are pharmacists required to mark prescribing dates and prescribed amounts on the labels?

2. What are some of the patient factors involved in non-compliance particularly in the elderly?
    a. What percentage of 78 year olds can read a prescription label clearly?
    b. Do you think that Mrs. A. could tell you the name, purpose and dosage of each medication?

3. What can the physician do to increase compliance in elderly patients?
    a. Can you design a drug dosage schedule sheet with large printing that would help such a patient?
    b. Which instruction leads to better compliance; 'Take one every 6 hours . . .' or 'Take one before meals three times daily plus one at bedtime . . .'?
    c. What is chromal confusion? (In Canada and the USA, all of Mrs. A.'s medications are white compressed tablets which will confuse her).
    d. What would be your patient education programme to improve Mrs. A.'s compliance?

D. H. Johnson, Toronto

TONY H.   AGED 2½   **110**

1. What are the possible diagnoses?
    a. What is the difference between marasmus, marasmic-kwashiorkor and kwashiorkor?
    b. What are the common presenting symptoms?

2. Are there differences in the management of these conditions?
    a. What is treatment directed at?

3. How do you explain the resurgence of this condition in an otherwise well-fed and affluent society?
   a. What are some of the problems of working parents?

Footnote: Many Chinese families in Hong Kong need to have both the parents working and the children are left to the care of the grandparents, whose lack of knowledge of nutrition leads to a resurgence of the above conditions.

N. C. L. Yuen, Hong Kong

111 MRS. PATRICIA M.   AGED 36   HOUSEWIFE

1. Is there any chance of a wombless woman conceiving?
   a. Are there recorded cases in which, through a fistula in the vaginal vault there was meeting of sperm and ovum?
   b. If such a conceptus could be implanted as an ectopic, how long might it live?
   c. Might it present a danger to life?

2. How can the doctor get her to face reality?
   a. Look out the window and say 'The last time something like this happened, wise men were led by a bright star'?
   b. Say something about good and bad spirits and how the wicked ones can often be very plausible?
   c. Play for time and say you cannot determine any sign of pregnancy yet but that it might be too early and to come back next month?

R. T. Mossop, Harare, Zimbabwe

112 SIMON L.   AGED 35

1. How far should the responsibility for regular follow up and management of long term disease rest with the patient?
   a. Should a doctor assume responsibility or should he put the onus on the patient?
   b. What organizational facilities might a practice need to detect defaulters?
   c. How might the doctor respond to a patient defaulting on treatment?

2. What factors should be considered before starting a patient on long term medication?
   a. Does the fact that the disease is asymptomatic have any relevance?

b. What factors affect compliance?

c. How far should the patient be involved in the decision?

3. How far is a general practitioner entitled to interfere with a specialist's proposals for therapy?
   a. Should the general practitioner always follow the regimen proposed by the specialist?
   b. Can specialist care sometimes be harmful to the patient?

J. C. Hasler, Oxford

MR. E.W.   AGED 56   MARINE ENGINEER   113

1. What constitute 'good' GP records?
   a. Legibility?
   b. Notes about every consultation regardless of its importance?
   c. Easy retrieval of relevant information at every consultation?
   d. Ruthlessly filleted so all folders are kept slim?
   e. A4 or does what is written matter more than what it is written on?
   f. Problem orientated records?

2. How would you ensure your own records were of a high standard?
   a. Disciplined regular summarizing and filleting of records?
   b. Can ancillary staff help?
   c. Would the use of summary and other special cards help?
   d. Use of external tags?

3. What is compliance and how can it be improved?
   a. How many patients don't take their prescribed medicines?
   b. What reasons do patients give for not following 'doctor's orders'?
   c. Would written instructions or information sheets help?

A. J. Moulds, Basildon, UK

D. L.   AGED 13   STUDENT   114

1. How does a family physician clinically assess normalcy in a child?
   a. Is the description of the other members of the family sufficient to reassure us about this child's size?
   b. What milestones are assessed in infants and children?
   c. Are there useful guidelines to follow?
   d. What factors might have influenced the family to enquire about David's size?
   e. Do you think the adopted child is a factor?
   f. What about pubertal concerns; are they realistic at this age?

    g.   Do you think mother or father might be the concerned parent?
    h.   What is the Singh Index?

2.   What do you think about the family physician's role in this patient's care?
    a.   Should he have sought a consultation sooner?
    b.   What routine tasks might or should he do before referral?
    c.   What pressure does he feel re referring versus not referring this child – will it do more good than harm?
    d.   How might the physician deal with David personally at this point?

3.   What might you expect from the Growth & Development Clinic?
    a.   Are there specific blood tests?
    b.   What organs might be measured?
    c.   What other observations do you think are in order?
    d.   What information, request, concern would you as the family physician convey to the consulting paediatrician?
    e.   How common is the problem?
    f.   When is treatment in order?
    g.   Is there a treatment?
    h.   What measurements might be made?

C. A. Moore, Hamilton, Canada

115   MRS. SARAH J.   AGED 68   WIDOW

1.   What are the lessons which should be learnt from this case?
    a.   What would have been the probable course of events if the diagnosis had not been made before the patient's departure overseas?
    b.   Does the general practitioner have a responsibility to offer more than the patient requests?
    c.   Is it desirable for a patient of this age to present for periodic examination in the absence of significant symptoms?
    d.   If it is, how frequently should examination be recommended?
    e.   How often do you find significant problems in routine check-up?

2.   What are the factors which prompt a patient to seek medical advice for an illness?
    a.   Why might the decision to go to the doctor be delayed?
    b.   What role can the general practitioner play in fostering his patient's awareness of the need to seek early advice?
    c.   Has the general practitioner any responsibility in training his patients in the 'self care' of minor self-limiting ailments?

    d.   What are the possible dangers associated with this policy?

    e.   What benefits might accrue as a result of a more rational use of primary health care services?

J. G. P. Ryan, Brisbane

MR. P.B.   AGED 30   BUSH FLIER   **116**

1. What are the problems?
    a.   What are the diagnostic criteria for diabetes?
    b.   What are the complications of diabetes that should be screened for or considered?
    c.   Will he require insulin?

2. What about his flying licence?
    a.   Will he have to go to hospital?
    b.   Should diabetics fly airplanes?
    c.   How do you feel about confidentiality of medical information?
    d.   What responsibility do private physicians have to (i) governmental agencies; (ii) patients; (iii) society?

3. What questions will his wife have when she appears with him at subsequent visits to the family doctor's office?
    a.   What should his diet be like?
    b.   Will it affect their sex life?
    c.   Will he be able to work and support them?
    d.   Should they still plan to have children?
    e.   What do they do at diabetic day clinics?
    f.   What about athletics?

P. R. Grantham, Vancouver

MR. S.   AGED 60   TRAIN DRIVER   **117**

1. How does the general practitioner manage the identity crisis that this man now faces, not only in his own mind but the image that he now presents to his family and work mates?
    a.   Should the GP become involved in the restoration of status so desperately sought by the patient?
    b.   Can the GP influence the consultant's opinion?
    c.   Are statutory medical examinations done by non-involved medical officers valid?
    d.   What is the real purpose of these examinations?
    e.   Should there be a judicial appeal mechanism which could examine medical opinion on fitness for work?

2. Is this man a risk as a train driver?
   a. How many accidents are due to sudden cardiac or cerebrovascular episodes?
   b. Should there be defined standards set, known to employers and employees, unions and medical officers which define fitness for work for various jobs?
   c. Can therapy increase or decrease risks?

3. Should the doctor advise the patient to accept the findings?
   a. How can doctors prepare people for retirement?
   b. Is this attitude on the doctor's part incompatible with his role of promoting positive health and rehabilitation?
   c. What measures can help those unable to cope with retirement?

P. F. Gill, Hobart

118   MRS. Q.R.   AGED 42   OFFICE MANAGER

1. Are you justified in discussing a patient's health with others without his or her knowledge?
   a. Can you discuss this information with employers, family, friends or the police?
   b. Is it justified if it is to the patient's benefit?

2. If you obtained Mrs. Q.R.'s permission what information would you send to the personnel manager?
   a. Should employers have confidential medical information in their employee's records?
   b. Is a note stating she is in good health adequate?
   c. Are regular health examinations a useful industrial screening procedure?
   d. Are annual examinations a useful routine procedure?
   e. Are executive health examinations beneficial?

3. Can a pre-employment physical examination screen out employees who might later develop industrial diseases?

4. If a patient developed a serious medical problem which he wished kept secret would you notify others?
   a. Would you notify his family?
   b. If he was a danger to himself or others would you notify his employer?
   c. Are any illnesses a contraindication to some types of employment?
   d. Are epileptics safe to work in all areas?

e. Should persons recovered from a heart attack work in strenuous or stressful situations?
f. Is a history of back pain a contraindication to heavy lifting?

E. V. Dunn, Toronto

WADE D.   AGED 4   119

1. Physical examination confirms that Wade has a mid-systolic murmur which is best heard over the upper praecordium. What characteristics of the murmur and what associated findings would enable you to assess its significance?
   a. What is the likely significance of a grade II mid-systolic murmur accompanied by a clicking sound over the aortic area?
   b. If a systolic murmur is heard over the pulmonary area what information can be gained by auscultation during inspiration and expiration?
   c. What non-invasive investigations are most likely to identify the mechanism of Wade's murmur?

2. What important issue does this incident raise for Wade and his parents?
   a. What information should be given to Wade's parents regarding his murmur?
   b. How is this information best provided?
   c. How should Wade's parents use this information?
   d. What risks does Wade run in the event of an unexpected hospital admission?

W. L. Ogborne, Sydney

MR. K.J.   AGED 37   PLUMBER   120

1. Describe the correct technique of recording blood pressure.
   a. In what position(s) should the patient be?
   b. How should the cuff be applied?
   c. When should non-standard cuffs be applied? Why?
   d. At what rate should the cuff be inflated and deflated?
   e. How often do you detect an auscultatory gap? Do some patients always have it?
   f. At what point do you record the diastolic pressure?

2. What other information would you wish to obtain?
   a. About what factors in the family history would you enquire?
   b. About what factors in the past history would you enquire?
   c. What features on physical examination would suggest end-organs are being adversely affected?

d. What features might suggest his hypertension is secondary to some other disorder?

3. What investigations would you perform?
   a. When are the following investigations indicated? Blood urea and creatinine, electrolytes, uric acid, urine microscopy and culture, cholesterol and triglycerides, ECG, chest X-ray, IVP, renal arteriography, urinary catecholamines?

4. How would you manage this case?
   a. When would you initiate treatment?
   b. Which drug(s) would you use?
   c. Is it better to use high doses of one or two drugs or lower doses of multiple drugs?
   d. Does dietary therapy, i.e. control of obesity and salt intake, have a place?

5. What are the long term benefits of treating hypertension?

6. Should general practitioners screen all patients for hypertension?

H. C. Watts, Perth, Australia

121 MRS. J.B.   AGED 49   HOUSEWIFE

1. Should she have a hysterectomy?
   a. What are the risks and benefits of such an operation?
   b. Is a referral to a gynaecologist indicated if she still refuses surgery?
   c. To what extent does referral to a gynaecologist predetermine her management?

2. Is the iron deficiency adequately rationalized by fibroids and menorrhagia?
   a. Should she have further investigations?

3. How should the physician act if the patient says, 'You are my doctor. I will leave it up to you'?
   a. To what extent should patients participate in medical decisions?
   b. How should a physician react when a well-informed patient acts contrary to his advice?
   c. How should a physician react when a poorly-informed patient acts contrary to his advice?

E. Domovitch, Toronto

MRS. JANICE L. AGED 28 HOUSEWIFE

1. How will you conduct the immediate portion of the consultation?
   a. Who has the power in the doctor–patient relationship?
   b. Do you think doctors and patients should be on a first name basis?
   c. Is a 'routine' examination sometimes used by the general practitioner to avoid the patient's 'real' problem?

2. What circumstances create this kind of patient story?
   a. Is this situation a common occurrence?
   b. What kinds of behaviour do patients find difficulty in exhibiting during a consultation (such behaviours may be part of their normal make-up)?
   c. Are our non-verbal messages necessarily congruent with our verbal messages?
   d. Are our verbal and non-verbal messages good indicators of our inner thoughts and feelings?
   e. How valid are patient criticisms of general practitioners that we don't care, we don't take time, we don't listen, and we don't understand?

3. What is the implication of her story for the practice you are working in?
   a. Who has responsibility for the outcome described by Janice the year before – your colleague, Janice, both of them?
   b. Is it necessary to explore with Janice why the vaginal examination and Pap. smear were apparently her best option a year ago?
   c. Will you discuss this case with the colleague involved in the earlier consultation?
   d. What is the value of 'feed-back' in inter-personal relationships?
   e. How do you feel about getting feed-back about your clinical cases?

M. W. Heffernan, Melbourne

MRS. LOUISE A. AGED 47 SOCIAL WORKER

123

1. What is your immediate assessment of her condition?
   a. Can scalp lacerations cause hypovolaemic shock?
   b. What is the most likely explanation of this woman's shock?
   c. How do you detect internal haemorrhage in an unconscious patient?
   d. What intracranial injuries are likely to be present?

2. What immediate action would you take?
   a. What are the indications for intravenous infusion or blood transfusion in head injuries?
   b. What are the dangers of intravenous infusion in head injuries?
   c. What other essential actions must be taken in this case?
   d. Why is a nasogastric tube so widely used in the management of head injuries?

W. E. Fabb, Melbourne

124 MRS. JANICE B.   AGED 70   HOUSEWIFE

1. How would you handle this situation?
   a. What assessment would you carry out?
   b. What immediate treatment would you employ?
   c. What further treatment and investigations need to be done?

2. What do you need to do about the refusal of a blood transfusion?
   a. Have you talked to the daughter who is the registered staff nurse?
   b. If she also refuses for her mother to have blood, are there any further steps you can take?
   c. Should you seek a legal opinion?
   d. Has a consent form been signed absolving the hospital from any negligence?

3. What are some other aspects that have to be considered when a Jehovah's Witness patient requires a blood transfusion?
   a. What is the age of the patient?
   b. If the patient is a minor, have the parents the right to say the child cannot have a blood transfusion?
   c. Can anyone countermand this order of the patient or the parents?
   d. If the patient would like the blood transfusion and the parents refuse, who has the right in this case?
   e. Are there any situations in which blood can be given to a person who is not a minor and yet who is a Jehovah's Witness?
   f. What are the laws in your state/country regarding blood transfusions?

M. D. Mahoney, Brisbane

125 MR. VICTOR R.   AGED 28   COUNCIL WORKER

1. What injuries would you suspect?
   a. What cervical spine injuries would you expect to find?
   b. What injuries to the soft tissues may have occurred?

2. What would you do for this man?
    a. What precautions would you take during physical and radiological examination?
    b. What sequence of steps should be carried out in the assessment of cervical spinal injuries?
    c. What is the value of taking initial anteroposterior, lateral and odontoid views?
    d. What are the indications for X-ray of the cervical spine in patients presenting with neck pain and stiffness following injury?
    e. What signs of spinal cord damage would you look for in this man?

W. E. Fabb, Melbourne

MR. R.C.   AGED 24   DRAFTSMAN   126

1. What are the diagnoses?
    a. What is the usual mechanism of injury in quadraplegia?
    b. What are the factors causing this man's shock?

2. What first aid measures would you adopt?
    a. What are the priorities in first aid?
    b. Have you yourself attended a first aid course?
    c. What responsibility has a GP/family doctor in first aid?

3. How should this man be evacuated and where to?
    a. What are the chances of full recovery in this case?
    b. Providing the cottage hospital has a physiotherapist available could this man be managed there?
    c. How would you manage his fluid replacement?

4. What measures can be taken to reduce accidents such as this?
    a. How important is education?
    b. How important is legislation?
    c. How important is law enforcement?
    d. How important is punishment?

R. W. Roberts, Ravensthorpe, Australia

T.H.   AGED 3   MALE CHILD   127

1. What should your initial management be in a case like this?
    a. What is the correct manoeuvre to perform to try to remove the obstruction caused by the popcorn?
    b. What can you do if these means fail?
    c. Is parental consent necessary?

2. Was tracheostomy the correct move, or could some other manoeuvre have been performed?
   a. Is this the kind of skill a family physician should have?

J. K. Shearman, Hamilton, Canada

128 MR. BILL S. AGED 50 ENGINEER

1. What are some of the thoughts that will be going through your head?
   a. What would suggest he is having a heart attack?
   b. What would suggest airway obstruction?
   c. Are there any other causes that you should consider?

2. What should be your next step?
   a. Is it an appropriate time to take a history? If so, to whom would you talk?
   b. Does the patient require immediate treatment? If so, what signs would indicate this?

3. You have ascertained that he has been eating some meat and has had some wine. The assumption is that the meat has stuck in his throat.
   a. What should you do next?
   b. Are you able to remove the meat from his throat?
   c. What is the appropriate manoeuvre that should be performed?

4. What is the incidence of death in people who have choked on food?
   a. How many die because people – onlookers – do not know what to do?
   b. Should everyone be taught this manoeuvre, e.g. anyone undergoing first aid courses, or at schools?
   c. Should there be any follow-up on Mr. S. once this situation has occurred?

M. D. Mahoney, Brisbane

129 DARYL A. AGED 4

1. What diagnostic hypotheses are in your mind?
   a. How would you distinguish between croup due to viral laryngotracheobronchitis and epiglottitis?
   b. What features in this child suggest epiglottitis?
   c. How common is epiglottitis? Is there a seasonal variation?
   d. Is the story consistent with inhaled foreign body?

2. How would you establish a diagnosis?
   a. What physical examination would you carry out to distinguish between viral croup and epiglottitis?

b. In what sequence would you examine the child?
c. What part of the examination carries special risks in epiglottitis? Under what circumstances should it be avoided?

3. How would you manage the situation?
   a. If epiglottitis was your provisional diagnosis, what would you do immediately?
   b. What would you tell the parents?
   c. What is the usual infecting organism in epiglottitis and what is the antibiotic of choice?
   d. If viral croup was your provisional diagnosis, what would you do?
   e. What would you tell the parents?

4. What complications must be avoided?
   a. How do you avoid the complication of airway obstruction in epiglottitis?
   b. How do you manage incipient total obstruction?

W. E. Fabb, Melbourne

MR. C.K.   AGED 52   BUILDER   130

1. What emergency investigations should be performed?
   a. Should an electrocardiogram be performed?
   b. Is an X-ray of chest for heart size necessary?
   c. What blood tests are necessary?

2. What emergency medical treatment would be administered?
   a. Should morphia be administered intravenously?
   b. Is frusemide advised in this patient?
   c. Is verapamil necessary to control the tachycardia?
   d. What immediate steps would you take?

3. What is the most likely diagnosis?
   a. Will the electrocardiogram show evidence of a pericardial effusion?
   b. Is electrocardiography of help in diagnosis?
   c. Do the signs of distended neck veins, dyspnoea and supraventricular tachycardia in a case of pulmonary carcinoma point to a definite diagnosis?
   d. Should you record an electrocardiogram before commencing treatment?
   e. What would an echocardiogram show?

B. M. Fehler, Johannesburg

131 MR. F.R.   AGED 45   BUSINESS MAN

1. What is the likelihood that a patient will survive such an event?
   a. Should the general public be skilled in CPR?
   b. Is there a target population to learn CPR?
   c. What is the role of paramedics?
   d. When is defibrillation used?
   e. What is the prognosis in such a case?

2. What are the risk factors in such a patient?
   a. Are personality types, eating habits, lack of recreation and smoking, really risk factors?
   b. What other risk factors real or apparent are there?
   c. Do certain occupations put people more at risk?
   d. What is the evidence to support such a hypothesis?

3. What residual effects seem apparent and what might you expect in this case?
   a. Why does he seem apathetic about his business?
   b. Does he fear for his life?
   c. Has he had a major personality change?
   d. How unusual is it for independent, hard-driving people to react in such a paradoxical fashion to adversity?
   e. What is the role of his family physician in this instance – for the patient – for the family?
   f. What particular step seems most imminently important?

C. A. Moore, Hamilton, Canada

132 ERNEST C.   AGED 70

1. What do you say to Mrs. C.?
   a. What instructions do you give her?
   b. What is the likely diagnosis?
   c. How is his past history related to the present?

2. What would you take with you on a home visit to Mr. C.?
   a. What drugs and why?
   b. What else and why?

3. You visit at home and he dies within 5 minutes of your arrival. What would you do?
   a. What do you say to Mrs. C.?
   b. What actions do you take?
   c. What was the likely cause of death?

J. Fry, Beckenham, UK

MRS. C.S.   AGED 68   HOUSEWIFE

133

1. How do you establish your diagnosis?
   a. Are blood investigations necessary?
   b. What conditions must be ruled out?
   c. Can the diagnosis only be made by ECG or will this confirm the diagnosis?

2. How do you stop this present attack?
   a. What procedures can be performed on the patient at the bedside?
   b. What medication is used intravenously if the above treatment fails?

3. What advice do you give the patient?
   a. To attempt to prevent attacks.
   b. To stop attacks without the help of a physician.

4. What complications can occur?
   a. From doctor's medication to stop the attack?
   b. If the attack is not converted to normal sinus rhythm?

B. M. Fehler, Johannesburg

MR. C.   AGED 34   COMPANY EXECUTIVE

134

1. What are the possible causes of the tachycardia?
   a. List the possible causes.

2. What simple test may help to decide the nature of the rapid rhythm? How would the various possible causes respond to such a manoeuvre?
   a. What response would carotid pressure produce in:
      – sinus tachycardia
      – paroxysmal atrial tachycardia
      – atrial flutter
      – atrial fibrillation

3. During the test the rate suddenly changes to 100 per minute. What is your presumed diagnosis?
   a. In what condition will a rate of 150 suddenly alter to 100?

4. What treatment will you prescribe?
   a. Will reassurance help?
   b. How will you advise him?
   c. Will you prescribe drugs and if so for how long?

J. R. Marshall, Adelaide

35 **MISS J.C.** **AGED 16** **STUDENT**

1. What is the most likely diagnosis?

2. What is the most likely cause?
   a. Is there likely to be underlying pathology?
   b. How does exercise play a part?

3. What is the appropriate management?
   a. Name four different vagal manoeuvres?
   b. Name four different drugs you may use, their sequence and dosage.

D. S. Muecke, Adelaide

136 **MRS. F.S.** **AGED 79** **WIDOW**

1. What are the likely diagnoses?
   a. What is the mechanism of a transient ischaemic attack and what is its management?
   b. What is the natural history of an embolism in the brachial artery and what is its treatment?
   c. Is there likely to have been a recent episode of myocardial infarction? Is it important to know whether or not there has been?
   d. How would you differentiate TIA from embolism?

2. What are the possible social consequences of each of your differential diagnoses?
   a. What advice would you give to this patient concerning car driving if she has had
      – an embolism of the brachial artery?
      – a transient ischaemic attack?
   b. What are the implications of Mrs. F.S.'s preference for your partner's care following her husband's death?
   c. In what ways might these ideas affect your management of Mrs. F.S.:
      – on that Sunday morning?
      – later?

4. Do you have any comments on her present medication?
   a. What do you know about elderly patients and their need for both a diuretic and low-dose digoxin?
   b. How do you deal with a partner of whose prescribing you disapprove?
   c. At what intervals would you have been seeing Mrs. F.S. if she had been your patient over the past ten years?

d. With particular reference to the elderly what are the advantages and disadvantages of chlorthalidone compared to
   - frusemide?
   - bendrofluazide?

P. Freeling, London

BABY M.H.   AGED 14 DAYS   137

1. What possible causes for these symptoms should be considered?
   a. Are there any congenital abnormalities which could cause a baby of this age to rapidly become ill?
   b. What possible sites of infection could cause serious sepsis in a baby of this age?

2. How do you recognize a seriously ill baby?

3. How would you arrive at a more precise diagnosis in this case?
   a. What symptoms would you enquire about?
   b. What physical signs would you look for?
   c. What investigations would you consider performing?

4. How often do you make a correct diagnosis from information given in a telephone call?
   a. What alerts you to a serious disorder on receiving a telephone call?
   b. After hours, what is the most common time or times that you receive calls?
   c. Do some conditions for which you are called out of hours have a common time of onset and/or seasonal distribution?
   d. What are the most common disorders for which you are called out, out of hours?

H. C. Watts, Perth, Australia

DONNA L.   AGED 2   138

1. What diagnostic hypotheses would you entertain?
   a. What is the diagnostic significance of the pale, feverish, quiet child?
   b. What serious conditions would you want to confirm or exclude?

2. How would you establish a diagnosis?
   a. What further history would be helpful?
   b. What physical signs would you seek to confirm or deny your suspicions?
   c. What investigations are appropriate for suspected meningitis or meningococcal septicaemia?

3. How would you manage the situation?
   a. If meningitis was confirmed, what would be your immediate management? What antibiotic(s) should be used before culture results are available, by what route, and for how long?
   b. If meningococcal septicaemia was confirmed, what would be your immediate management? What antibiotic(s) should be used before sensitivities are available, by what route and for how long?
   c. What is the outlook in these conditions?
   d. What would you say to the mother?
   e. What arrangements does your practice make for handling such emergencies?

W. E. Fabb, Melbourne

139 **RODNEY O.   AGED 12 MONTHS**

1. How would you manage this situation?
   a. What would alert the doctor that the condition is more serious than a simple febrile illness?
   b. Are any investigations necessary at this stage?
   c. Is mere observation sufficient reason to hospitalize?

2. What other illnesses besides meningitis may cause neck retraction, or meningismus?
   a. What infecting organisms may be present despite the administration of penicillin?
   b. What are the likely causes of the abdominal rash?

G. M. Dick, Hobart

140 **TOM   AGED 12   SCHOOLBOY**

1. What was the syndrome this boy suffered from?
   a. What organism was basically responsible?
   b. What environmental conditions predispose to this condition?

2. What is the best treatment of meningococcal meningitis?
   a. What is the explanation of the purpura?
   b. What is the usual cause of death in this condition?
   c. Do you think the doctor should have administered penicillin in the first instance?
   d. What are the arguments against the wholesale use of penicillin or other antibiotics?

J. G. Richards, Auckland

DEBBIE G.　　AGED 3　　　　　　　　　　**141**

1. How would you manage this situation?
   a. What is the effect of ingestion of ferrous sulphate?
   b. How would you ascertain how many had been ingested?
   c. What treatment would you give to Debbie and her mother?

2. What measures would you institute after the crisis was over to avoid such a situation in the future?
   a. What medications and poisons do children of this age commonly ingest?
   b. How do you manage these poisonings?
   c. What instructions would you give mother about the safe storage of drugs and poisons?

3. What do you do in your practice to avoid accidental poisoning amongst your patients?
   a. Do you check on drug and poison storage during home visits?
   b. Are any health education pamphlets available for patient instruction about poisoning?
   c. What packaging techniques minimize poisoning with medications?

W. E. Fabb, Melbourne

MRS. LOUISE A.　　AGED 48　　HOUSEWIFE-CLERK　　**142**

1. What are some of the characteristics of this doctor–patient relationship?
   a. How prevalent in the community is Louise's view of general practitioners?
   b. What in this consultative process has caused Louise to become suspicious of the general practitioner's role?
   c. Is this doctor–patient relationship of an appropriate kind?
   d. Are the 'messages sent' necessarily 'those received'?

2. What are the implications of this statement for:
   - day-to-day general practice?
   - the vocational training of general practitioners?
   - the vocational training of other specialties?
   a. Do medical schools train their graduates in communication skills?
   b. Are home visits cost-effective?
   c. Can a home visit be therapeutic of itself?
   d. What can be learnt from home visits?
   e. What criteria can be used to determine the need for a home visit?

M. W. Heffernan, Melbourne

143 MRS. R.   AGED 82

1. What are your working diagnoses?
   a. How do you differentiate between myxoedema coma and accidental hypothermia?
   b. What specific blood tests will help establish the diagnosis?
   c. What are the possible complications of hypothermia?
   d. Explain the reasons for her muscle rigidity and abdominal tenderness.

2. What is your first priority in treatment?
   a. What are the advantages and disadvantages of rapid rewarming?
   b. Should you prescribe any drugs?

3. What essential information should you find out from the neighbours and relatives?
   a. What drugs increase the risk of hypothermia?
   b. What can be done to prevent this happening again?

G. Williams, Iowa City

144 MR. C.R.   AGED 31   BUSINESSMAN

1. What steps are important in the management of seriously ill patients?
   a. Can you usually arrive at a differential diagnosis after a complete history and physical examination?
   b. Are laboratory tests of any value without clinical direction?
   c. It has been said that the diagnosis is the most important part; one can always look up the treatment. Is this true in the case of this patient?
   d. Is it always best to try to explain the total clinical picture on the basis of a single diagnosis?

2. What essential data are required to determine the treatment of this patient?
   a. Does it matter if it is a cold or a warm agglutinin?
   b. Is it common for the basic pathophysiology to be so important as a guide to therapy?
   c. How much of our therapy is superficial and automatic, without even thinking of the nature of the underlying disease process?

3. What is the role of the family physician after he has called in a consultant?
   a. Does he continue to struggle with the clinical problem or does he move into the background?

b. What does he do if he disagrees with the consultant's diagnosis or management?

c. Should he hesitate to call a second consultant if the problem is still unresolved?

d. How important is it to 'hang tough' when treating a seriously ill patient?

e. If you were the patient, would you want your family doctor to 'hang tough' until you were better?

R. L. Perkin, Toronto

BABY G. AGED 5 MONTHS   **145**

1. Who should decide which cases need to see the doctor quickly and which can safely wait?
   a. The doctor – as he is the one who takes the ultimate responsibility?
   b. The receptionist – as she is trained to make exactly this kind of decision?
   c. The patient – as she is the only one aware of all the circumstances?

2. Are barriers between patients and GPs necessary?
   a. What advantages do they have for patients?
   b. What advantages do they have for doctors?
   c. Why should receptionists be called 'dragons' when they are only obeying the doctor's orders?

3. What possible explanations are there for Mrs. G.'s behaviour?

4. What are the principles of management of nappy rash?
   a. What advice should be given?
   b. What creams should the mother be expected to buy herself?
   c. What prescription only medication might be needed?

A. J. Moulds, Basildon, UK

MRS. P.J. AGED 29 TEACHER   **146**

1. What are the patient's main two problems?
   a. In the patient's mind which is the major problem?
   b. Is the solution mainly in the patient's or the doctor's hands?
   c. Which is the most difficult problem to solve?
   d. Is the solution of this mainly in the patient's or the doctor's hands?

2. What types of patient problems need doctor orientation solutions and what need patient orientation solutions?
   a. In whose heads respectively does the necessary information mainly reside for solving this patient's two problems?

F. Mansfield, Perth, Australia

147   **MR. H.C.**   **AGED 60**   **RETIRED GENERAL MANAGER**

1. What immediate steps would you take in such a situation?
   a. How would you immobilize such a patient?
   b. What tranquillizing agent is suitable to be given by injection to such a patient?

2. How would you manage him after his discharge from the hospital?
   a. How do you determine his suicide potential?
   b. Discuss the role of anti-depressants, tranquillizers and hypnotics in a depressed patient.
   c. What is the role of the family in his aftercare?

3. What are some of the problems associated with high rise flats?

F. E. H. Tan, Kuala Lumpur

148   **MR. S.T.**   **AGED 40**   **OCCUPATION UNKNOWN**

1. Can you treat a patient against his will?
   a. Under what circumstances can you treat a patient without consent?
   b. What if patients refuse consent for their children?
   c. If Mr. S.T. loses consciousness can you then treat him as you feel necessary?

2. What is informed consent for treatment?
   a. Do you have to tell the patient everything?
   b. Is a signed consent always necessary for treatment?

E. V. Dunn, Toronto

149   **MR. B.S.**   **AGED 44**   **BUSINESSMAN**

1. What responsibilities are involved when a primary care doctor is committed to continuity of patient care?
   a. What sort of patients should a general practitioner continue to see even when not on duty?

    b.   What other resources are available to assist a general practitioner when dealing with an 'out-of-hours' social-psychiatric emergency?

    c.   Should this sort of problem be dealt with initially solely by the general practitioner?

2.   How often does change in life circumstance induce psychiatric illness?

    a.   What particular stresses occur in a family after the arrival of a new child?

    b.   How can the stresses involved in a new job be minimized?

    c.   At what stage should the patient's immediate superiors at work be notified about the patient's personal problems?

    d.   What are the particular dangers inherent in developing a compulsive and obsessive approach to work?

    e.   How can these dangers be minimized?

3.   What immediate help does this man require?

B. H. Connor, Armidale, Australia

MRS. A.B.   AGED 34   HOUSEWIFE   **150**

1.   What would be the basis of your discussion with the woman in the car?

    a.   Would you discuss treatment for her with the husband present or absent?

    b.   What attitude on your part may entice her into the hospital for observation?

    c.   Why could you be somewhat optimistic about eventually treating her in hospital appropriately?

2.   What would be your management of the problem once she was admitted to hospital?

    a.   How could you obtain more precise information about the alleged overdose?

    b.   What observation could you initiate?

    c.   What immediate treatment may be useful at this stage and possibly acceptable to the patient?

3.   What long term management would you suggest?

    a.   If on the next day she has recovered, what would be an appropriate preventive strategy?

    b.   If a joint husband and wife interview is undertaken by you, how would you assist them in changing their behaviour to prevent a similar occurrence?

    c.   Is a formal psychiatric referral indicated here?

T. D. Manthorpe, Port Lincoln, Australia

151 MISS A.G.   AGED 30   BUYER

1. To what conditions are the single as opposed to the married members of the population more susceptible?
   a. What do you understand by the phrase 'the smiling depressive'?
   b. What subjects would you broach with a patient who presents a very minor complaint after not attending for a prolonged period?
   c. What are the particular risks run by female alcoholics?
   d. At what times are patients more likely to make suicide attempts?

2. What is the differential diagnosis of sore throat?
   a. How do the clinical appearances of a sore throat correlate with the causative agent?
   b. What are your criteria for treating a sore throat with antibiotics?
   c. What complications would you look for in infectious mononucleosis?

3. What is the principal danger of paracetamol overdosage?
   a. What is the usual hospital treatment of paracetamol overdose?
   b. What are the principles of emergency treatment of any overdose?
   c. Was this likely to be a genuine suicide attempt?

T. A. I. Bouchier Hayes, Camberley, UK

152 MR. & MRS. H.   AGED 40

1. Whose side are you on anyway?
   a. Will mother or father make a better single parent?
   b. What, if any, consideration should be given to the children's opinion?
   c. How does the family doctor express an opinion in court?
   d. Who most effectively resolves marital conflicts: the individual parties, friends, family, doctors, clergy, counsellors, judges?

2. Is mother mentally ill?
   a. How can sincerity of a suicide attempt be assessed?
   b. Would you request a psychiatric consultation for mother?
   c. How would you determine severity of depression?
   d. Discuss the ambulatory management of depression.

3. Is father a good risk for a second marriage?
   a. How does an orchidectomy affect fertility?
   b. What is the natural history of seminoma?

c. What patterns of (in)fidelity exist in modern marriages?
d. What is likely to happen to father re his: (i) marital status; (ii) longevity?

P. R. Grantham, Vancouver

SUSAN   AGED 19   SCHOOL LEAVER

153

1. In sharing information with colleagues, what considerations need to be taken into account?
    a. Does written permission by a patient require to be witnessed?
    b. How far into the future, if at all, might such written permission apply?
    c. In Susan's case, where you feel the crisis has resolved, but its disclosure might prejudice her chances of employment, would you refer to the episode?

2. Overdose with paracetamol, even if not associated with a fatal outcome, may cause structural damage. Which organs may bear the brunt?
    a. Susan's notes contain a biochemical report two weeks after the self-poisoning episode: 'GGTP 55 International Units'. What does this mean, and what is its bearing on the clinical and ethical situation vis-a-vis the medical report requested by the occupational health doctor?

3. What is meant by the term 'adolescent crisis'?
    a. Who and/or what services might help Susan cope at this time in her life?

J. D. E. Knox, Dundee

MRS. B.C.   AGED 31   HOUSEMINDER

154

1. What is the incidence of carcinoma of the ovaries in family practice?
    a. What is the natural history and prognosis of ovarian carcinomas?
    b. What is the difference between incidence and prevalence?
    c. What would be the predictive value of Mrs. C.'s symptoms and signs for carcinoma of the ovary and other genito-urinary tract carcinomas?
    d. What would be the predictive value of a hard small mass in the adnexa for any other condition?

2. What possible interactions could have occurred between the doctor and Mrs. C. on informing her of her diagnosis?

    a.   What influence, if any, would the doctor's own self-awareness have on these interactions?

    b.   How much of what the doctor should discuss may be initiated by the patient?

    c.   What counselling technique or techniques would you use in this situation?

3.   On diagnosis, should the doctor initiate 'care of the dying'?

    a.   What are the stages patients are said to go through in a terminal illness?

    b.   How far would you proceed to get patients to be aware of these if they constantly deny their illness?

    c.   What are the advantages and disadvantages of transplanting a model of management into family practice?

    d.   How would you apply the model of 'care of the dying' to a 51 year old woman who has just been diagnosed as having angina?

4.   What changes in family dynamics could you expect in this situation?

    a.   Do you think the doctor was 'right' in trying to involve the children?

    b.   How would he set about it?

    c.   Do you really feel 'they knew nothing'?

    d.   What would be your plan of action at the consultation which took place six months later?

J. H. Levenstein, Cape Town

155 MISS J.C.   AGED 80   RETIRED SECRETARY

1.   How would you manage her when she returned for the result of the barium swallow?

    a.   How reliable is a barium swallow in diagnosing carcinoma of the oesophagus?

    b.   Are there any other conditions which should be considered in the differential diagnosis?

    c.   Should efforts be made to persuade her to have endoscopy (where she previously refused) and perhaps surgery?

    d.   What is her prognosis with and without surgery?

    e.   If she asks whether she has cancer, what would you say?

2.   How would you organize her terminal care in your practice?

    a.   What symptoms is she likely to develop and how would you manage them?

    b.   What facilities do you have to care for the terminally ill?

3.   Should patients with malignancy be told their diagnosis and prognosis?

a. If so, when and how?
b. If not, why not?

H. C. Watts, Perth, Australia

MR. G.T.   AGED 48   COMPANY DIRECTOR   **156**

1. Do you think patients should be told when they are suffering from cancer?
   a. Who should tell them?
   b. At what stage is it best to be told?
   c. Does the absence of direct questions mean that the patient does not want to know more?
   d. Is the patient likely to find it easier to talk to the doctor on his own?
   e. Should a doctor insist on seeing a patient alone?

2. Do you think this particular situation was made more difficult by the fact that the doctor was a woman?
   a. What feelings can develop in patients in relation to a doctor of the opposite sex?
   b. How should the doctor recognize these feelings and deal with them?

3. How important is peace of mind to the dying patient?
   a. How can it best be achieved?

4. How would you have managed this situation?

G. Strube, Crawley, UK

R.C.   AGED 6   PRE-SCHOOL   **157**

1. What are the main problems involved?
   a. What can you do to make the parents understand the problem?
   b. What would persuade you to have the child admitted to
      - your hospital?
      - the metropolitan hospital?
   c. Are you comfortable with death?

2. What assistance can you mobilize?
   a. How often should you visit the patient?
   b. What place has sedation and/or anti-depressants in handling parental anxiety?
   c. What would your reaction be to a request for a referral to a faith healer?

R. W. Roberts, Ravensthorpe, Australia

158   MR. J.B.   AGED 72   RETIRED LABOURER

1. What is the likely diagnosis?
    a. What is the prognosis?
    b. What is the morbidity of definitive surgery?
    c. Do you agree with the decision not to undertake surgery?
    d. Is there an aetiological agent?
    e. Is this disease on the increase or the wane?

2. What are the emotional stages you might expect the patient and his wife to undergo?
    a. How should a physician cope with this?

3. What resources are available to assist in keeping a patient at home?
    a. Could you devise a group of services to include nursing and medical assistance, psychosocial support, nutrition and household needs?
    b. Do you think it is cost efficient?

4. What are the relative merits of a patient being allowed to die at home versus in the hospital?
    a. Is there an advantage to the patient or the spouse?
    b. What are the disadvantages?
    c. What are the problems versus the advantages of dying in the hospital?
    d. What is the attitude of nursing staff and resident staff to pain release.
    e. Do you think it would be difficult to engage the hospital staff in cooperating with the family's decision not to have intravenous therapy and for the patient not to be resuscitated?
    f. What are the ethics of a no resuscitation order?

5. What is the family physician's role at home and in the hospital?
    a. What are the unique attributes a family physician should possess in undertaking such a task?
    b. Are there other health care professionals and institutions which might be helpful?
    c. What is the usual attitude of physicians towards analgesia for dying patients?

C. A. Moore, Hamilton, Canada

159   R.T.   AGED 40   SOLICITOR (MARRIED, YOUNG SON)

1. What determines whether pneumonia is fully investigated?
    a. Was the triad of symptoms referred to initially relevant to the pneumonia? If not, what does it suggest?

   b.   What historical facts may suggest that a pneumonia could be unusual?

   c.   What special tests will assist your understanding of this problem?

2. How might carcinoma of the lung be identified when associated with pneumonia?

   a.   Is haemoptysis in chest conditions specific for a neoplasm of the bronchus?

   b.   How might examination of sputum and pleural fluid aid diagnosis?

3. To whom and by whom should treatment options be presented and discussed?

   a.   Should treatment options be discussed with the patient, his wife, both together?

   b.   Who should present and discuss options?

   c.   What would determine, if anything, that you advised a particular course of action, or inaction?

4. What will influence your management of impending, inevitable death in this relatively young man?

   a.   Would you be able to discuss impending death with the patient? Do you feel you should?

   b.   Would you recruit any assistance, if so what?

   c.   How would you help the wife and child to cope?

   d.   How would you decide whether to manage the terminal phase of illness at home or in hospital?

W. D. Jackson, Launceston, Australia

MR. F.   AGED 53   SHOP ASSISTANT   160

1. Why did the GP not refer the patient for a chest X-ray on the first consultation?

   a.   Should all patients with haemoptysis be referred for chest X-ray immediately?

   b.   Did the delay in having the chest X-rayed have any effect on the outcome of treatment?

2. How should the GP have managed the situation when confronted by the patient's wife?

   a.   To what extent was the patient's wife's anger being displaced from her husband's condition onto the GP?

   b.   To what extent should the GP have attempted to justify his actions?

   c.   What is the importance of accepting the patient's angry feelings?

    d.   What other feelings might the patient's wife also have been experiencing, and how best could they have been elicited by the GP?

3. How would you manage this situation further?
    a.   Should the GP visit the patient at home or hospital of his own accord?
    b.   In what way will the GP be able to give medical help to the patient?
    c.   What feelings can the patient be expected to experience?
    d.   How can the GP be of assistance to the patient in helping him deal with these feelings?
    e.   What is the GP's future role in relation to the patient's family?

S. Levenstein, Cape Town

161 THE E. FAMILY

1. What is meant by 'responsibility' in general medical practice?
    a.   What is implied by 'responsibility' to the patient and his/her family?
    b.   What is meant by responsibility to colleagues?
    c.   Should the general practitioner attempt to defend his colleague for the obvious physical finding missed?
    d.   What role can the general practitioner play in the education of those of his colleagues practising in the 'technical specialties' in the significance of responsibility to the whole family and not just to the patient's pathology?

2. What is the role of the general practitioner in terminal care?
    a.   What particular problems were likely to be encountered in this family?
    b.   How should the general practitioner help them through their anger, even though it may not necessarily have been verbalized?
    c.   How can the general practitioner help the daughter overcome her feelings of guilt and reluctance when she wished to marry and leave the male members of the family caring for themselves.

D. A. Game, Adelaide

162 MRS. MARY M.   AGED 75   PENSIONER

1. How should she be treated?
    a.   What are the possible causes of her chest infection?
    b.   Is this patient likely to respond to antibiotics?

2. Are there any grounds for withholding antibiotic therapy?
   a. What factors might determine a decision not to prescribe antibiotics?
   b. Is such a decision ethically justifiable?

3. What are the main causes of dementia in elderly patients?
   a. What are the mistakes that can be made in making a diagnosis of senile dementia in the aged?
   b. What is meant by 'pseudo-dementia' and how can it be treated?
   c. How should demented patients who are aggressive or violent be controlled?
   d. When taking a history from an elderly patient whose mental competence is suspect, what questions should the patient be asked?

J. G. P. Ryan, Brisbane

MRS. ROSE Y.   AGED 61   HOUSEWIFE   163

1. What should have been the general practitioner's response to the patient's request to be taken off the chemotherapy?
   a. How much control should be exerted by the patient over her own treatment?
   b. What must the general practitioner have done if he acceded to her request?
   c. Is there any question of medical ethics involved in agreeing to cease the treatment?

2. If specific therapy is ceased, what overall treatment plan must be followed by the general practitioner in the ensuing months?
   a. What are the principal fears of the dying patient in this situation?
   b. Assuming that the patient is being nursed in the home, what ancillary services could be mobilized to help in caring for her?
   c. What are the considerations that might make the doctor decide to transfer the patient to hospital?
   d. What principles should be followed in the treatment of pain in terminal illness?

J. G. P. Ryan, Brisbane

MRS. C.   AGED 76   164

1. How would you cope with this patient's request?
   a. What are the pressures on the doctor to make a diagnosis of depression?
   b. In what sense of the word is the patient depressed?

c. Could anti-depressants be of any help?
d. What could one have given Mrs. C. if one had agreed to her request?
e. Has the patient a right to euthanasia?

2. Although sick, her sudden death was unexpected – or was it?
    a. Was her death on entering hospital sheer coincidence?
    b. What kinds of feelings might the doctor experience?

3. Could this outcome have been changed in any way?
a. To what extent should a patient's family be involved in severe illness if they have not previously shown concern?
    b. How often is non-compliance associated with a death wish?

A. L. A. Reid, Newcastle, Australia

165 PENNY   AGED 11

1. What would you send?
    a. What are the indications for sedatives in the acutely bereaved?
    b. Do they merely postpone grief?
    c. If not R_x Doctor, R_x who else might be indicated?

2. Why is considerable criticism levelled at the family physician/general practitioner in relation to the bereaved?
    a. Why might only two GPs have visited the surviving relatives of 22 consecutive acute deaths at a casualty unit?
    b. How soon should a GP visit the recently bereaved?
    c. Should such visits be charged for or are they part of vocation?

3. Is grief a natural physiological process?
    a. What indications do you recognize as distinguishing 'normal' grief from 'pathological' grief? How would you manage it?
    b. Is the feeling of a 'real' presence normal?
    c. What would be your approach if someone 'confided' in you that her husband 'still visited their home', or a daughter said 'Mum still makes Dad's bed and he died six months ago'?

4. What would you do if the mother reported six months after her husband's death that the child was still sleeping badly and was also having some behaviour problems?
    a. How long do most people suffer significant feelings of grief – 2 months, 2 years, 10 years?
    b. What support systems are, should be, available during mourning for the bereaved?
    c. Why do doctors so rarely use them when necessary?

A. J. Radford, Adelaide

MR. NICHOLAS P.   AGED 16   **166**

1. What is the importance of a normal grief reaction?
   a. Should this be modified by drugs or social strictures?
   b. Is the incidence of physical disease higher following bereavement: can you recall examples from your own experience?

A. G. Strube, Crawley, UK

MRS. G.N.   AGED 53   SHOPKEEPER   **167**

1. What is this person trying to say?
   a. Is she angry about the medical care?
   b. Does she feel guilty about her husband's death?
   c. Is she likely to be suffering a bereavement reaction?
   d. Has she come to terms about her husband's death?
   e. Is she really as ignorant as she sounds?

2. Has the medical profession failed in the management of this problem?
   a. Is patient education about the reasons for death important?
   b. Should someone have taken the responsibility to call on the bereaved and, if so, whom?
   c. Do we generally cope well with the question of death?

3. How should Dr. Z. manage this problem?
   a. Should he follow up this problem personally?
   b. Should he discuss the conversation with other members of the team?
   c. Should he call on the patient or advise one of the doctors to call?

J. E. Murtagh, Melbourne

MRS. LUCY O.   AGED 24   HOUSEWIFE   **168**

1. What immediate reactions might you anticipate from the mother?
   a. Why are guilt feelings so strong following a cot death?
   b. What psychological responses, other than guilt, are usual in such cases?
   c. What might mother want to do with or to the dead baby?

2. What would you do immediately?
   a. Would you give reassurance; if so, how?
   b. How would you comfort Mrs. O.?
   c. What advice would you give her, especially about viewing and holding the baby?
   d. What support would you arrange?

e. What would you do with the dead child?
f. What are the medicolegal implications of cot death?
g. What is your attitude to the use of hypnotics and tranquillizers in such circumstances?

3. What long term reactions should you anticipate?
   a. How long does it take parents to 'get over' a cot death?
   b. What bereavement reactions might you expect?
   c. When might the memory of this tragedy be particularly prominent?
   d. What are the common reactions of friends and relatives to the parents, and particularly the mother, after a cot death?
   e. What are the usual reactions of siblings after cot death?
   f. How do the family dynamics change as a result of cot death?

4. What follow up would you organize?
   a. What community support is available for parents following a cot death?
   b. What is your role as a family doctor in the follow up? How long would you follow up this family?
   c. How would you manage the parents' bereavement reactions?
   d. What advice would you give about another pregnancy?
   e. How would you identify and manage the reactions of the siblings?
   f. What opportunities does such a tragedy present for preventive care and health promotion?

W. E. Fabb, Melbourne

169   MRS. H.K.   AGED 34   HOUSEWIFE

1. What are your criteria for diagnosing primary infertility?
   a. What are the possible causes of primary infertility?
   b. Devise a plan for the investigation of an infertile couple.
   c. How might a couple go about (a) fostering, (b) adopting a baby?
   d. What are the factors of particular importance in the antenatal care of the elderly primigravida?

2. What does this mother's behaviour illustrate?
   a. Who is really the patient when this precious baby is presented constantly to the doctor?
   b. What are the functions of the various members of the primary care team in the care of the well baby?
   c. What resources are available to guide the inexperienced mother?

3. Of what syndrome is this baby's death an example?
   a. What have been considered to be the possible causative mechanisms of the sudden infant death syndrome?

b. What are the 'risk factors' for cot death?
c. What are the likely reactions of the parents to this tragedy?
d. What support can be given to parents who have lost children by cot death?

T. A. I. Bouchier Hayes, Camberley, UK

MRS. MARGARET K.   AGED 36   HOUSEWIFE   **170**

1. Discuss cardiopulmonary resuscitation.
   a. What application could it have had in this situation, solo or with aid?
   b. How well is the general community aware of the need to be properly trained in these techniques?

2. How would you handle Margaret in this situation?
   a. Assuming that he died from a massive coronary occlusion, would you assure her that she could not have saved her husband's life?
   b. Would you offer to obtain the post-mortem report?
   c. Discuss temporary sedation and coping with grief reactions.
   d. What contacts would you arrange for her in the ensuing days and weeks?
   e. Do anti-depressants have a place in Margaret's treatment? If so, how would you use them?
   f. What organizations in the community could be helpful to her in the present crisis?
   g. Her children are 6 and 8 years of age. They are currently with their grand-parents. What advice can you give regarding their handling over the next few weeks and months?

3. Discuss the impact and consequences of sudden death in a family.

K. C. Nyman, Perth, Australia

MR. O.M.   AGED 91   PENSIONER   **171**

1. What are the possible causes of death?
   a. What is the mechanism by which heat causes death?
   b. How could this man's fall have caused his death?

2. In your examination how do you determine how long a body has been dead?
   a. What is the significance of the body temperature?
   b. What is the significance of rigor and hypostasis?
   c. What other signs do you look for to determine the time of death?

3. Can you issue a death certificate?
   a. What are the legal requirements when issuing a death certificate?
   b. What are the legal stipulations to determine a coroner's case?
   c. How do you activate the mechanism for a coroner's case?
   d. What material should you put in your statement to the police?

D. S. Pedler, Adelaide

172 MISS A.   AGED 81   PENSIONER

1. What does the family doctor take into account in 'diagnosing' death?
   a. What factors determine your estimate of the time of death?
   b. What are the clinical signs of death?

2. What medico-legal implications are there in Miss A.'s case?
   a. Should the family doctor issue a death certificate?
   b. Might the issue of homicide arise?
   c. What is the position regarding cremation in this instance?

3. What assistance can the family doctor provide for Miss A.'s sister?
   a. Does the fact that Miss A.'s sister is already under treatment for arthritis by another doctor's practice influence your management decisions?
   b. What legal requirements must be met by those involved at the time of death of a person?

J. D. E. Knox, Dundee

173 MISS M.N.   AGED 18   SHOP ASSISTANT

1. List in rank order the level of efficacy of the usual methods of contraception.
   a. The newer forms (post 1975) of IUCD are easier to insert and have greater efficacy. Why?
   b. Every IUCD should be removed if pregnancy occurs. Why?
   c. The earlier the better. Why?
   d. What to do about the IUCD you can't find?

2. Pill failure does occur. List the reasons.
   a. Why does concomitant antibiotic therapy decrease efficacy of OCs? (at least 2 reasons).
   b. When did you last recommend that a female patient on OC, for whom you prescribed antibiotics, consider additive (e.g. condom) contraceptive methods during, and especially for two weeks after, the course?

c. Which other drugs also decrease efficacy of OCs?
d. What regime of OC medication is usually an effective contraception for the non-taker who presents 'the morning after the night before'? Nausea and vomiting are a complication of this procedure. Which OC group decreases these symptoms?
e. What alternative effective contraceptive process can be offered in lieu of OC in this situation?

3. List the contraindications (relative and absolute) for giving OCs. There are over 15 of each!
a. What is the increase in relative risk for a significant cardiovascular episode for pill takers over 35, over 40?
b. Acne is a significant problem for a number of adolescent girls. Why are OCs sometimes helpful, indeed they may remove the need for long term antibiotics? Which one would you choose? Why?
c. What are the options and advice you would offer to a 47 year old who has insisted up till now on remaining on the pill and now thinks she might stop?

A. J. Radford, Adelaide

MISS I.J.   AGED 20   STORE CLERK   174

1. What are the relatively effective birth control modalities?
a. Discuss the use of the pill, IUD, foam, diaphragm, rhythm method and other types of birth control.
b. How does the partner fit in to her plans?

2. Does I.J. have absolute contraindications to any of these methods?
a. How do the hormones in the pill affect acne and migraine?
b. Is migraine a contraindication to the pill?
c. Is there a relationship between the IUD and pelvic inflammatory disease?
d. What are the long term risks of the pill. Is this worse with cigarette smoking?

3. How can you help I.J. to decide what is best for her?
a. Should she have all the knowledge available?
b. Does the patient's personality affect success in using various birth control methods?

4. How would you follow-up the patient with each method you might use?

E. V. Dunn, Toronto

175 **THREE MISSES**

1. Are all these young women suffering from similar problems?
    a. In what way does the demand for sleeping pills, nerve pills, or headache pills point to a similar diagnosis?
    b. How does the request for repeat prescription of oral contraceptive alert the doctor to other problem areas?

2. Should any of these patients achieve their initial expectations?
    a. How does the doctor manage to promote a positive healthy life style to these girls?
    b. What are the dangers in prescribing sleeping pills, nerve pills or headache pills in this age group?
    c. Is a full gynaecological history and examination necessary?
    d. How often is a pelvic examination and cervical cytological test warranted?

3. What problems has the doctor at these interviews?
    a. How does he cope with the time factor at these interviews?
    b. How does this doctor achieve his goals in competition with a less conscientious colleague?
    c. How far can the doctor attempt to change environmental factors?

G. M. Dick, Hobart

176 **MISS C.M.   AGED 15   SCHOOLGIRL**

1. What are the legal and moral implications of advising this girl on contraception?
    a. What is the age of consent in law?
    b. Should you inform her parents before complying with her request?
    c. If not, what risks is the doctor taking?

2. What further questions would you wish to ask her?
    a. What features in the family or personal history represent contra-indications to prescribing oral contraception?
    b. What is the incidence of pregnancy in girls below 16 years of age?
    c. What are the special risks of termination of pregnancy in this age group?

3. What examination would you perform and why?
    a. Is hypertension a contraindication to prescribing oral contraception?
    b. What is the significance of a Class III cervical smear in this context?

   c.   What action would you take if she was found to have a Class III smear?

4. If you decide to prescribe an oral contraceptive, which product would you choose?
   a.   What is a 'low dose' oral contraceptive?
   b.   What are the advantages and disadvantages of the progesterone-only pill?

5. What routine surveillance procedures would be appropriate?
   a.   Is it necessary to perform a breast examination, pelvic examination and cervical smear each year?
   b.   Is it necessary to check the blood-pressure? If so, should it be done monthly, quarterly, six-monthly, annually or every 5 years?
   c.   Is it necessary to weigh the patient regularly?
   d.   What other side effects should you be aware of?

E. C. Gambrill, Crawley, UK

DIANA W.   AGED 15   177

1. What are the pros and cons of putting a teenager on an oral contraceptive?
   a.   What are the ethical and legal hazards involved?
   b.   What are the risks of using oral contraceptives in this age group?

2. How do you supervise patients on oral contraceptives?
   a.   How often would you perform a pelvic examination and cervical smear and why?
   b.   How often would you measure the blood pressure and why?

3. How would you respond to the mother's request?
   a.   At what age are children treated as adults in the eyes of the law?
   b.   Would you keep the mother's intervention confidential?
   c.   Would you inform the mother if you decided to prescribe the pill?

J. C. Hasler, Oxford

MISS J.E.   AGED 15   SCHOOLGIRL   178

1. Is confidentiality an outdated concept?
   a.   What advantage does it have for doctors?
   b.   If patients can be libellous in their comments about doctors, why shouldn't doctors be able to reply?
   c.   Is gossiping to other doctors a breach of confidentiality?

    d.   Does confidentiality actually have any standing in law?

    e.   Shouldn't parents be entitled to know about and consent to any medical care their children need?

2. Should you prescribe the pill for her?
    a.   Do her parents' views matter?
    b.   Is she at risk of having an unwanted pregnancy?
    c.   Would the risk of bad publicity if her parents find out influence your decision?
    d.   Would it be easier to send her to a family planning clinic?

3. What factors should be considered before starting a young girl on the pill?
    a.   What medical contraindications exist?
    b.   Is her menstrual history really relevant?
    c.   Are any baseline measurements or investigations necessary?

A. J. Moulds, Basildon, UK

179   JANET R.   AGED 15   SCHOOLGIRL

1. What is the family doctor's professional responsibility to a legal minor?
    a.   Does Janet have a 'right' to contraceptives?
    b.   Does prescribing a contraceptive imply that the doctor is sanctioning sexual promiscuity?
    c.   Should the doctor insist on receiving parental permission?
    d.   Are there any other implications to the doctor's decision?

2. What other factors could affect the doctor's response to her request?
    a.   What personal factors in the doctor?
    b.   What personal factors in the patient?
    c.   What factors in her family?
    d.   What cultural factors in society?

3. What are the special risks of teenage pregnancies?
    a.   For the pregnant teenager?
    b.   For the foetus during pregnancy?
    c.   For the infant during the first year of life?
    d.   For the unmarried father?
    e.   How do these special risks influence the family physician's decisions in prescribing contraceptives to legal minors?

4. What other problems of adolescents are relevant to the family physician?
    a.   Physical problems?
    b.   Emotional problems?

   c. Social problems?
   d. Sexual problems?
   e. Drugs and other addictions?
   f. What are some possible implications of these problems on the family physician's management of Janet?

Z. Cramer, Tel-Aviv, Israel

HIGH SCHOOL STUDENTS   **180**

1. Is it appropriate to manage this problem over the phone?
   a. Who is the patient?
   b. Are you prepared to treat people you don't know?
   c. What about the rights of parents?
   d. Should 17 year olds expect physician confidentiality?
   e. Should they not go to their regular doctor?

2. How effective are the various methods of contraception?
   a. What special contraceptive needs do teenagers have?
   b. How effective is morning after pill (MAP) therapy?
   c. What is the dosage regimen?
   d. What are the contraindications?
   e. How do you get the pills to the patient on Sunday?

3. Should doctors give sex education lectures in schools?
   a. Does sex education affect behaviour?
   b. What is the role of other professionals?
   c. Should sex education be compulsory in schools?

P. R. Grantham, Vancouver

MRS. R.D.   AGED 22   HOUSEWIFE   **181**

1. What is 'consent' and how does it affect our day to day work?
   a. What do the terms implied and informed consent mean?
   b. Are there any situations where doctors can act without a patient's consent?
   c. By not asking for the coil to be removed had the patient then given her consent to its fitting?
   d. Who gives consent for the treatment of the under aged?

2. What right has the gynaecologist, rather than the patient, to make the final decision about sterilization?
   a. Who knows the patient's mind best?
   b. Is a 35 year old with one child more 'entitled' to sterilization than a 20 year old with 4 children?

    c.   If doctors are the arbiters for social operations then are the views of the doctor a patient sees more important than the patient's actual circumstances in determining whether the operation is carried out?

3. How would you proceed to manage the patient's gynaecological symptoms?
    a.   Should the coil be removed and, if so, what about contraception?
    b.   Should the gynaecologist be given the opportunity to reassess his handling of the case?

A. J. Moulds, Basildon, UK

182 MR. G.P.   AGED 33   ARCHITECT

1. What constitute acceptable indications and contraindications for sterilization?
    a.   What is the relative effectiveness of various forms of contraception?
    b.   Would oral contraceptives affect management of her tumour?

2. How can marital health be assessed?
    a.   Does illness alter roles within families?
    b.   What is the natural history of marriage today?
    c.   Should physicians be advocates for marriage – or for individuals – or either?

3. Who should be sterilized here, if anyone?
    a.   What techniques of sterilization are currently employed?
    b.   What are the side effects of (i) tubal cautery or ligation (ii) vasectomy?
    c.   How do physicians avoid taking sides?

P. R. Grantham, Vancouver

183 MRS. S.C.   AGED 29   HOUSEWIFE

1. Is immediate post-partum tubal ligation generally a good idea?
    a.   Are there circumstances, social or otherwise, when a sterilization procedure should not be performed in the immediate post-partum period?
    b.   Are there circumstances, social or otherwise, when a sterilization procedure should be performed in the immediate post-partum period?

2. On whom should a sterilization procedure be performed?

a. What is the difference in cost (procedure, anaesthesia and hospital stay) of Fallopian tubal ligation compared with vasectomy?

b. What is the difference in loss of time from usual daily activity, work or home, in Fallopian tubal ligation versus vasectomy?

c. Can you think of situations where sterilization of the female would be much preferred over sterilization of the male?

d. Can you think of situations where sterilization of the male would be much preferred over sterilization of the female?

3. What might be the explanation for Mrs. C.'s apparently good mood?

a. Is it possible that Mrs. C. is angry at her physician?

b. Is it possible that Mrs. C. is angry at the physicians caring for her daughter?

c. Is it possible that Mrs. C. is angry at herself?

d. Is it possible that Mrs. C. is depressed?

G. G. Beazley, Winnipeg

MR. ARAN W.   AGED 29   BUS DRIVER   184

1. Do you agree with the doctor's attitude?

a. Should sterilization of either party always be discussed jointly? Apart from ethics is this good medical practice?

b. Discuss the pros and cons of sterilization at the age of 29 years.

2. Assuming you have a joint consultation, what points would you make?

a. Would you advise for or against?

b. Would you bring up all factors that could cause later regrets? How would you do this?

c. If you detected hesitancy in either party, how would this influence your advice?

d. Would you discuss fully alternative contraceptive measures?

e. Describe vasectomy and its possible after-effects in lay terms.

3. Discuss your attitude to 'reversal procedures' for sterilized patients.

a. If sterilization is done on carefully selected patients for the right reasons, should reversals be necessary?

b. What factors influence the success rate in such procedures?

K. C. Nyman, Perth, Australia

MRS. G.E.   AGED 35   HOUSEWIFE   185

1. What is the possible explanation of the mother bringing the child for frequent visits to her family physician, for what seemed like minor, inappropriate problems?

a. Should this child be investigated thoroughly for a rare disease?
b. Should the family physician seek consultative help and if so, why?
c. Should the family physician suspect other potential problems in this family?
d. Should additional information be sought from other family members, and if so, who?
e. Can you suggest how the doctor might address this confounding problem of multiple, seemingly inappropriate visits?

2. What are the issues surrounding male/female sterilization?
a. How should the doctor respond to a request for sterilization?
b. Is male or female sterilization more common?
c. What is the incidence of failure?
d. Can it be reversed?
e. What is the follow-up for the assurance that the vasectomized patient is sterile?
f. Could the pregnancy test be falsely positive?
g. Are there early and late failures?

3. Is the physician performing a failed sterilization, legally cupable?
a. How do we know if the father has fathered this woman's baby, if she is pregnant?
b. How would you approach this subject of paternity with the patient?
c. How does the physician performing the vasectomy cover himself legally?
d. What is informed consent?
e. What should the physician do if he senses that he is potentially legally liable?

4. What are the implications of this woman's membership in Right to Life?
a. Will the patient consider abortion?
b. What will be the effect of this unwanted child on the family and the marriage?
c. If she has an abortion, what long-term emotional effects could it have on the mother?

C. A. Moore, Hamilton, Canada

186 MRS. T.G.　　AGED 23　　RECEPTIONIST

1. What are the possible causes of infertility in this case?
a. In examining both partners what evidence are you seeking for normal hormonal status?

b. What are the most likely female causes of infertility in this case?

c. What proportion of cases have combined male and female factors?

2. What would be the initial investigations of this couple?
   a. How do you determine whether this lady is ovulating?
   b. How do you assess her hormonal state?
   c. What criteria are necessary for a proper collection of seminal fluid and how many collections are necessary?

3. What other aspects of management should be adopted in this case?
   a. What psychological effects is this infertility likely to have on each partner?
   b. How are these psychological effects likely to affect their sex life?
   c. How are the investigations likely to effect the psychological state of each partner?

D. S. Pedler, Adelaide

MRS. C.B.   AGED 27   HOUSEWIFE   187

1. What would you do next?
   a. What would you do about the cervical discharge?
   b. What other investigations would you wish to make on this young woman, and in what sequence.

2. Would you want to see her husband, if so when?
   a. Would you investigate husband and wife in parallel or check out one partner first?
   b. You find the husband azoospermic and certain other signs suggest he may have Klinefelter's syndrome. Ought you try to prove this, if so how?
   c. Would you tell him and/or his wife about this?
   d. With this knowledge, under what circumstances would you pursue investigation of his wife?
   e. What options could you present to this couple who are very keen to have children?

3. If you find no barriers to conception how would you structure future management?
   a. They ask you about artificial insemination (AI) – what answers do you have?
   b. They opt for a try at AI but when discussed with the wife's parents they became embroiled in a bitter ethical debate – where do you stand in this?
   c. Wife is finally pregnant by AI – are there any special hazards?

W. D. Jackson, Launceston, Australia

188 SALLY T.   AGED 23   HOUSEWIFE

1. Is it appropriate for a general practitioner to attempt to deal with this problem?
   a. What are the prerequisites for a successful outcome?
   b. What are the principal causes for sexual dysfunction for which no physical cause can be found?
   c. What are the principal causes of the tension headache and how does it differ from a typical migraine headache?
   d. What treatment may be used in the management of tension headache?

2. If he attempted to solve the sexual problems in this marriage, how would the general practitioner go about it?
   a. What might help the patient lose her inhibitions?
   b. What modern techniques might be effective in this situation?

3. What are some of the factors that might lead to failure of this treatment plan?

J. G. P. Ryan, Brisbane

189 MRS. J.B.   AGED 29   HOUSEWIFE

1. How common are sexual problems in the general population?
   a. What are the organic and behavioural bases of frigidity and impotence?
   b. How might a patient's reluctance to discuss sex influence the presentation of symptoms?
   c. What can you do as a physician to help people feel comfortable to consult you about their sexual problems?
   d. What is the Plissit model of sexual therapy?

2. How well founded are this patient's fears that her vagina is just 'too small' for her husband?
   a. Do you think it worthwhile to investigate with this patient the normal range of sexual functions and dysfunctions?

3. How would you intervene to help this patient?
   a. What about the vulval lesion?
   b. Who should manage the psychological components of the problem?
   c. When should you refer to a specialist?

K. F. Weyrauch, Charleston, SC, USA

MR. DOUG M.   AGED 28

190

1. What is the normal physiology of penile erection?
   a. What is the psycho-pathophysiology going on here?

2. What examination would you do?
   a. Are hormone assays indicated?

3. What treatment plan would you offer?
   a. What help would you expect from exogenous testosterone?
   b. Would your treatment plan work if the couple had already broken up?

D. H. Johnson, Toronto

MR. O.P.   AGED 32   LAWYER

191

1. Is this a normal sexual response for a man of this age?
   a. What factors could affect performance?
   b. Do elderly patients have more problems?

2. What are the common male sexual psychological changes with age?

3. What is the most probable cause for the second episode of impotence?
   a. How does fear of performing affect performance?
   b. Is this a common occurrence?
   c. What diseases can cause impotence, what medications?

4. Does Mr. O.P. require chemotherapy, long term sexual counselling or reassurance?
   a. Is past performance a good indication?
   b. How effective is reassurance?
   c. Would you immediately refer him for intensive sexual counselling?

E. V. Dunn, Toronto

MR. W.T.   AGED 48

192

1. What is the likely cause of this man's reduced libido?
   a. Does libido change with age? If so, at what age?
   b. Are there any likely physical causes?
   c. Would you expect him to experience the same problem with a girl friend?

2. Why does he come to the doctor about it?
   a. What influences a patient in his choice of confidante?
   b. Whom else might he have chosen?

3. Should doctors expect to be able to deal with this sort of problem?
   a. What other agencies are available for referral?
   b. What is the incidence of sexual problems in the population?
   c. What proportion of people with sexual problems need referral?
   d. What is the prognosis?

G. Strube, Crawley, UK

193 MR. ROBERT R.   AGED 51

1. Is this a common problem of the male in his 50s?
   a. To what extent are such problems psychological?
   b. Can physical tiredness be the main factor?
   c. Discuss the 'male menopause'.
   d. What medical conditions can cause impotence?

2. Is the condition reversible?
   a. Can drug therapy really achieve much or is the placebo effect its main value?
   b. If you do use drugs, which are of value and in which case?
   c. Have good books and information leaflets a place in treatment? Which would you use?

3. Would you arrange to see this patient's wife?
   a. Would a joint consultation be useful?
   b. Would you discuss sexual technique?
   c. Would you offer instructive literature?

4. What advice would you offer to the patient?
   a. Is reassurance and urge for patience enough?
   b. Is it in fact common for men to become impotent at this age? Is this usually temporary?
   c. What specific counselling on sexual behaviour could be of value to him?
   d. Would you refer him to a psychiatrist, a 'sexual therapist' or a physician, – or would you refer the couple to any of these?

K. C. Nyman, Perth, Australia

194 J.G.   AGED 55   CLERK

1. Give your assessment of J.G. and the likely pathologies.
   a. What physical causes may be responsible?
   b. What psycho-pathology might be present?

QUESTIONS AND SUB-QUESTIONS

2. How do you manage the situation?
    a. What explanations do you give J.G.?
    b. What clinical examination would you carry out?
    c. What investigations would you arrange?

3. He comes back to see you for the results of the investigations saying
    that his frequency and aching have cleared but he is still impotent.
    Why is he impotent and what do you do about it?
    a. What is impotence?
    b. What are its causes?
    c. What is its treatment?
    d. How successful is it likely to be?

J. Fry, Beckenham, UK

MR. JOHN P.   AGED 52   ELECTRICIAN   195

1. What are the causes of secondary impotence?
    a. What are the effects on potency of failure to satisfy his partner?
    b. How might middle-aged couples react to an imbalance in libido?
    c. What are the possible effects of the menopause on sexual
        relations?
    d. How has the Women's Liberation Movement affected male
        partners?
    e. How can lack of knowledge of facts of sex affect potency?
    f. What effects has media relaxation of sex taboos had on gener-
        ations reared in a more puritanical environment?

2. What are the factors involved in female orgasmic dysfunction?
    a. How many women achieve orgasm in coitus without clitoral
        stimulation?
    b. How important are upbringing and cultural environment?
    c. What aspects of sexual ignorance are important?
    d. What are the effects of misconceptions about female
        masturbation?
    e. What is the relationship between pelvic congestion unrelieved by
        orgasm and chronic pelvic pain?

3. How should this couple's sexual dysfunction be treated?
    a. What is the Masters and Johnson three stage sensate focus
        programme?
    b. What is meant by non-genital pleasuring, genital pleasuring and
        non-demanding coitus?
    c. How can the development of oral stimulation techniques help?

D. G. Chambers, Clare, Australia

196   MR. J.S.   AGED 57   UNEMPLOYED/WIDOWER

1. What concerns or questions might this man wish to voice?
   a. Will he be able to achieve an erection?
   b. Will his sex drive be reduced?
   c. Will he develop gynaecomastia?
   d. Will his voice change?
   e. Will he eventually experience a lot of pain?

2. What is the prognosis in this case in terms of life expectancy?
   a. If he had not had the orchidectomy would his prognosis have been worse?
   b. What drugs might have been tried if Mr. S. had refused orchidectomy?
   c. Would any of these drugs have offered a better prognosis than orchidectomy?
   d. Are there other drugs which might now be added which would improve the prognosis?

3. Could this disease have been cured if discovered earlier?
   a. What is the best screening test for carcinoma of the prostate?
   b. What laboratory investigations are also of some use as screening tests for carcinoma of the prostate?
   c. What percent of prostatic nodules palpated on rectal examination are positive for carcinoma of the prostate?
   d. Is it likely that a solitary prostatic nodule can cause impotence?

G. G. Beazley, Winnipeg

197   MR. H.H.   AGED 46

1. How can society best help the patient with multiple sclerosis?
   a. What facilities are there in your community to help this kind of patient?
   b. What kind of facilities should there be in the ideal world?
   c. What is the role of the family physician in this patient's total care?

2. Why do you think this man's leg fractured with such apparent ease? (prior to this major fracture, he sustained a tibial plateau fracture in the same leg by bringing his leg down too hard and after this hospital admission, he sustained an above knee femoral fracture while receiving physiotherapy).
   a. How can he avoid such incidents in the future?

3. How can we help this man with his sexuality?
   a. Do you think this man is liable to be impotent?

b. What kind of sexual advice can you give to help a disabled person?
c. What are your attitudes to sex and the disabled person?

J. K. Shearman, Hamilton, Canada

MR. C.S.Y.   AGED 26   BARTENDER   198

1. Identify the problems presented by this patient.
   a. What evidence do you have to suggest that the asthma may be psychogenic in origin?
   b. Discuss the terms 'intersexuality', homosexuality', 'transexuality' and 'transvestism'. Which terminology or terminologies refer to this patient?

2. What further history would you like to obtain from this patient?
   a. How would his family history assist you in your management?
   b. How could the attitude of his homosexual partner have brought about the request for advice regarding a transexual operation and his asthma?

3. What would you look for in particular at physical examination?

4. How do you propose to manage this patient?
   a. What are the controversial aspects of sex reassignment surgery?
   b. What is your community's view towards homosexuality?

F. E. H. Tan, Kuala Lumpur

DORIS J.   AGED 18   CIRCUS HAND   199

1. What other history would support your suspected diagnosis?
   a. What other symptoms might suggest gastroenteritis as the diagnosis?
   b. What else do you want to know about her gynaecological history?
   c. What is the relevance of a detailed sexual history?
   d. What are the symptoms of early pregnancy?

2. How would you confirm the diagnosis?
   a. What are the physical signs of early pregnancy?
   b. What does the urine pregnancy test measure?
   c. How should the urine specimen be collected?
   d. If the urine pregnancy test is negative, what is the most likely diagnosis and why?

    e.   What investigations other than a urine pregnancy test might you do?

    f.   If the pregnancy test is negative what will you advise?

3.   What factors affect the management of this patient?
    a.   Is termination of pregnancy just another form of contraception?
    b.   How might her religious beliefs affect the situation?
    c.   What is her current legal situation regarding termination of pregnancy?
    d.   What problems might there be with continuation of the pregnancy?
    e.   Who else might you involve in discussing the situation?

4.   What preventive measures are relevant to this patient?
    a.   What form of sex education is appropriate?
    b.   What issues help you decide what form of contraception to advise?

R. P. Strasser, Melbourne

200   MRS. E.R.   AGED 36   HOUSEWIFE

1.   What are the possible diagnoses?
    a.   Does the presence of a large fibroid preclude vaginal delivery?
    b.   What are the problems associated with an ovarian cyst in pregnancy?
    c.   Assuming pregnancy prior to her arrival two months ago, should she be offered termination of her pregnancy?

2.   What investigations would you order?
    a.   Should all pregnancies have an ultrasound scan?
    b.   What are the indications for amniocentesis?
    c.   Assuming she has twins, what is the most appropriate confirmatory investigation, and when?

3.   What are the possible risk factors in this patient?
    a.   What are the problems associated with an elderly primigravida?
    b.   Should an elderly primigravida be delivered by a specialist obstetrician?

R. W. Roberts, Ravensthorpe, Australia

201   MS. E.F.   AGED 17   STUDENT

1.   What are the abortion laws in your country?
    a.   How would you manage this patient if abortion was illegal?

b. How would you manage this patient if abortion was legal?
c. How would you manage this patient if you believed abortion was morally or religiously wrong?

2. Is unwanted pregnancy an accident or illness?
   a. If unwanted pregnancy is an illness what preventive measures could you, as a family physician, have initiated in this patient or in patients generally?
   b. Are pregnancies in women under the age of 21 on the increase or decrease in the world?
   c. Discuss possible reasons for your answer to the above question.
   d. Do family planning clinics help all those at risk?

3. Are there any risks to putting a young girl on oral contraceptives?
   a. Are there any alternatives to oral contraception for birth control in this age group and what are their advantages and disadvantages?
   b. If Ms. E.F. was not pregnant, how would you manage the situation?

J. H. Levenstein, Cape Town

MISS N.   AGED 15   SCHOOLGIRL   202

1. How would you advise this girl in the management of her pregnancy?
   a. How would you advise her father to cope with this problem?
   b. How would you advise her mother to cope with this problem?
   c. How would you advise her sister to cope with this problem?

2. If her father refused to allow her to abort the pregnancy, what would be your main objective in subsequent management?
   a. What is the impact of therapeutic abortion on a 15 year old?
   b. What are the physical risks of therapeutic abortion?
   c. What are the emotional risks of a therapeutic abortion?

3. What are the risks of an unwanted pregnancy in a 15 year old?
   a. Should this be considered a low, moderate or high risk pregnancy?
   b. Should you manage the pregnancy or should it be managed in a high risk pre-natal unit?
   c. In this situation, should the girl be told to keep the baby, or give the baby up for adoption?
   d. Ethically, is the physician bound to treat a 15 year old pregnant girl as an adult, or the child of her parents?

W. W. Rosser, Ottawa

203 R.D.   AGED 18   WAITRESS

1. As a family physician, how do you approach the topic of adolescent sexuality?
    a. What attitudes do adolescents commonly hold towards sexuality?

2. What is your responsibility towards the patient, her mother, the unborn child?
    a. How frequent is adolescent pregnancy today?
    b. What forms of birth control are available to adolescents and what are the risks, benefits, effectiveness of each?

3. How will you manage the present visit and her mother's concerned inquiries?
    a. How do you approach the question of abortion?
    b. What techniques are available at different gestational ages?
    c. What is the legal, ethical climate surrounding abortion in your community?

K. F. Weyrauch, Charleston, SC, USA

204 MAUREEN T.   AGED 19   STUDENT TEACHER

1. What comments would you make to Maureen's mother?
    a. Should the situation be discussed at all without Maureen's permission?
    b. What would be a suitable way to have such a discussion?

2. Should you arrange a full discussion with Maureen and her boy friend?
    a. Is it the doctor's role to point out the responsibilities of parenthood and what it means to such young parents?
    b. What support can the community offer these people?
    c. What could be the effect on their careers?

3. How would you react to a request for termination?
    a. What are the associated legal problems?
    b. What are the associated medical problems?
    c. What complications or psychological sequelae commonly follow terminations?

4. Should you arrange other opinions for Maureen if you feel that you are basically prejudiced in her case?
    a. Where would you send her?
    b. Would her religious convictions be a major issue?

c. Could her mother's acceptance of the pregnancy completely change the situation?

d. How could this be achieved?

K. C. Nyman, Perth, Australia

MISS G.G.   AGED 24   MENTALLY RETARDED   **205**

1. What options are there for the management of this pregnancy?
   a. Who should be involved in making a decision about the continuation or termination of the pregnancy?
   b. Whose formal consent might be required if a therapeutic abortion was proposed?
   c. If this pregnancy is carried to term, what options might there be for the custody of the child?

2. What contraceptive measures might be adopted in the future?
   a. Should all mentally retarded females undergo Fallopian tubal ligation when they enter their reproductive years?
   b. Would this patient qualify for tubal ligation?
   c. Whose formal consent might be required if a tubal ligation was proposed?
   d. How would you obtain 'informed consent' in a situation like this?

3. Is it generally accepted that all babies born to mentally retarded mothers should be apprehended?
   a. Would you allow this woman to keep her baby?
   b. Can you think of situations where a mentally retarded individual could care for a baby?
   c. Are babies born of unions in which both parents are mildly retarded likely to be of lesser intelligence than either parent?

G. G. Beazley, Winnipeg

MRS. K.L.N.   AGED 25   HOUSEWIFE   **206**

1. How would you answer her?
   a. Is it possible from the history to know who is responsible for this pregnancy?

2. Should she request termination of pregnancy, how would you advise her?
   a. What are the dangers of termination of pregnancy at 16 weeks maturity?
   b. What do you think are the likely reasons for the patient to request termination so late in her pregnancy?

3. What medico-legal problems may arise after the delivery?
   a. How are you able to confirm the paternity of the child after delivery?
   b. If her husband confronts you and tells you that he suspects that his wife has been unfaithful, how would you manage the situation?

F. E. H. Tan, Kuala Lumpur

207 MRS. K.W.   AGED 28   HOUSEWIFE

1. Who decides how a patient should be treated?
   a. Is it the patient and her family?
   b. Is it the hospital or the unions?
   c. Is it the doctor?
   d. Is it the air ambulance system?
   e. Should the church be involved?
   f. Is it the organization or person who gets paid for carrying out the treatment or the organization (e.g. health or government fund) which pays for the treatment to be carried out?

2. How does a retarded child affect a family?
   a. How extensively should a retarded child be investigated to determine the cause of the retardation?
   b. How should the siblings be helped when considerable time must be spent on a specially affected child in a family?
   c. What support services should be available for a family with a handicapped child? Should they be financial, residential, paramedical or ambulance services?

3. How does a history of subfertility affect the management of subsequent pregnancies?
   a. What form of delivery should be advised when a mother is subfertile?
   b. What investigations are needed – which partner first?
   c. What marital counselling might be needed when a couple are infertile?

B. H. Connor, Armidale, Australia

208 MRS. D.C.   AGED 32   HOUSEWIFE

1. What do you understand by the rhythm method of contraception?
   a. What methods of contraception are available?
   b. What are the failure rates of the various contraceptive methods?
   c. What is the morning-after pill?
   d. What factors would you take into consideration in counselling a couple about contraception?

2. What are the laws governing the therapeutic termination of pregnancy?
   a. What are the possible early and late complications of first trimester abortion?
   b. What are the current national trends for birth rate and termination of pregnancy?
   c. If termination is refused or decided against, what special risks would you consider?
   d. What agencies might you enlist to help in the care of a family in which a child is considered to be at risk?

3. What are the common presentations of anxiety?
   a. With what other conditions might anxiety be confused?
   b. What do you understand by non-verbal communication?
   c. What are the complications of the use of tranquillizers in the treatment of anxiety?

T. A. I. Bouchier Hayes, Camberley, UK

MRS. L.H.   AGED 35   HOUSEWIFE

209

1. What are the real issues behind this request?
   a. Would the woman really want an abortion?
   b. Could an abortion be detrimental to her and the marriage?
   c. What are the social pressures to seek an abortion?
   d. What has really caused the husband to react in this manner?
   e. Would the birth control techniques be a significant problem?

2. Should the doctor comply with this request?
   a. Should we comply 'carte-blanche' with reasonable requests for abortion?
   b. Do we tend to take the soft option too readily?
   c. Should we try to influence these people to seriously reconsider their decision?
   d. Are there strong grounds for this family to have another child?

3. How would you manage this problem?
   a. Should you endeavour to involve the husband in discussions and decision making?
   b. Should you refer her for another opinion?
   c. Should her age be a factor favouring abortion?
   d. Is it hazardous procuring an abortion in the second trimester?
   e. Do psychiatric opinions generally tend to show a significant bias in favour of abortion?

J. E. Murtagh, Melbourne

210   MRS. A.T.   AGED 39   HOUSEWIFE

1. How do you confirm a pregnancy?
    a.   What are the symptoms and physical signs?
    b.   Would you perform an immunological pregnancy test – blood or urine?
    c.   For pregnancy tests on urine, what precautions do you take in collecting the specimen and what are the pitfalls in the test?

2. What are the risks of pregnancy in this case?
    a.   To the mother?
    b.   Of foetal abnormality?
    c.   To the family?

3. How would you manage this case?
    a.   What advice would you give to her?
    b.   Is termination justified?
    c.   How do your own views affect your decision making in these problems?

4. What are the legal requirements which have to be met before termination is justifiable?

5. What are the long term effects of termination and the risks involved to the mother?
    a.   Physical risks?
    b.   Are there long term psychological sequelae following termination?

6. What form of contraception would you advise subsequently?

H. C. Watts, Perth, Australia

211   MRS. N.L.   AGED 23   SCHOOLTEACHER

1. What factors need clarification before accurate advice can be given?
    a.   Is she really pregnant?
    b.   Can German measles be diagnosed clinically with confidence?
    c.   If it is German measles, was her nephew infectious when he was staying with her?
    d.   Could she have had German measles without knowing?

2. How would you interpret the possible rubella antibody results that might be revealed by serological testing?
    a.   What is the range of the incubation period of rubella?
    b.   What should you do if there is no detectable rubella HI antibody?

   c.   Does rubella HI antibody detected in serum taken within 10 days of contact exclude rubella from having occurred earlier in the pregnancy?

3.   If she has caught rubella how would you explain the risks of pregnancy?
   a.   What are the features of congenital rubella?
   b.   What are the chances of the baby being born undamaged?

4.   Under what circumstances is abortion legal?

A. J. Moulds, Basildon, UK

MRS. D.   AGED 30   TEACHER   212

1.   What would be your approach to her problem?
   a.   Was the pregnancy exposed to the radiation?
   b.   What are the hazards of such an exposure and the likely outcome?
   c.   Would you recommend termination of pregnancy?
   d.   What precautions do radiologists take to avoid such problems?

2.   Her infuriated husband wishes to take legal action against both the general practitioner and the radiologist and wants you to testify. Do you pacify and attempt to talk him out of it or express willingness to testify?
   a.   Is there medical negligence in this case?
   b.   Would you return her to the other general practitioner and try to avoid testifying altogether?
   c.   Is it possible to determine that the foetus suffered the effects of irradiation?

3.   How could such a situation be prevented?
   a.   What are the indications for radiology in obstetrics?
   b.   What measures are available to reduce the hazards of irradiation?

F. E. H. Tan, Kuala Lumpur

SARAH P.   AGED 32   213

1.   How might the doctor manage the consultation?
   a.   What kind of anxieties and feelings should he anticipate in the patient?
   b.   How is a prostaglandin termination carried out?
   c.   What are the chances of this foetus being affected?

2. By what methods can meningomyelocoele be detected in a foetus?
   a. What is the reliability of alphafoetoprotein blood levels?
   b. When can they be done?
   c. How can suspicions from high levels be confirmed?

3. What kind of problems does the birth of a baby with meningo-myelocoele present?
   a. What legal problems must the doctors be aware of?
   b. What treatment is available?
   c. What feelings do the parents commonly experience?

J. C. Hasler, Oxford

214 MR. J.M.   AGED 27   MEDICAL STUDENT

1. What important family history would need to be obtained?
   a. What information would lead you to consider a subsequent pregnancy at risk?

2. How would you explain the benefits versus risks and indications for amniocentesis to this medical student and his wife?
   a. What are some of the factors that might be leading J.M. to demand amniocentesis?

3. How would you counsel them if they had **no** risk factors in their family and personal history?

P. Boiko, Charleston, SC, USA

215 MRS. B.   AGED 21   HOUSEWIFE

1. What is the most likely aetiology of this problem?
   a. Was the heat and condition of the household an important factor in this woman's illness?
   b. Could pregnancy have played any role in this woman's illness?
   c. Why was this an acute emergency? How acute was the emergency and what steps would you take to cope with this problem effectively?

2. What were the risks in moving this woman to the hospital?
   a. Could the condition be aggravated by the move?
   b. Are there any steps to be taken prior to the move that would reduce the risks?
   c. What drugs carried in one's bag might be of value in this situation?

3. How might this situation have been prevented?
   a. Would health education prevent this problem?

b. Would more frequent physical examination and screening by physicians prevent this problem?
c. What is the surgeon most likely to find on surgical intervention?
d. What is the next step in management of this case as soon as the patient arrives in hospital?
e. What role does the physician's personal comfort and well-being play in influencing our decisions in management of patients?

W. W. Rosser, Ottawa

MISS LOIS D.   AGED 23   SALES ASSISTANT   216

1. What are the major obstetrical risks at this stage?
   a. What drugs, instruments should routinely be carried in a doctor's bag in order to cope with such an emergency?
   b. Will Lois need a curettage?
   c. If you decide not to admit her locally:
      – what factors need to be considered so that she can be transported safely to the chosen centre?
      – who will you refer her to?
      – what are the objectives to be attained during the convalescence?
      – will you generate a 'cover story' that will allow adequate explanation for the referral and, for the time being, allow Lois and her family to be free of the local consequences of this unplanned pregnancy?

2. What history do you need at this point?
   a. What are the common causes of maternal death?
   b. What are the family likely to know of Lois's condition?

3. What family and social dynamics need to be considered?
   a. Will you let her convalesce in the local hospital?
   b. What would you do regarding the father of the child?
   c. What role will you adopt with regard to the parents?
   d. What role will you adopt with regard to Lois?
   e. Will you conduct/arrange a post-mortem on the products of conception? Where?

M. W. Heffernan, Melbourne

MRS. J.W.   AGED 35   HOUSEWIFE AND PART-TIME   217
                             TEACHER

1. What is the cause of post-partum depression?
   a. What is the place of medication in these cases?
   b. Is the pain threshold lowered when people are suffering from depression?

    c.   Should patients who suffer one attack of puerperal depression be advised to become pregnant again?

2.   What complications of pregnancy can be treated at home?
    a.   How is it possible to determine the difference between liquor and urine?
    b.   What complications are associated with premature loss of liquor?
    c.   When should consultant help be sought in this situation?

3.   How is it possible to balance the needs of the husband and wife when counselling a married couple?
    a.   How is a wife's depression reflected in her husband?
    b.   What can a primary care physician do to help a husband who is under apparently unavoidable stress at work?
    c.   How does a professional woman cope with home responsibilities without damaging her career prospects?
    d.   How can a primary care physician encourage a married couple to enjoy doing things together?
    e.   What proportion of counselling time should be spent with the husband and wife together and when should this be done in the couple's own home?

B. H. Connor, Armidale, Australia

218   MRS. B.S.   AGED 29   HOUSEWIFE

1.   Should confinements be conducted in isolated country hospitals?
    a.   What special skills are required by the general practitioner working in this sort of situation?
    b.   What consultant cover should be organized to help general practitioners in isolated country hospitals?
    c.   What special preparation might be required for a woman who is to be confined in her own home town local hospital?

2.   What special assistance might be available to help with this unexpected emergency?
    a.   How would radiography help?
    b.   What specialist help might be obtained by telephone?
    c.   How could the maternity ward staff help?
    d.   How many doctors should be present at the delivery?

3.   How should this delivery be conducted?
    a.   What information should be given to the patient?
    b.   Should she be sedated?
    c.   Would an intravenous drip be of assistance?
    d.   Should the patient have an episiotomy?

e.   Would forceps be useful in this situation?
f.   What resuscitation might be required for the baby?
g.   Should the husband be permitted to stay for the confinement?
h.   What type of anaesthesia would you use?

B. H. Connor, Armidale, Australia

MRS. H.B.   AGED 26   FILM CLERK   **219**

1. What are the diagnostic possibilities?
    a.   What are the diagnostic features of a threatened abortion?
    b.   What are the diagnostic features of an incomplete abortion?
    c.   What are the diagnostic features of a missed abortion?

2. What investigation might be carried out?
    a.   At what stage in pregnancy does a urine pregnancy test normally become positive?
    b.   At what stage in pregnancy does a urine pregnancy test normally become negative?
    c.   Would it be important to do coagulation studies in this situation?

3. Who else might you wish to talk to?
    a.   How might you involve her husband?
    b.   What problems commonly requiring the help of a consultant obstetrician are peculiar to the evacuation of the uterus containing a dead foetus?

G. G. Beazley, Winnipeg

MRS. DENISE S.   AGED 25   **220**

1. What is your further management?
    a.   How would you confirm intra-uterine death?
    b.   At what point do you advise her of your suspicions?
    c.   How soon should active intervention be undertaken?

2. What reasons can you suggest for this and the preceding intra-uterine death?
    a.   What investigations would you consider necessary of the patient, her husband and the conceptus when it is available?
    b.   It is common to console a mother after spontaneous abortion with the suggestion that there was some lethal foetal abnormality. Is this appropriate here, or in any circumstance, especially those in which extensive investigation has proved negative?

3. What advice would you give about further pregnancies?
    a. What factors would influence your response to questions about the possible outcome of another pregnancy?
    b. What factors would you outline to the parents in helping them to a decision about whether to try again?
    c. What is 'reassurance' and how can you offset the disappointment and perhaps reproach when it is ill-founded?

J. A. Stevens, Ulverstone, Australia

221 MRS. P.M.   AGED 26

1. As she is only in early labour is there any point in getting up to see Mrs. P.M.?
    a. What questions would you ask the mother?
    b. What examination would you make?
    c. Would you rupture the membranes?

2. If you can't feel movements and can't hear the foetal heart what will you say to the mother and her husband?

3. The labour results in a stillbirth and baby and placenta are normal. What matters are there to discuss with the parents?
    a. What can you say about future pregnancies?
    b. What will you discuss about the grieving process?
    c. What funeral arrangements are common for stillbirths?

F. Mansfield, Perth, Australia

222 MRS. X.Y.   AGED 32   HOUSEWIFE

1. Could this condition be serious?
    a. Are pains in the calf common in pregnancy?
    b. Does unilateral swelling always suggest a serious cause?
    c. What condition more commonly causes localized pain and tenderness in the leg of a pregnant woman that the serious one suggested above?
    d. Is the latter serious and how is it treated?

2. How would you determine if any pathology existed?
    a. What clinical signs would help in elucidating the seriousness of the problem?
    b. What investigation is mandatory to make an absolute diagnosis?

3. What would be considered optimal management?
    a. Should this woman be hospitalized?

b. Should this woman be hospitalized if a DVT is found on venogram?

c. If a DVT is found, should anticoagulant treatment be commenced?

d. If anticoagulant treatment is considered, which of the two anti-coagulants would you favour
   – warfarin?
   – percutaneous heparin?

T. D. Manthorpe, Port Lincoln, Australia

MRS. A.B.   AGED 18   HOUSEWIFE   223

1. What physical findings would you anticipate?
   a. Would you expect this patient to appear acutely ill?
   b. Would a few 4 mm erythematous lesions showing a bluish-white centre on the left leg, right thumb, and left second toe be of any significance?
   c. Would pelvic findings of right adnexal tenderness and a moderate yellowish-white discharge appearing in the cervical os and vaginal vault be of any significance?
   d. What would the differential diagnosis be for a right knee which is swollen, warm, and tender on movement?
   e. Would it help to know that the right ankle shows definite swelling and capsular tenderness, as do the right second, third, and fourth metatarsophalangeal and proximal interphalangeal joints?

2. What are the essential problems in the problem list?
   a. Fever and chills?
   b. Skin lesions?
   c. Vaginal discharge?
   d. Pregnancy?
   e. Joint symptoms?

3. How would one proceed to obtain efficient use of the laboratory in this case?
   a. Would a sedimentation rate of 30 mm per hour and a negative test for antinuclear antibodies be helpful?
   b. Would a Gram stain or culture of the skin lesion aspirate be expected to be diagnostic?
   c. Should a sample of the right knee synovial fluid be obtained? What would be the expected findings?
   d. Would a series of blood cultures be expected to be helpful or diagnostic?
   e. Would a Gram stain of the vaginal secretions be helpful?
   f. Would aerobic or anaerobic (Thayer-Martin) vaginal cultures be helpful or diagnostic?

4. What epidemiological and therapeutic measures would be helpful?
   a. Would it be helpful to find out the patient's relationship with her husband?
   b. Should a careful review of extramarital sexual contacts by both parties be sought?
   c. Would it be important to interview and examine such contacts?
   d. Would it be important to prevent cross contamination of the patient's skin lesions?
   e. If antibiotics are indicated, what would be first and second line drugs?

L. H. Amundson, Sioux Falls, SD, USA

224 MRS. MARTHA M.   AGED 35   LAWYER

1. What are some of the important issues you would be thinking about?
   a. Does it matter that she is seven months pregnant and perhaps needs removal of the lump?
   b. What if it is cancer – what should be done about the pregnancy?
   c. Is a family history of breast cancer important?
   d. Will the method of treatment chosen be determined by the fact that Mrs. M. has five other children?
   e. What might be the importance to her condition of the timing of her menarche, being on the pill, and breast feeding her other children?

2. What would you do?
   a. What would you say to the patient at this stage?
   b. What treatment would she require?
   c. What do you do about the 7 month pregnancy?
   d. What other examination would you perform?

3. What are the effects of pregnancy on breast cancer?
   a. Should the mother be allowed to continue with the pregnancy?
   b. What do you tell the husband who is waiting outside the door?
   c. What are the possible methods of treatment for a 35 year old woman with breast cancer who is not pregnant?
   d. Does the fact that she is pregnant alter the prognosis?
   e. What do you say when she asks can she breast feed this baby after his/her birth?

M. D. Mahoney, Brisbane

225 MRS. NERIDA C.   AGED 41   HOUSEWIFE

1. What are the most important issues to be considered at this stage?
   a. How do you assess the severity of the spina bifida deformity?

    b.   What other deformities may be present?

    c.   How do you determine when to operate?

    d.   How will you assist the parents to cope with this baby?

2.   How are the parents likely to react at this stage?

    a.   How can you help the parents cope with their feelings of anger and guilt?

    b.   Should an amniocentesis have been performed during the pregnancy?

    c.   How do you as their doctor cope with their feelings of anger with you for not having diagnosed the condition before birth?

    d.   What can you say to comfort the parents when they feel helpless and depressed at the thought of the years ahead?

    e.   Is it normal for the parents to have these feelings?

3.   What are the legal, moral and ethical issues involved with a baby with spina bifida?

    a.   Do you believe in euthanasia?

    b.   Should the baby be left to die or should the baby, if he gets an infection, be declined antibiotics?

    c.   If the baby does have surgery straight away, are you condemning him to a life of misery?

    d.   What do you think about the case in America where a court judge ordered a doctor to perform an operation on a baby when the parents had refused permission, (the baby had a spina bifida deformity)?

4.   What are the facilities for children with spina bifida in your state/country?

    a.   Is there a Spina Bifida Association which supports parents?

    b.   What is the prognosis for a child with spina bifida?

    c.   If the parents were to have another baby, what is the likelihood of them having another affected child?

M. D. Mahoney, Brisbane

NEWBORN BABY GIRL   **226**

1.   What emergency services should be available to help isolated rural communities?

    a.   Should the transport services be confined to air ambulance services?

    b.   Who decides the priorities for emergency services and their availability – the doctor, the politicians, the ambulance staff?

    c.   How should this baby be transported?

2.   What can be done immediately to help the baby?

    a.   How would a chest X-ray help?

b. What use would antibiotics and intravenous glucose be?
c. How could specialist help be obtained despite the lack of air ambulance transport?

3. What important preparations can be made before the trip by air ambulance?
a. How should the baby's temperature be controlled?
b. What oxygen concentration should be maintained?
c. What should be done for the parents of the child?

B. H. Connor, Armidale, Australia

227 R.T. AGED 2 WEEKS

1. How would you feel if you were in Dr. P.'s place? How would you feel if you were Mr. and Mrs. T.?
a. How could Dr. P. effectively deal with these parents while also diagnostically evaluating the baby?

2. What causes of jaundice in a 2 week old would you want to investigate by further history, physical examination and/or laboratory data?
a. Is jaundice in a 2 week old an emergency problem that needed to be dealt with that day or could Dr. P. wait a week until their regular doctor returned?

3. How can you ask about alcohol history without putting a patient (in this case Mrs. T.) on the defensive?

P. Boiko, Charleston, SC, USA

228 MISS M.T.R.   AGED 18

1. What is the probable underlying pathology in the breast?
a. Can cancer ever present like this?
b. Could the lump contain pus?
c. What criteria help select the choice of antibiotic?
d. If an antibiotic is given, what should be done if there is no improvement after 2 days?
e. If an antibiotic is given, what should be done if there is partial improvement after 3 days?
f. Will the induration ever disappear?

2. What possible anxieties have assailed this patient's psyche in the last month?
a. What pressures influence an unmarried adolescent to proceed with pregnancy?

b. What pressures influence an unmarried adolescent to keep her baby?
c. What part do the breasts play in female self-image?
d. What importance do teenage mothers attach to their breast feeding?

3. What potential for health education/preventive medicine exists in this consultation?
   a. When should oral contraception commence after childbirth?
   b. What criteria help select the choice of an oral contraceptive?
   c. Should her claim that pregnancy started while she was on the pill influence advice on contraception?
   d. How does one assess her ideal weight?
   e. How does a GP assist his patient to achieve weight loss?
   f. How does a history of 20 cigarettes daily affect the issue?
   g. What clues lead to a suspicion of child abuse?
   h. What clues lead to a suspicion of promiscuity?
   i. What are the benefits of breast self-examination properly undertaken?

D. Levet, Hobart

MR. & MRS. ANTHONY A.   AGED 40 AND 45 RESPECTIVELY   **229**
MR. A.   STOCKBROKER,   MRS. A.   JOURNALIST

1. What are 'surrogate' mothers and what are the implications of using surrogate mothers?
   a. What are the laws in your state/country relating to the use of surrogate mothers?
   b. What are the laws relating to artificial insemination?

2. What are the legal, moral and ethical issues that need to be raised with the parents?
   a. How would Mrs. A. feel if her husband is able to be the father of a child and Mrs. A. is not able to be the actual mother of the child but will be looking after the child as if it were her own?
   b. How would they be able to select a surrogate mother who will be appropriate to be the mother of the child?
   c. What would happen if there was something wrong with the child when it was born?

3. What are some of the issues that need to be considered with 'test tube baby' research?
   a. What do you think about frozen embryos being kept in a store bank?
   b. What does the Church, the Law and the Medical Profession think about the test-tube research?
   c. Is it leading to a 'Brave New World' situation?

M. D. Mahoney, Brisbane

230 STEPHEN G.   AGED 14

1. What significance would you place on a 14 year old boy coming to consult you alone?
    a. Elaborate on the social pathology underlying Stephen's problems.
    b. What is likely to happen to the family set-up?

2. Why has Stephen come to consult you at this time?
    a. What are Stephen's fears?
    b. What are his mother's fears?

3. What diagnosis would you make?
    a. What conditions would have to be considered?
    b. What is the likely natural history?
    c. What investigations would you carry out?

4. How would you manage the case?
    a. What would you tell Stephen?
    b. How would you communicate with his mother?
    c. What therapy would you suggest?

J. Fry, Beckenham, UK

231 MRS. C.D.   AGED 55   HOUSEWIFE

1. Why has she presented at this time with these headaches?
    a. Is it really migraine?
    b. Does she believe there could be a more sinister cause?
    c. What is the most probable diagnosis?

2. Is there anything else you would like to know about Mrs. D. or her headaches at this stage?
    a. Why is she so apprehensive?
    b. How much influence does stress have on such headaches?
    c. How much help can you give a patient with such frequent headaches?
    d. What treatment will most benefit her?
    e. What produces cluster headaches?

3. How far should one investigate such a patient?
    a. Is there a need for X-rays of the skull?
    b. How significant is a normal skull X-ray?
    c. What features would you expect to find on CNS examination during an attack?

W. F. Glastonbury, Adelaide

MRS. E.B.   AGED 52   HOUSEWIFE

232

1. What distinguishes migraine from other common types of headache?
   a. Is the pattern always the same?
   b. Is a prodrome always essential for the diagnosis?
   c. What is the duration of an untreated headache?
   d. Is vomiting common?
   e. What is a cluster headache?

2. How do you treat migraine headache?
   a. Do you treat it right away or wait?
   b. Are ergot preparations better than ordinary analgesics?
   c. What route of administration is best?
   d. What is the role of rest? Quiet? Darkness?
   e. What about hypnosis? Acupuncture?
   f. Do all migraine sufferers need psychotherapy?

3. Can migraine be prevented?
   a. What preventive medications are available?
   b. When are they indicated?
   c. What are their side effects?

4. What are the cross-relationships of migraine?
   a. Is there usually a family history?
   b. What is the relationship between migraine headache and the birth control pill?

R. L. Perkin, Toronto

MISS ANGELA T.   AGED 18   NURSE

233

1. What sort of conditions would you be considering?
   a. Would the pill be responsible?
   b. Should cerebral thrombosis be considered?
   c. What evidence would point to cerebral tumour?
   d. Has she been having any other symptoms that need to be elicited either from herself or from members of the family or work-mates?
   e. What would be the features of migrainous hemiplegia?

2. How urgent are her symptoms and signs?
   a. Are there any symptoms and signs which would suggest that the patient could be treated without further investigation?
   b. What symptoms and signs would necessitate urgent admission to hospital?

3. What are the next steps now she has been admitted to hospital?
   a. What would your immediate management of this patient be?
   b. Are further investigations required and if so, what should be undertaken?

4. All the investigations were done and no pathology found. The numbness and weakness had disappeared in a couple of days. What would you do now?
   a. What would you say to the patient about the possibility of future attacks?
   b. What advice would you give about her lifestyle?
   c. Should she continue nursing?

M. D. Mahoney, Brisbane

234 MISS MARIE W.   AGED 27

1. Who is the patient?
   a. On whom should the doctor focus attention?
   b. How should the migraine be handled?
   c. How should the tension headache be handled?

2. What is the problem?
   a. How does a dependent role in the man affect the issue?
   b. To what extent does the insecure relationship affect the issue?

3. How can it be resolved?
   a. What is your management of alcoholism?
   b. How can Miss W. help him to seek treatment?

4. What are the facilities for assisting alcoholics in your neighbourhood?
   a. How do you persuade an alcoholic who denies his problem, to seek help?

R. M. Meyer, Johannesburg

235 MR. P.M.   AGED 52   SENIOR RESEARCH SCIENTIST

1. How extensively should headaches be investigated?
   a. What specific investigations should be done for a person suffering from migraine?
   b. What is the place of a CT scan in cases of recurrent headache?
   c. When should a myelogram be performed in these cases?
   d. How would a therapeutic trial of medication assist in determining the cause of the headaches?

2. What sort of tensions could be contributing to this man's headaches?
   a. What family pressures might be a factor in causing tension in this man?
   b. How does a physically fit adult cope with the threat of sudden premature retirement?
   c. What is the community expectation of someone nearing retiring age?

3. How can migraine be prevented?
   a. How does tension relate to migraine?
   b. What dietary management might be necessary in a patient with migraine?
   c. Should this patient be referred to a pain clinic?
   d. What services are offered by a pain clinic which cannot be provided by a well-trained general practitioner?

B. H. Connor, Armidale, Australia

B.F.   AGED 5   PRE-SCHOOL   236

1. What is the differential diagnosis?
   a. Is headache a common symptom in childhood?
   b. What is the usual manifestation of migraine in childhood?
   c. What intracranial tumours occur in childhood?

2. What would be your next step?
   a. How would you facilitate fundoscopic examination in this child?
   b. What place has chemotherapy in primary intracranial neoplasms in childhood?
   c. What are the other forms of treatment available for intracranial neoplasms?

R. W. Roberts, Ravensthorpe, Australia

MARY S.   AGED 15   237

1. How did the doctor arrive at a diagnosis of premenstrual syndrome?
   a. What are the features of premenstrual syndrome?
   b. What other conditions can it be confused with?

2. What features might have alerted the doctor to the diagnosis at the initial consultation?

3. Why did the headaches occur only premenstrually?
   a. What causes the headaches associated with intracranial tumours?
   b. What are their characteristics?

4. What would you have done in this case at the first consultation?
   a. In what circumstances would you undertake further investigation or refer someone complaining of headache?

5. What are the likely effects of stress such as anxiety about examinations on a girl of 15?
   a. How would you treat such symptoms?

G. Strube, Crawley, UK

238   MR. C.H.   AGED 70   RETIRED

1. What are the likely diagnoses?
   a. How would you confirm or exclude Paget's disease of the skull? What treatment is available?
   b. How would you confirm or exclude temporal arteritis? What treatment is available?
   c. What generalized condition is often associated with temporal arteritis?

2. What are the possible risks in this situation?
   a. Why does blindness occur in temporal arteritis? Is it reversible?
   b. What underlying conditions should be excluded?
   c. How far would you investigate the patient before commencing treatment?

3. How do you cope with the likelihood of error by a colleague, especially if the patient is aware of the implications?
   a. What are the essential features of a good record system?
   b. What would you say to your colleague?
   c. How can a doctor protect himself from the risks of complaint and litigation?

E. C. Gambrill, Crawley, UK

239   MRS. VERA U.   AGED 38

1. What is your differential diagnosis?
   a. Does the fact that it occurred during stress help you to differentiate?
   b. If her neck is supple, does that satisfy you that this is likely to be a tension headache?
   c. What characteristic of this headache makes you suspect that this is not a tension headache?

2. What pathology are you worried about here?
   a. What diagnostic test(s) would you do?

b. Why do subarachnoid haemorrhages often occur during emotional or physical strain?
c. What is the natural course if the initial leak from a Berry aneurysm is missed?

D. H. Johnson, Toronto

J.M.   AGED 14   SCHOOLBOY   **240**

1. What conditions should be considered?
    a. What other enquiries would you make?
    b. What would one look for during examination?
    c. What advice would you give on likely further developments of the condition in the next 24 hours?

2. How would you manage this case?
    a. What complications are possible in mumps?
    b. When would these be likely to occur?
    c. What problems might be expected in a female of the same age?
    d. What are the consequences of this condition in persons over the age of 40?
    e. What specialties could be involved in the long term from complications of mumps?

E. J. H. North, Melbourne

MR. F.O.   AGED 35   DAIRY FARMER   **241**

1. What are the likely causes?
    a. Should any investigations be repeated?
    b. If so, when?
    c. What might they show?
    d. What other workers are likely to suffer from this problem?

2. How is the disease contracted?
    a. Why are dairy farmers and abattoir workers suspected?
    b. How are they contaminated?
    c. What significant role do pigs have in transferring the disease?
    d. What time of the year is the disease more prevalent?
    e. Why is this so?

3. Are there any complications to be expected?
    a. Are others likely to contract the condition?
    b. How can the problem be treated?
    c. What is the likelihood of recurrence?
    d. Is the condition notifiable?
    e. How do you notify infectious diseases?

E. J. H. North, Melbourne

242 **MR. LELAND G.**   **AGED 52**   **SCHOOL PRINCIPAL**

1. What is your differential diagnosis?
    a. What cultures or smears would you take?
    b. What other tests might be helpful?

2. If Gram negative diplococci are found on scrapings from the rash, what treatment would you institute?
    a. Would you investigate or treat his wife?
    b. Would you recommend any preventive measures with staff or children he has been in close contact with at school?

D. H. Johnson, Toronto

243 **MISS M.N.**   **AGED 27**   **NURSE**

1. What else might you have thought about if you had been the first doctor?
    a. Why mightn't she have been taking anti-malarials?
    b. If one is not sure of the malarial status of, or the presence or absence of chloroquin resistant strains in a country, should one not check in any case from the local health authority?
    c. Every minute may magnify the mortality of falciparum malaria. True or false?
    d. What is the first aid (immediate) procedure(s) if malaria is on the differential diagnosis list?

2. What are the common causes of a PUO acquired on travel?
    a. Which ones are associated with a rash?
    b. Which ones require paired titres?
    c. Which ones are dangerous to others?
    d. Which ones can appear weeks or months (or years) after return home?
    e. Why has the incidence of malaria in western countries increased recently?

3. This patient nearly died of cerebral malaria – she had over one in eight red cells parasitized. What could have been done to prevent her getting to this state?
    a. Before she left – by you?
    b. While she was there – by her?
    c. When she returned – by her?
    d. When she returned – by the doctor?

A. J. Radford, Adelaide

MR. A.B.   AGED 50   BUS DRIVER   **244**

1. What are the possible diagnoses, and on which would you focus in the first instance?
    a. At what levels do you begin to treat blood pressure? Do you vary these with the patient's age? Do you have a systematic protocol for the management of symptomless hypertension? What is the meaning of the terms 'case-finding' and 'population screening'?
    b. What, if any, characteristics of a headache would lead you to suspect it was
        – emotional in origin?
        – truly associated with hypertension?
        – due to a 'brain tumour'?
        – a result of the accident?
        – of sinus origin?

2. What problems does this consultation present in terms of the doctor's responsibility to the community?
    a. What are the laws regarding fitness to drive,
        – a public service vehicle?
        – a private vehicle?
    b. Given that the laws as to fitness to drive can pose problems as regards the confidentiality of your consultations with a patient:
        – List four conditions which may pose these problems other than those in your differential diagnoses for Mr. A.B.
        – What is your attitude to breaching confidentiality in each of the conditions, including those in Mr. A.B.'s differential list?
        – If your attitude does differ, why?

3. What significance do you attach to the patient's not having consulted for 10 years?
    a. In what ways are patients who do not consult likely to differ from
        – those who consult occasionally?
        – those who consult very frequently?
    b. What do you understand by the terms 'the sick role' and 'illness behaviour'?
    c. What will you say to Mr. A.B. if your eventual diagnosis is:
        – tension headache?
        – symptomless hypertension requiring long-term treatment?
        – benign prostatic enlargement?
        – malignant prostatic change?

P. Freeling, London

245 ELIZABETH C.   AGED 17   SCHOOLGIRL

1. Are some headaches due to undemonstrable pathology in the neck which is amenable to resolution by manipulation?
   a. Could it be due to
      – disc pressure on the dura?
      – pressure on a nerve root?
      – minor displacement of a facetal joint with resultant muscular spasm?
   b. Would any of these show on an X-ray – even with myelography?
   c. Why do some of the ghastly looking cervical vertebrae often seen on X-ray appear to cause minimal or no symptoms?
   d. Is it possible that symptoms may arise from the apparently normal areas rather than those with obvious osteoarthritic or disc degenerative changes?
   e. Is there a synaptic connection between the cervical nerves and the 5th nerve ganglion?

2. What is the rational place of tranquillizers in 'tension headache'?
   a. Are they given to reduce awareness so that the patient does not complain so much?
   b. Do any have a muscle relaxing effect?
   c. Do they make patients more liable to accidents in the same way as alcohol?
   d. If one of your patients on a tranquillizer had a serious accident would you feel a twinge of conscience?
   e. Is diazepam – for example – addictive?

3. How does the doctor react to being put on the spot?
   a. What is the patient's problem?
   b. Would you defend your initial treatment?
   c. What explanation, if any, would you give?

R. T. Mossop, Harare, Zimbabwe

246 ELIZABETH C.   AGED 23   (NOW ELIZABETH G.)   HOUSEWIFE

1. How was it possible that she could hide from a number of doctors that she was taking drugs for so long?
   a. Are there subtle clues which might make an experienced doctor suspect oral drug addition which may have been missed in this case?
   b. Is there a case for closer control of over-the-counter drugs?
   c. How might this be achieved?

2. Why would she continue taking analgesic drugs after her headaches had gone?

a. Is there a sharp differentiation between physical and psychological addiction?

b. What sort of record have we in weaning drug addicts from their addiction before irreversible changes have taken place?

3. What is the place of chronic dialysis?
   a. In a developed country?
   b. In the third world?
   c. If the patient continues to take the offending medication?
   d. Where does renal transplant come in?
   e. What are the contraindications and what are the possible effects in the long term of renal transplant?

R. T. Mossop, Harare, Zimbabwe

MR. RONALD B.   AGED 20   INVALID PENSIONER   247

1. What general attitude should you adopt to this young man?
   a. Should you encourage him to train for a job and discontinue his pension?
   b. What advice would you offer about living at home?
   c. Should you stress the importance of leading a normal life?
   d. Could it be helpful to interview his parents. If so what points would you make?

2. What prohibitions and precautions are necessary in an epileptic?
   a. What specific advice would you give about driving?
   b. What would be your recommendations about sport?
   c. What particular careers could be dangerous for him?

3. Are there any community facilities which could help him?
   a. What is the specific role of the Epilepsy Association?
   b. Could youth groups such as YMCA be useful to him?

4. He complains that his current medications make him drowsy. How would you deal with this?
   a. What is the value of blood tests to assess circulating levels of drugs? Should you ever allow them to alter your clinical judgement of a case?
   b. Should you attempt reduction of long-standing therapy in this case? What criteria do you use for reduction or cessation of therapy in an epileptic?
   c. Would it be helpful to have a neurological opinion?

5. Ronald tells you he fears female entanglements, because he is afraid to marry with his disability. How would you counsel him?

a. To what extent is epilepsy hereditary?
b. Is normal sexual activity bad for an epileptic?

K. C. Nyman, Perth, Australia

248 MRS. JOAN M. AGED 36 HOUSEWIFE

1. Have I really got epilepsy? How do you know?
   a. Well has she? Are you satisfied or what additional evidence can you obtain?
   b. Should she continue anti-convulsants?

2. Would the drug have cured me? What should I do now; a friend who has epilepsy tells me that some drugs are very dangerous.
   a. What alternatives would you use and in what order of preference?
   b. Is she right about the dangers of anti-convulsants? What? Which?

3. We live four miles out of town, how am I going to get the shopping or the children to school? Can I still drive the tractor on the farm?
   a. Should she drive at all?
   b. Should she surrender her licence?
   c. Should you advise the authorities if she elects to go on driving?
   d. What other precautions and advice should you offer?
   e. What should you tell her about the possibility of the children manifesting the disease?

J. A. Stevens, Ulverstone, Australia

249 MASTER A.L. AGED 15 MONTHS

1. What is the significance of this episode?
   a. Does this severe attack indicate an underlying cerebral problem such as epilepsy?
   b. Will this attack cause some permanent brain damage?
   c. Will it be possible to reassure his anxious parents about an optimistic outcome?
   d. How predictable are similar attacks?
   e. At what age do febrile convulsions in children usually subside?

2. How would you manage this problem?
   a. Should a conservative 'wait and see' approach be adopted?
   b. Should the child be referred immediately to a neurologist?
   c. Should an EEG be arranged at this stage?
   d. Would you prescribe a long-term anticonvulsant?

3. What advice would you give to the parents?
   a. Would you reassure the parents that this is a temporary problem and will soon subside?
   b. Would you reassure the parents that the child is normal and that these convulsions are relatively harmless?
   c. What advice would you give the parents about coping with future episodes of fever and infections?
   d. What advice would you give the parents about coping with a convulsion at home?
   e. How accessible should you make yourself to this family?

J. E. Murtagh, Melbourne

MRS. J.S.   AGED 27   UNIVERSITY TEACHER OF A FOREIGN LANGUAGE   **250**

1. What are the pros and cons of progestogen-only pills for contraception in a nursing mother?
   a. On what grounds do you select between the various 'combined' contraceptive pills for individual patients?
   b. What are the advantages and disadvantages of an intra uterine contraceptive device for Mrs. J.S.?
   c. Mrs. J.S. had an episiotomy which extended by tearing. At this examination the wound at the introitus is not completely healed. What advice and explanation would you give Mrs. J.S.?

2. What conditions may be represented by mother's description of Natalie's twitching?
   a. Would you wish to investigate Natalie now or only see her to examine her?
   b. In what way, if any, will mother's observation affect your later decisions concerning immunizing Natalie?
   c. What is your approach to the long-term management of a child who has had a single febrile convulsion?

3. What do you understand by the term 'role' as it is used in psychology and sociology?
   a. Does the pre-conception conflict between Mrs. J.S. and her husband affect your decisions concerning any of the previous questions?
   b. What is the legal position concerning the protection of women's employment status?

P. Freeling, London

251   **MR. W.H.**   **AGED 28**   **DUSTMAN**

1. What are the likely causes of uncooperative behaviour in general practice?
   a. What kinds of psychiatric illness can produce this picture?
   b. What organic alternatives must be considered?
   c. What immediate treatment or management would you suggest?

2. What does the wife mean by a 'fit'?
   a. What further questions would you ask of her?
   b. How would you follow up the case now?
   c. Can you relate this episode to his previous history?

3. Could this dramatic episode have been prevented?
   a. What hints of organic disease are given?
   b. The hospital make a diagnosis of malignant glioma; what do you tell the wife, and the patient?

J. Grabinar, Bromley, UK

252   **MRS. V.L.**   **AGED 58**   **HOUSEWIFE**

1. What would be your strategy for further definition of the problem?
   a. What additional history would you try to obtain?
   b. Would you rely on her answers?
   c. To whom might you turn for additional history?
   d. Which parts of the physical examination would be of most importance?
   e. What investigations would you perform if your physical examination was essentially normal?

2. What might be the cause of the weakness?
   a. What are the mechanisms of spread of cancer of the colon?
   b. What is the most common mechanism of spread of cancer of the colon?
   c. Which organ is most likely to be involved in haematogenous metastasis?
   d. Which other organs might be involved in haematogenous metastasis?

3. What might be the cause of the seizure?
   a. When do alcohol withdrawal seizures ('rum fits') occur with respect to cessation of drinking?
   b. How would you distinguish a withdrawal seizure from delirium tremens?

c. Is it possible that the seizure is related to a focal intracranial lesion?

d. If so, what kind?

G. G. Beazley, Winnipeg

CHERYL M.   AGED 30   HOUSEWIFE

253

1. What explanations might have been suggested as a cause for these fits?
   a. Despite repeated questioning Cheryl denied that she had been forgetting to take her tablets. How could this have been checked?
   b. With all tests normal and a guarantee that Cheryl had been taking her tablets regularly as prescribed, what possible explanations for her fits must now be considered?

2. Cheryl continued to be a problem. She complained of 'feeling awful', of experiencing sexual difficulties with her husband, of not being able to do her housework and of falling about the house. She frequently presented to the surgery with facial bruising which she said was due to hitting the wash basin when she 'passed out in the bathroom'. How could these symptoms and signs be best explained?
   a. What would be the value of a joint consultation with Cheryl and her husband?
   b. What investigations could be performed to clarify the situation?
   c. What could explain Cheryl's continued fitting?

3. Cheryl's continuing ill health and the recurrence of seizures 8 years after she began effective therapy led to the discovery that her serum phenytoin and carbamazepine levels were homeopathic and that she had not been taking her drugs regularly. What is the likely explanation of her behaviour?
   a. What side effects of analeptic drugs might cause a patient to discontinue them?
   b. What alternative medication should be considered to control Cheryl's fits and to ensure that she will comply with her therapy?
   c. How can one be sure that the patient's symptoms and signs are due to the anti-convulsant therapy and not due to mental deterioration?

W. L. Ogborne, Sydney

MRS. F.P.   AGED 34   NURSE

254

1. What are the hazards of anti-convulsant therapy seen in this patient?
   a. How frequently does phenytoin cause a rash?

    b.   What is the risk of oral contraceptive failure when combined with carbamazepine?

    c.   What specific monitoring must be carried out with carbamazepine therapy?

    d.   Are there any increased chances of genetic malformation with anti-convulsants?

2.   What is the most likely cause of this patient's grand mal attacks?
    a.   How frequently should further investigations be performed?
    b.   When could she undergo a trial without anti-convulsants?

3.   What genetic counselling is necessary for this patient?
    a.   What is the most likely cause of her Mongoloid child?
    b.   How can Mongolism be detected in pregnancy?
    c.   What substance is elevated in the amniotic fluid with neural tube defects, and what are the accuracy rates for prediction?
    d.   At what stage of pregnancy can these changes be detected?
    e.   What emphasis needs to be placed on permanent contraception?

4.   What psychological history would throw light on this patient's behaviour?
    a.   What depressive elements are to be seen in this patient?
    b.   What anxiety and areas of guilt should be explored?
    c.   What is her attitude to doctors?
    d.   Despite her nursing knowledge, why has she such reticence in matters relating to her own health and domestic affairs?

G. M. Dick, Hobart

255   MISS C.   AGED 16   UNEMPLOYED

1.   What questions is it necessary to ask?
    a.   Is the pill required only to 'regulate' periods?
    b.   How can one find out about the possibility of pregnancy in this situation?
    c.   How much do the parents know; is this part of their anxiety?

2.   What are the reasons for her menstrual problems?
    a.   What is the appropriate management of menstrual irregularity at age 16?
    b.   Is the pill appropriate in a situation like this?
    c.   If she needs contraception what are the problems, and how may they be solved?

3.   Why is she suffering from nausea?
    a.   What are the features for and against a simple stomach problem?

b. Could she, in spite of the pill and the bleeding, be suffering from 'morning sickness'?
c. Can anxiety cause as much nausea and vomiting as this?
d. Could the pill be the cause of the nausea?

4. Why is she still having epileptic fits?
    a. How would you check compliance?
    b. Do blood estimations of drugs reflect the true position?
    c. Could drug interaction be a problem?

A. L. A. Reid, Newcastle, Australia

MISS PAULINE V.   AGED 36   SALESWOMAN   256

1. What possible problems are present in Miss V.'s case?
    a. What is the probable cause of her blackouts?
    b. What evidence is there to support a diagnosis of renal colic?
    c. What can be said about her sexual orientation?
    d. What is her psychological state?
    e. How could her social problems relate to her illness?

2. How can Miss V.'s case be assessed?
    a. Can a cerebral space occupying lesion be definitely excluded?
    b. Does her normal intravenous pyelogram exclude renal colic?
    c. Does haematuria positively indicate urinary tract pathology?
    d. How can haematuria be proved to be a patient induced artifact?
    e. Does her high serum uric acid support a diagnosis of renal colic?

3. How should Miss V. be treated?
    a. What grounds are there for certifying her for an invalid pension?
    b. How can she be helped to come to terms with her ambivalent sexuality?
    c. What should be done about her hyperuricaemia?
    d. How should her hysterical behaviour be handled?

D. G. Chambers, Clare, Australia

MR. X.Y.   AGED 32   PRIMARY SCHOOL TEACHER   257

1. What additional information should be sought?
    a. Can all the necessary information be deduced from a good account of the incident by an eye witness and a complete examination?
    b. Would a history of similar attacks influence your line of reasoning?
    c. Is the history of anxiety both at home and at work significant?

2. Is this condition a medical emergency?
   a. Should immediate transport (several hours by ambulance) to a large base hospital be considered?
   b. Should you commence any immediate treatment?
   c. Providing all systems appear normal (BP, pulse, colour, urine) apart from the abnormalities described above, is time on your side?

3. How would you manage this condition using only the resources of the country hospital and yourself?
   a. Would you leave the patient under close observation in the hospital while you went on consulting?
   b. Are there any additional investigations that you would consider absolutely necessary to arrive at a diagnosis?
   c. Is there a way you could communicate with this patient?

T. D. Manthorpe, Port Lincoln, Australia

258 MR. J.S. AGED 47 JEWELLER

1. What is the likely diagnosis?
   a. Is this condition a specific problem? If so, what is this syndrome called?
   b. What are other possibilities?

2. What investigations would be appropriate?
   a. Is this a condition that can be diagnosed clinically in the office?
   b. What simple investigations can be done in the office?
   c. Is there any risk in assuming that this condition is a specific syndrome without need for further investigation?
   d. Are expensive investigations justified in this case?

3. How would you manage the problem?
   a. How would you explain the cause to the patient?
   b. Is there any preventive advice you could offer?
   c. When would you see the patient again?

T. D. Manthorpe, Port Lincoln, Australia

259 MR. CLAUDE K. AGED 65 RETIRED FISHERMAN

1. What significant fact was overlooked at the time of the first examination?
   a. In the absence of physical signs on examination what might the doctor have done in an attempt to avoid the emergency situation which developed?

b. What is the most common cause of syncope seen by the general practitioner, and in what circumstances do syncopal attacks most often occur?

c. In which other common abdominal emergencies is syncope likely to be a feature?

d. What are the ways by which abdominal aortic aneurysm may be diagnosed by the general practitioner?

2. Often syncope may be confused with an epileptic seizure. What are the implications of an error in diagnosis by the general practitioner?

a. What evidence would be important in making a firm diagnosis?

b. What action should the general practitioner take when a teenager is suspected of having an epileptiform seizure for the first time?

J. G. P. Ryan, Brisbane

MRS. M.W.   AGED 55   **260**

1. What other investigations are necessary, now or later?
   a. What other haematological tests may be desirable?
   b. Could menorrhagia account for the anaemia, despite three months amenorrhoea?
   c. What lesions could cause blood loss from the GI tract?
   d. Could X-ray of the stomach and bowel exclude GI cancer or are other investigations necessary?

2. How should this situation be managed?
   a. Does the holiday have to be postponed?
   b. Would giving a transfusion interfere with any subsequent investigations?
   c. What explanations must be given to the patient?
   d. How many litres would be needed to raise the Hb from 5 to 12 g/dl?

3. Are there any obligations to her original doctor?
   a. If she wishes to change doctors, does the original doctor need to be informed?

G. M. Dick, Hobart

MR. A.H.   AGED 62   **261**

1. What is the biochemical mechanism of reactive hypoglycaemia following partial gastrectomy?
   a. What advice did the doctor give the patient about his diet?
   b. What other malabsorption states can follow partial gastrectomy?

2. What other conditions could have caused attacks of unconsciousness
    in this man?
    a. What further investigations might help in diagnosis?

A. G. Strube, Crawley, UK

262 MR. ROBERT J.   AGED 46   MECHANIC

1. What problems could Mr. J. have had?
    a. Can alcoholics become hypoglycaemic?
    b. What damage can occur to the liver in alcoholism?
    c. What damage can occur to the pancreas in alcoholism?
    d. What are the symptoms of chronic pancreatitis?

2. What are the possible roles of his wife in his illness?
    a. What precipitating factors can make alcoholics go on binges?
    b. How often do wives collude to hide a husband's alcoholism?
    c. What is the effect of alcohol on the male libido?
    d. Do daughters of alcoholics marry alcoholics?

3. What treatment does he require?
    a. How can he reduce the risk of further hypoglycaemia?
    b. How would you advise the wife to cope with any
        hypoglycaemia?
    c. What is the treatment of alcoholism?
    d. What treatment agencies for alcoholics do you have access to?
    e. How effective is the treatment of alcoholism?
    f. What is the treatment of alcoholic hepatitis and pancreatitis?

D. G. Chambers, Clare, Australia

263 MRS. O.H.   AGED 78   WIDOW

1. What is the likely cause of her problem?
    a. Can oral hypoglycaemics cause coma?
    b. Should all unconscious patients be regarded as hypoglycaemic
        until proven otherwise?
    c. Should the doctor be capable of performing a domiciliary blood
        sugar?
    d. Is depression likely to be a significant problem? Overdosage?
    e. Is the chronic infection likely to produce this complication?

2. Who should take responsibility for this home visit?
    a. What motivated the patient's doctor to refuse a home visit?
    b. Was the daughter's doctor correct in making the house call?
    c. Should the daughter's doctor have immediately contacted the
        patient's doctor?

    d.   Would it have been appropriate to call an ambulance and hand over the problem to the hospital?

3. Who should take responsibility for the patient's ongoing management?
    a.   Should the attending doctor continue the management?
    b.   Should he contact the patient's doctor to continue management?
    c.   Should the patient be returned to the care of the specialists?
    d.   Should her medication be changed?

J. E. Murtagh, Melbourne

MR. E.S.B.   AGED 21   UNEMPLOYED UNSKILLED   264

1. Is the diagnosis likely to be functional or organic?
    a.   What specific questions would be asked about the symptoms of 'dizziness' and feeling unwell?
    b.   What specific questions would be asked in relation to his social background?
    c.   Is it necessary to perform a physical examination?

2. Examination reveals a sweaty, febrile patient with scattered rhonchi, crepitations and a degree of bronchospasm throughout the chest. Does this change your earlier diagnosis?
    a.   Could this patient have a functional and organic illness?
    b.   What are the likely diagnoses?

3. What further investigations are indicated in this case?
    a.   Is a chest X-ray necessary?
    b.   Are any haematological investigations required?

4. Is counselling of any use here?

D. U. Shepherd, Melbourne

MR. WILLIAM L.   AGED 59   CHEMICAL ENGINEER   265

1. What is the most likely cause of this patient's symptoms and of the physical findings?
    a.   What is the relationship between the dizziness and the wearing of bifocal spectacles?
    b.   What is the relationship, if any, between the paired quadrantic visual defect and the complaint of dizziness when wearing spectacles?
    c.   In the light of the physical findings what other information would be helpful in elucidating the cause?
    d.   What investigations would be helpful in localizing the lesion?

2. What is the overall management plan for this patient?
   a. Should this patient continue to drive his motor car?
   b. What is the relationship between the symptoms and signs and the previous stresses experienced at work?
   c. What contribution could an ophthalmologist make to this patient's management?
   d. What specific drug therapy might be employed?

W. L. Ogborne, Sydney

266 MRS. M.S.   AGED 72

1. What is the differential diagnosis of this condition?
   a. Is there always a preceding history of head injury?

2. How important was the doctor's previous knowledge of the patient in arriving at the correct diagnosis?
   a. Could her past history influence the diagnosis?
   b. What are the causes of organic dementia?

A. G. Strube, Crawley, UK

267 MR. C.G.   AGED 80   RETIRED CIRCUS AERIALIST - WIDOWER

1. What causes of his attacks should be considered?
   a. Cardiovascular?
   b. Central nervous system?
   c. Vestibular?

2. How would you attempt to determine the cause?
   a. How important is the history in determining the cause?
   b. What physical findings would you look for?
   c. What special investigations should be done?

3. Would you treat his hypertension?
   a. Is there evidence that treatment of systolic hypertension in the elderly will lessen the probability of strokes and other complications?

C. T. Lamont, Ottawa

268 MR. COLIN H.   AGED 45   BANK OFFICER

1. You are asked directly whether he should consider early retirement. What factors would influence your advice?
   a. Discuss the association of stress and TIAs.

b. Should his financial ability to retire be of major relevance?

c. Would a family history of cerebro-vascular accidents or coronary artery disease be important?

d. What are the dangers of early death or disablement in patients with TIAs?

e. He has several months of accumulated sick leave due to him. How would you suggest he use this?

2. Colin asks what activities he should avoid?
   a. Would you advise against driving a car?
   b. Would you offer specific advice about diet, exercise, smoking, alcohol and sexual activity?
   c. Would you advise a change of job?

3. What treatment would you recommend?
   a. During an actual TIA is any treatment helpful?
   b. What role do aspirin or dipyridamole play in therapy?
   c. Which patients are suitable for surgery in this condition?
   d. Is it true or false that in some cases TIAs are self-limiting?

K. C. Nyman, Perth, Australia

MRS. Y.B. AGED 63 ACCOUNTANT 269

1. What is the most likely diagnosis?
   a. What are the other possibilities?
   b. What role does diabetes play in the aetiology?
   c. What role does hypertension play?
   d. Is the history or the physical examination the more important?

2. How would you confirm the diagnosis?
   a. Is a lumbar puncture indicated?
   b. Should such patients all have a brain scan?
   c. Should all such patients have a CT scan?
   d. Should all such patients have an angiogram?

3. How would you treat this patient?
   a. What is the role of surgery?
   b. In medical treatment, is aspirin effective in females?
   c. What alternative drugs may be used?
   d. What do you tell the patient?
   e. What do you tell the family?

4. What is the prognosis?
   a. Do all such patients progress to a completed stroke?
   b. What is the life expectancy?

R. L. Perkin, Toronto

270 **MR. G.S.** **AGED 46** **UNIVERSITY PROFESSOR**

1. What is causing the pain in his knees?
   a. What is the significance of the peripheral arterial calcification?
   b. What management is available for arteriosclerotic obliterative disease?
   c. What management is available for osteoarthritis of the knees?
   d. Is further investigation indicated or can you depend on the clinical diagnosis?

2. What advice do you give regarding exercise at work and recreation?
   a. Is exercise helpful in emotional disorders, peripheral vascular disease or osteoarthritis?
   b. What alternatives to exercise could be incorporated into his lifestyle?
   c. What are his chances of having a stroke?

3. How do you feel about referral to a specialist?
   a. Does diet modification offer anything?
   b. What neurological investigation is indicated? Why?
   c. Should he see a cardiologist? Why?
   d. Discuss the procedures available for investigation of arteriosclerotic obliterative disease.

4. What nutritional advice do you give?
   a. Whom should he consult about his diet?
   b. What is the significance of dietary fat, fibre, refined carbohydrate and salt?
   c. How can he effectively and comfortably plan on controlling his weight?

P. R. Grantham, Vancouver

271 **MRS. C.D.** **AGED 52** **HOUSEWIFE**

1. What could be the cause of this epileptiform seizure?
   a. What would you find during your physical examination?
   b. How certain can you be that this was an epileptiform seizure?
   c. What procedure would be of assistance to you?
   d. What could the final diagnosis be?

2. What investigations and diagnostic procedures would you advise?
   a. How far would you go with investigations following the original attack and later with the second attack?
   b. Would a lumbar puncture be performed?
   c. Would a neurologist and neurosurgeon's report be of assistance to you?

3. What would you advise the family and patient?
   a. What medicolegal problems arise?
   b. Can the patient live a normal life?
   c. What medications would be advised?

B. M. Fehler, Johannesburg

MR. W.C.   AGED 81   RETIRED GOLDMINER   272

1. What morbid processes are involved?
   a. What blood vessels are involved?
   b. What are the possible causes of his failing vision?
   c. Was admission to hospital a mistake in view of the onset of the patient's hemiparesis?

2. What investigations are warranted in this case?
   a. At what stage should a glucose tolerance test be carried out?
   b. Do you routinely dilate pupils to enable adequate fundoscopic examination?

3. What is the most appropriate treatment?
   a. How important is physiotherapy?
   b. Can this man eventually go home?
   c. Assuming he can, how can you assist him?

R. W. Roberts, Ravensthorpe, Australia

MRS. W.H.   AGED 37   MOTHER (EX NURSE)   273

1. How do you proceed when presented with a patient who has alarming symptoms?
   a. How much do you tell the patient right away?
   b. Do you attempt to arrive at a diagnosis quickly or sit back and observe the natural history of the disease process for a while?
   c. How much reassurance to the patient and family is appropriate in such a situation?

2. What are the important skills for managing patients with chronic incurable disease?
   a. What is the role of nurses and other health professionals?
   b. How do you tap the resources of community agencies?
   c. Are home visits important in the care of such patients?
   d. How much do you tell the patients?

3. How do you deal with the family and home situation?
   a. Do you sometimes need to speak to family members apart from the patient?

    b.   What is meant by 'preventive counselling' especially as it applies to the children of an incurably ill patient?

    c.   How can community agencies, other family members and friends be utilized to support the nuclear family in such situations?

R. L. Perkin, Toronto

274   GAIL M.   AGED 22   PHARMACIST'S ASSISTANT

1. What would make you suspect that the first incident was physical disease?

    a.   Do pharmacist's assistants run any special risks?

    b.   Does the complete symptomatic recovery help with the diagnosis?

2. Are there any further investigations that would assist you in resolving this case?

    a.   Is it necessary to have any kind of proof to diagnose multiple sclerosis?

    b.   With such a diagnosis what would you tell the patient?

    c.   What sort of occupation would you suggest to your patient?

    d.   Is it necessary for you to inform any prospective employer who inquires as to her condition?

    e.   In the event of Gale becoming engaged how would you counsel the couple?

R. M. Meyer, Johannesburg

275   MR. C.D.   AGED 45   PROCESS WORKER

1. What diagnosis is most likely?

    a.   What are the causes of this condition?

    b.   What will be the outcome?

    c.   What therapy can be given?

    d.   Does medical intervention halt the disease?

2. What iatrogenic causes could present like this?

    a.   Can phenothiazines cause these symptoms?

    b.   Is there any specific antidote to this?

3. If the patient's father had the same symptoms prior to his death, what advice would you give the patient's son?

    a.   Assume he is 20 years old and has a girlfriend, should he marry, should they have children?

    b.   If the disease is an autosomal dominant, what proportion of the children are affected?

c. At what stage would you expect the patient's son to show symptoms if he carried the chromosomal defect?

A. Himmelhoch, Sydney

MR. J.H.   AGED 103   SPANISH AMERICAN WAR VETERAN   276

1. Do you agree with this recommendation?
   a. What are the indications for a permanent pacemaker?

2. What type of myocardial infarction is most likely to cause complete heart block?
   a. What drugs are used to increase heart rate?
   b. What drugs are contraindicated?

C. T. Lamont, Ottawa

MR. ANDREW G.   AGED 22   UNIVERSITY STUDENT   277

1. What are the diagnostic possibilities?
   a. What is the commonest cause of this presentation?
   b. Are the features consistent with corneal foreign body, corneal ulcer or abrasion, episcleritis, pterygium, stye or allergic conjunctivitis?
   c. Is this presentation consistent with herpes simplex keratoconjunctivitis? What features does this condition exhibit on examination?

2. How will you distinguish between these possibilities?
   a. What is your diagnostic approach to the unilateral red eye?
   b. Do the unilateral symptoms rule out bacterial conjunctivitis?
   c. What is the place of culture of the excretions from the conjunctival sac?

3. What management is appropriate for each cause of the unilateral red eye?
   a. What are the principles of management of bacterial conjunctivitis?
   b. What antibiotics are used, how often and for how long?
   c. What hygienic measures would you advise?
   d. How would you manage other causes of a unilateral red eye?
   e. If Andrew G. has bacterial conjunctivitis, what opportunity does this situation provide for preventive care?

W. E. Fabb, Melbourne

278 HARRY L.   AGED 40   SCIENTIFIC OFFICER

1. What constitutes an epidemic?
   a. What predictors are available to give the family doctor prior warning of an epidemic?
   b. How do family doctors adjust their ways of working to meet the additional burdens caused by an epidemic?

2. What factors influence the doctor's decision to follow up a patient?
   a. How does 'follow-up' determine the volume and nature of the family doctor's work?
   b. If a decision is made to follow up, what factors determine the time interval between contacts?

3. Does Harry suffer from a potentially serious eye condition?
   a. What further information (if any) might the doctor need to make an appropriate management decision in Harry's case?
   b. What (if any) ophthalmological diagnostic/therapeutic agents do family doctors have readily available on their home visits?

4. What needs to be done to help Harry?
   a. If consultant services are indicated, how may they be mobilized in the case of a patient bed-bound at home?

J. D. E. Knox, Dundee

279 MR. GEOFFREY B.   AGED 24   MOTOR MECHANIC

1. What specific enquiries would you make concerning the possibility of traumatic injury?
   a. What are the typical accidents in a motor repair workshop which cause eye injuries?
   b. What protective gear should be available?
   c. How important is vision testing in such cases?

2. If he revealed that he had been using an emery wheel to take the rough off a weld, what would you specifically look for?
   a. What are the characteristics of an emery wheel eye injury?
   b. What is the importance of the rust ring in such injuries?

3. How do you manage a ferrous foreign body in the cornea from an emery wheel?
   a. How would you remove the metallic fragment?
   b. How would you deal with the rust ring?
   c. Would you use antibiotics; if so, which, how often and for how long?
   d. What is the value of an eye pad?

e. How do you determine whether the patient should have time off work?

f. What opportunity does this accident provide for preventive care at a personal and workshop level?

g. What follow up would you arrange?

W. E. Fabb, Melbourne

MR. DARRYN E.   AGED 38   SHEETMETAL WORKER   280

1. What is the likely diagnosis?
   a. What accidents typically result in intraocular foreign bodies?
   b. What are the most common intraocular foreign bodies?

2. How would you assess this patient?
   a. What are the physical findings with an intraocular foreign body?
   b. How would you exclude an intraocular foreign body if you were in doubt in this case?

3. How would you manage this problem?
   a. What immediate treatment would you give?
   b. What is the ophthalmic surgeon likely to do?
   c. What opportunities does this situation present for preventive care at a personal and workshop level?

W. E. Fabb, Melbourne

MRS. JESSICA F.   AGED 63   HOUSEWIFE   281

1. What diagnostic hypotheses would you entertain?
   a. What are the diagnostic features of acute glaucoma? What precipitating factors could be responsible?
   b. How is acute glaucoma distinguished from iritis?
   c. Are there any other diagnostic possibilities?

2. What steps would you take to investigate this problem?
   a. What special tests are essential?
   b. Would you use a tonometer in acute glaucoma?
   c. Is vision testing necessary?

3. What emergency measures would you be anticipating may have to be carried out?
   a. What would **you** do immediately?
   b. What would you expect the ophthalmic surgeon to do?
   c. When the emergency situation has been dealt with, what follow up measures and preventive care would be appropriate following an attack of acute angle closure glaucoma?

W. E. Fabb, Melbourne

282   **MR. T.C.**   **AGED 28**   **PROOFREADER**

1. What main types of hypertension should be considered in this case?
   a. What are the salient features of essential hypertension?
   b. What features of this case make renovascular hypertension a possibility?
   c. What investigations are necessary?
   d. Are there significant physical findings that help to rule out coarctation of the aorta?
   e. What are the features of malignant hypertension that should be sought?

2. What compliance factors will be important in the management of this case?
   a. In what ways can anxiety and stress relate to a malignant phase of hypertension?
   b. How important will it be to encourage him to never start smoking, to limit his alcohol intake, and to ensure that his current weight of 185 lb does not increase?
   c. In light of current evidence, what dietary factors will be important in the management of this case?

3. What are the feared complications of sustained non-malignant hypertension?
   a. What factors make blindness a threat?
   b. What factors in this case make myocardial infarction a possibility?
   c. What are the risk factors which predispose to the development of a stroke?
   d. What therapeutic measures should be instituted in order to prevent hypertensive encephalopathy?

L. H. Amundson, Sioux Falls, SD, USA

283   **MR. JONATHON J.**   **AGED 23**   **BOOKKEEPER**

1. What conditions would you be thinking about which might have caused his blurred vision?
   a. What intraocular conditions can cause blurred vision or loss of vision?
   b. What neurological conditions may present in this way?

2. How would you investigate this problem?
   a. How would you check his visual acuity?
   b. How do you distinguish refractive errors from more serious causes of blurred vision?
   c. What ophthalmoscopic features would you seek?
   d. What other investigations would be appropriate?

3. If he told you that he had noticed some clumsiness in his gait whilst walking to work a couple of weeks ago, which cleared up in a few days, what would you suspect? What would you do to confirm or rule out your suspicions?
   a. What neurological condition does this suggest?
   b. How would you 'confirm' multiple sclerosis?
   c. What would you tell Mr. J.?
   d. What follow up would be appropriate?

W. E. Fabb, Melbourne

MR. D.W.   AGED 25   SOCIAL WORKER   284

1. What is the most likely cause of his visual loss?
   a. Did this result directly from the football injury?
   b. Did it result from the anaesthetic in any way?
   c. Should this have been found at the time of his admission to hospital?
   d. Should the intern have diagnosed it when Mr. W. complained of visual troubles?
   e. Would the prognosis have been better if it had been diagnosed 1 week ago?

2. What other conditions could cause these symptoms?
   a. What is the treatment of detached retina?
   b. What are the short and long term complications of detachment of the retina and its treatment?

3. Mr. W. is entitled to compensation for his leg injury. What about his eye injury?
   a. Would you be prepared to state in court that his eye injury is due to the football injury?
   b. How would you assess his long term disability?

4. Knee permitting, will Mr. W. be able to return to football?
   a. If so, when?
   b. Would you be in favour of him playing football again, even though he is a semi-professional footballer and his football earnings form a significant part of his income?
   c. His wife of 5 months wants to know when they can resume sexual relations?

W. F. Glastonbury, Adelaide

MRS. J.   AGED 27   MEDICAL SECRETARY   285

1. What are the signs and symptoms of acute retinal detachment?
   a. How do you diagnose acute retinal detachment?

479

b. How does a general practitioner manage an acute retinal detachment prior to receiving consultative help?

c. What advice could be given to the above patient concerning appropriate precautions and follow-up with her problem?

2. How can the risk of giving women undesirable drugs very early in pregnancy be reduced?

a. How would you advise this woman concerning the risk of teratogenic effects of Torecan (thiethylperazine)?

b. What is the risk of teratogenicity from a benzodiazepine early in pregnancy?

c. What steps might be taken during the pregnancy to reduce anxiety about foetal abnormalities?

3. How would you propose to manage labour in this situation?

a. Is an elective caesarean section indicated?

b. How might you manage a vaginal delivery in such a way as to reduce the risks of eye complications?

c. What are the advantages and disadvantages of caesarean section versus vaginal delivery and what are the perinatal and maternal risks of these two approaches in your community?

W. W. Rosser, Ottawa

286   MRS. H.J.   AGED 58   HOUSEWIFE

1. What is happening?
   a. Does she need new glasses?
   b. What test will give you a definite diagnosis?

2. What side effects can occur with chlorothiazide and propranolol?

3. What other side effects can occur with anti-hypertensive therapy?
   a. Why do people get gout when on anti-hypertensive therapy? Will it recur if the drug is stopped?
   b. Is hyperglycaemia common? Will the blood glucose revert to normal when the drug is stopped?

A. Himmelhoch, Sydney

287   MR. G.H.   AGED 75   RETIRED

1. What points are you looking for when examining the patient?
   a. What condition is suggested by headaches and visual loss?
   b. What other features can occur in this condition?

2. What investigation might give you the diagnosis?
   a. What is the value of arterial biopsy?

3. What is the management of the case?
   a. What is the natural outcome for people with temporal arteritis?
   b. Are any other vessels involved?
   c. Can blindness be prevented?
   d. Are non-steroidal, anti-inflammatory drugs effective?
   e. If you elected to use prednisolone, what dose would you commence with?
   f. What will be your guidelines for reducing or stopping therapy?
   g. If visual loss occurs, will it recover?

A. Himmelhoch, Sydney

LISA P.   AGED 9 MONTHS   288

1. What eye conditions merit such drastic treatment?
   a. What is the inheritance of a retinoblastoma?
   b. What are the long-term prospects?
   c. When she grows up, should she have children?
   d. Will there be any recurrence?

2. What reactions are possible from her parents?
   a. How much explanation of the condition should be offered?
   b. What special precautions are needed in caring for the child?
   c. What other professional workers can be put in touch with them?

3. How should her present problem be treated?
   a. What should her mother be trained to do regularly?
   b. How often should you see her?
   c. What advice can be given to prevent hazard to her remaining eye?

J. Grabinar, Bromley, UK

MATTHEW B.   AGED 2   289

1. What clinical examination would you make and how would you do it?
   a. How would you endeavour to gain his confidence? Are there any special techniques in examining small children?
   b. What regions would you examine? If he were uncooperative, what would be the minimum physical examination you would perform?
   c. In what way, if any, does such an examination differ from that which a junior hospital doctor would perform?

2. What is the most likely diagnosis?

3. What predisposing conditions might be associated with this disorder?
   a. Do adenoids influence the onset?
   b. Is allergy a contributory factor?

4. What is the most likely causative organism?
   a. Is it likely to be purely viral or bacterial or both?
   b. If bacterial, what is the most likely organism?
   c. To what antibiotics is *Haemophilus influenzae* most sensitive?

5. What medications would you prescribe?
   a. What would you give for pain relief?
   b. Would you always prescribe antibiotics? If so, which one? If not, when would you see him again?
   c. Do ear drops help? What are their dangers?
   d. Are nose drops or decongestants indicated? If so, what would you use, for how long and how often?

6. What advice would you give the parents?
   a. When should they contact you again?
   b. Should children with otitis media always be seen for review?
   c. What should they do if perforation occurs?
   d. Are there any serious sequelae of such an infection?

H. C. Watts, Perth, Australia

290 M.N.   AGED 3

1. What are this child's problems?
   a. Does a clinically clear chest exclude the cough as a significant symptom?
   b. Is the past history of similar attacks of any significance?
   c. Could there be a problem present which is aggravating the otitis media?

2. What immediate treatment is indicated?
   a. Does the appearance of the drums modify the treatment in any way?
   b. Will drug therapy suffice?
   c. Is any immediate surgical intervention necessary?
   d. What type of antibiotic is indicated?

3. What advice would you offer to the parents about future management?
   a. When would you see the child again?

b. What preventive treatment would you advise for the parents?
c. Is referral for a specialist opinion justified and on what grounds?

T. D. Manthorpe, Port Lincoln, Australia

JOHN F.   AGED 6   **291**

1. What is the diagnosis?
   a. What are the causal organisms?
   b. What is the natural history?
   c. What complications?

2. What would you do?
   a. What regional examination would you do?
   b. Explain the disorder to mum?
   c. What treatment and why?
   d. What follow-up?

J. Fry, Beckenham, UK

DAVID M.   AGED 3   **292**

1. Why was the cause not recognized?
   a. The pain was unquestionably present in the cheek. What explanation can you offer for this?
   b. What clinical clues might lead one to suspect otitis media?

2. What treatment would you have recommended if the diagnosis had been made in the first instance?
   a. General measures?
   b. Specific treatment?

3. Do you regard otitis media as a medical emergency?
   a. If so, do you think a doctor should get up at night and visit a child whose parents suspect he is suffering from otitis media?
   b. What organisms are usually responsible for otitis media?

4. Would you wish to follow up the child?
   a. What is the prognosis of a perforated drum?
   b. What complications may ensue?
   c. Does a perforated drum have any late consequences with respect to career choice?
   d. How successful is tympanoplasty? Does the procedure have any late consequences?

J. G. Richards, Auckland

293 JAMES H.   AGED 7   SCHOOLBOY

1. What problems have occurred?
   a. Why is earache more prevalent on the right side?
   b. How could this problem be prevented?
   c. Why is the ear painful now following relief with discharge?

2. How would you manage this problem?
   a. What are the complications of otitis media?
   b. How would you diagnose mastoid disease?
   c. What complications may occur?

3. Discuss the infection process in this case?
   a. Should antibiotics be given for a viral illness?

E. J. H. North, Melbourne

294 MASTER J.R.   AGED 3

1. Is this just another attack of otitis media and 'bronchitis'?
   a. Does he have an underlying precipitating source of infection?
   b. Is each attack clearing completely?
   c. What other underlying diseases could be responsible?
   d. What investigations are indicated?

2. What do you want to know about the social situation?
   a. Are the parents able to afford adequate food, clothing, etc.?
   b. Is he being neglected by his parents, i.e. is this some form of child abuse?
   c. Are his parents giving him his medication correctly?

3. What long term effects are taking place?
   a. Is this permanently affecting his physical development?
   b. What are the effects on his physical development?
   c. Are these attacks in any way detrimental to the parent's marriage?
   d. What are the effects on the siblings?

W. F. Glastonbury, Adelaide

295 MRS. S.K.   AGED 29   SCHOOLTEACHER

1. How would you clarify this problem?
   a. Personal and family history?
   b. Physical examination?
   c. Office tests and investigations?
   d. Additional tests requiring referral?

2. What are the implications on the family, of a child suffering from permanent hearing impairment?
    a. Implications for the child?
    b. Implications for the parents?
    c. Implications for the other siblings?
    d. Implications for family function as a psychosocial unit?

3. What facilities in the community can assist the family to cope with a child suffering from impaired hearing?
    a. What is the role of the family physician?
    b. What are the roles of the practice nurse, health visitor, public health nurse, social worker and other health professionals?
    c. What specialized medical services are available in the community, and in the regional hospital?
    d. What facilities are available in the kindergarten and school?

4. Could Ronnie's hearing disorder have been diagnosed at an earlier age, or perhaps been prevented?
    a. What is the incidence of hearing disorders among children?
    b. What factors may contribute to delay in diagnosis?
    c. What children are at special risk for developing hearing disorders?
    d. What tests may be used for early diagnosis?
    e. What health education measures could assist in shortening the delay before diagnosis, or in preventing hearing impairment?
    f. Of what value is premarital counselling or ante-natal care in preventing congenital hearing defects?

M. R. Polliack, Tel-Aviv, Israel

MR. C.K.   AGED 50   ENGINEER   296

1. What measures do general practitioners take to enable patients, who are new to a practice, to make the best use of the services they have to offer?
    a. Under the National Health Service regulations, what constitutes a 'temporary resident'?
    b. What documentation is necessary to secure payment for a 'temporary resident'?
    c. What areas in Mr. C.K.'s life would it be appropriate to explore at the **first** consultation he has as a 'temporary resident'?

2. Deafness is a relatively common presenting symptom in family medicine. In general, what are common causes of bilateral deafness?
    a. What is the likely cause for Mr. C.K.'s deafness?
    b. What 'medical measures' might have been deployed in managing Mr. C.K.'s problem?

c. What might specialist referral achieve in Mr. C.K.'s case – what is the specialist likely to do?

d. What degree of urgency should be accorded this referral?

e. What special risk might Mr. C.K. run were he to travel home by air?

3. Putting a patient on the 'sick list' is a common doctor activity. Viewed in sociological terms, what does this activity entail?

a. What reasons might there be to justify the action in Mr. C.K.'s case?

b. What details would the doctor enter on the sickness certificate?

J. D. E. Knox, Dundee

297   MR. G.   AGED 54   COMPANY DIRECTOR

1. What advice will you give him related to his current infection?
   a. What are possible problems if it is not settled prior to departure?
   b. Will any treatment help?
   c. Is there any place for antibiotics?

2. What will you advise him about immunizations in general?
   a. What immunizations are necessary?
   b. Are immunizations effective?
   c. How often do these require to be repeated?

3. What is your advice about malaria prophylaxis?
   a. Is prophylactic treatment necessary?
   b. If so
      – when should it start?
      – how long should it be continued?
      – what would you prescribe?

J. R. Marshall, Adelaide

298   MR. GERALD M.   AGED 71   RETIRED SCHOOLTEACHER

1. What are the likely contributing factors to his epistaxis?
   a. How important is hypertension in epistaxis?
   b. What changes occur in the blood vessels in the nose with age?
   c. From where do most epistaxes originate?

2. How would you manage this situation?
   a. How do you estimate the amount of blood he has lost?
   b. What immediate steps would you take?
   c. What would you do about the blood clot in his nose?
   d. How do you pack a nostril with an anterior bleeding point?

e. How do you pack a nostril with a posterior bleeding point?
f. What more radical measures are sometimes needed?

3. What follow up will be needed?
   a. If you pack the nostril, when would you remove the pack?
   b. What advice would you give about preventing further epistaxes?
   c. If the epistaxes recurred frequently, what would you do?

W. E. Fabb, Melbourne

G.P.   AGED 2½   299

1. Why is the above history unsatisfactory?
   a. In which bleeding diseases does family history offer useful infor-
      mation? His mother's brother had nosebleeds cured by cautery.
      Does this narrow the field of diagnosis?

2. What would your next move be toward effective management?
   a. What would be necessary to establish an accurate diagnosis?
   b. What specific deficiency would enable you to diagnose Von
      Willebrand's disease?
   c. How would you treat bleeding episodes?
   d. Could you treat without admitting the child to hospital each
      time?
   e. What problems might frequent hospital admissions pose, and
      for whom?
   f. How could his trouble be readily identified by other doctors who
      might have to assume responsibility for him in an emergency?

3. What are your intuitive feelings about this story?
   a. Do you often see frequent severe episodes of bleeding in small
      children without demonstrable cause?
   b. When are you as attending GP not reassured by other advice
      about your patient?

W. D. Jackson, Launceston, Australia

MR. C. CHAN   AGED 46   CHINESE RICE MERCHANT   300

1. What further examination and investigations are required to establish a diagnosis?
   a. What is the most significant sign or symptom in this condition?
   b. What is the most significant predisposing factor so far known
      about this condition?
   c. Does the fact that Mr. Chan is from the Chiu Chow Clan (a
      province of SE China) have any significance?
   d. What office procedures can be performed by the GP to establish
      the diagnosis?

2. What is the treatment of choice?
   a. Is surgery indicated?
   b. Is there any place for radiotherapy?

3. What is the prognosis?

Footnote: Naso-pharyngeal carcinoma is particularly common amongst the Southern Chinese, especially of Chiu Chow origin. A predisposing factor in this condition is thought to be salt-fish ingestion.

N. C. L. Yuen, Hong Kong

301 MR. N.M. AGED 41 SAW MILLER

1. Is another referral advisable and if so, to whom?
   a. Is a full sensitization workup by an allergist indicated?
   b. How effective are desensitization courses in 'allergic sinusitis'?
   c. Could his occupation be relevant to this condition?

2. Do simple radical antrostomies have a high success rate in chronic sinusitis?
   a. This man originally had a nasal polypectomy. What does this suggest?
   b. The X-rays originally showed no abnormality in the sinuses. How does this result affect the overall management?
   c. Is the protection of the patient from over zealous procedural therapies a proper role of the GP?

3. Are there any simple measures that may be helpful?
   a. How can a doctor help a patient come to terms with his condition?
   b. Is simple saline douching of value in chronic recurring sinusitis?
   c. How effective are oral decongestants in contrast to local decongestants?

T. D. Manthorpe, Port Lincoln, Australia

302 MR. F.M. AGED 42 INSURANCE AGENT

1. What would constitute an appropriate differential diagnosis of this man's respiratory symptoms?
   a. What are the usual underlying causes of acute sinusitis?
   b. What are the potential pulmonary complications of upper respiratory infections?
   c. What are the usual complications of self-medication for nasal, sinus, and upper respiratory infections?

d. What is the differential diagnosis of mechanical interference with upper respiratory toilet?

2. What are the ramifications of this man's heart murmur?
   a. What is the importance regarding the need to accurately classify this murmur?
   b. Would your recommendations for follow-up vary depending upon a diagnosis of rheumatic valvulitis, mitral valve prolapse syndrome, congenital defect, or functional murmur?
   c. How important would antibiotic prophylaxis be in the event that a sinus problem required any manipulative treatment (such as antral irrigation or dental work)?

3. What laboratory procedures would be of most value in assessing this patient's respiratory infection?
   a. Can sinusitis be diagnosed by X-ray?
   b. What would the likely sinus X-ray findings be if this represents acute maxillary sinusitis?
   c. Would a culture of the mucopurulent nasal material provide the aetiological agent for this man's symptoms?
   d. Would the finding on Gram stain and culture of the pneumococcus identify a likely aetiological agent?
   e. What factors in the clinical course of this patient would dictate an ENT consultation for antral irrigation or a dental consultation for an infected focus in a maxillary molar?

4. What are the expected outcomes of a general type screening examination, even for seemingly well-defined, localized problems such as upper respiratory infection?

L. H. Amundson, Sioux Falls, SD, USA

BETTY R. AGED 2   303

1. What was the most likely cause of her illness?
   a. What other causes must you consider?
   b. What complications might occur?
   c. What treatment would you prescribe for this child?
   d. How do you describe the probable clinical cause of the illness to the parents?

2. If this condition were due to an infective agent, what other clinical manifestations could be produced by it?
   a. What treatment is available for these?
   b. What long-term effects might follow an infection by this agent?

J. G. P. Ryan, Brisbane

304 **MR. Q.R.** **AGED 65** **RETIRED ENGINEER**

1. What is the doctor thinking?
   a. Was the doctor careless when he first inspected the tongue?
   b. What percentage of ulcers of the tongue are malignant?
   c. How regular should re-inspection be in such a case?

2. What does he say next to the patient?
   a. Is it ever sufficient to make such a statement as 'Let me see it again if you are not happy about it.'? If so, does a doctor have to give definite instructions about what to look for? Or does he say, 'See me again in so many weeks.'?

3. What does he say to the patient's wife, whom he knows will be ringing up after the consultation?
   a. Does the doctor make conscious efforts to regain these patients' feelings of respect for his clinical ability?
   b. How does the doctor cope with all the uncertainties such a tragedy create in his mind about his clinical acumen? How can he reassure himself about the contribution of the patient, given that the patient was neglectful in allowing matters to proceed as far as they did before coming back?
   c. Was the doctor right to advocate by-pass surgery at 63?

P. L. Gibson, Auckland

305 **DR. P.F.** **AGED 32** **UNIVERSITY LECTURER**

1. How specific can a general practitioner be when diagnosing viral respiratory infections?
   a. What is the differential diagnosis of a tonsillar exudate?
   b. What place has antibiotic treatment in these cases?
   c. How rapidly do viral respiratory infections spread to other family members?
   d. Will the same infection present in different ways in other members of the family?

2. What viral infections cause concern during pregnancy?
   a. Is antibiotic treatment useful in any of these cases?
   b. Are any viral infections particularly serious in the last months of pregnancy or for the new born baby?
   c. In this situation, if the other children in the family become ill, should they be separated from the newborn baby?

3. How does a nuclear family cope when the only wage earner in the family is ill?
   a. What resources are available to help a family with young children when several members of the family are ill at the same time?

b. What advice should be given to a patient who is recovering from a viral illness but who is concerned about getting back to a busy job?

B. H. Connor, Armidale, Australia

S.P. AGED 5   **306**

1. What would be key diagnostic elements in the history and physical examination?
    a. Is the family history of siblings with a similar condition of any help?
    b. What is the significance of none of the children having had basic immunizations?
    c. What is the signficance of a friable white exudate covering the tonsils?
    d. What is the significance of tender cervical adenopathy?
    e. What is the significance of palatal petechiae?

2. What factors would be helpful in making a positive diagnosis?
    a. What is the accuracy of the aetiology of tonsillo-pharyngitis by physical findings alone?
    b. What are the advantages and disadvantages of the office use of the strep. plate?
    c. Would it be helpful to screen other family members for streptococcal carrier state?
    d. In view of the immunization status, should other culture techniques be utilized?
    e. If this patient has streptococcal pharyngitis, what are first and second line drugs used for therapy?

3. What other physical findings might help confirm or exclude a streptococcal tonsillo-pharyngitis?
    a. Bullous myringitis?
    b. Rhinitis?
    c. Hoarseness?
    d. Injected conjunctivae?
    e. Dry, hacking cough?
    f. Liver and spleen enlargement?

L. H. Amundson, Sioux Falls, SD, USA

TRACEY N.   AGED 4   **307**

1. How would you manage the present complaint?
    a. Would you take a throat swab and blood investigations – if so with what requests?

b. What antibiotic would you advise and for what length of time?
c. How would you promptly lower the temperature?
d. Is this a 'new' attack of tonsillitis?
e. What reasons underlie tonsillitis of such frequency?

2. What advice would you give the parents?
   a. In regard to possible tonsillectomy?
   b. How to manage the hyperpyrexia and possible convulsion?

3. Would you refer the patient to an ENT surgeon?
   a. What history would make you refer patient to a surgeon?
   b. What complications can arise from tonsillectomy?
   c. What are indications for tonsillectomy?
   d. How much is recurrent tonsillitis a compliance problem?

B. M. Fehler, Johannesburg

308 MASTER A.T.   AGED 8   SCHOOLBOY

1. What immediate treatment is necessary?
   a. Would you suggest an antipyretic?
   b. Would observation suffice at present?

2. When should antibiotics be prescribed in an otherwise healthy child?
   a. If commenced, how long should antibiotics be continued?
   b. Are antibiotics routine treatment for tonsillitis?

3. What signs of complications would you look for?
   a. What would you expect to find in the ears?
   b. What would you expect to find in the chest?
   c. What would you expect to find in the blood picture?
   d. What would you expect to find in the urine?

4. At this age, and with this history, what other diagnoses are likely?

5. Is tonsillectomy indicated? If so, when?

D. U. Shepherd, Melbourne

309 DICK THOMSON   AGED 8   SCHOOLBOY

1. Would you prescribe an antibiotic?
   a. Are any laboratory investigations indicated?
   b. Which organisms cause tonsillitis/pharyngitis?
   c. Which antibiotic(s) would cover the likely bacterial causes of sore throat?

    d.   Which antibiotic is indicated in this case?

    e.   Even if this is a viral infection, why not prescribe an antibiotic?

2. Would you arrange a tonsillectomy?
    a.   What are the current indications for tonsillectomy?
    b.   Is a specialist opinion indicated?
    c.   What are the risks of tonsillectomy?

3. What other factors are there in managing this case?
    a.   What is Mrs. Thompson's understanding of Dick's illness?
    b.   How is the illness affecting Dick?
    c.   How will you deal with Mrs. Thompson's demand for a quick resolution of the illness?

R. P. Strasser, Melbourne

DAVID P.   AGED 10   SCHOOLBOY   310

1. What two problems face the doctor?
    a.   How would you cope with the father's anger?
    b.   At what stage of the consultation would you consider the father's anger?

2. What could be a differential diagnosis of David's condition given the few facts above?
    a.   Would you support your partner's diagnosis?
    b.   Would you suggest alternative diagnoses at this stage?
    c.   What would your treatment be?

F. Mansfield, Perth, Australia

MR. A.J.   AGED 25   UNIVERSITY STUDENT   311

1. What physical diagnoses would you consider to be likely?
    a.   To establish a working diagnosis in Mr. J.'s case, how extensive would you make your physical examination of Mr. J.? (i.e. out of the complete repertoire of 'the clinical examination', what items would you select as appropriate?)
    b.   What are the arguments for and against invoking laboratory assistance at this particular home consultation?

2. What problems, real or imaginary, may be inherent in this situation?
    a.   What special problems commonly face immigrants who fall ill in a 'foreign' country?
    b.   If, as seems possible, Mr. J. is suffering from an infection, in what ways might this influence the situation?

3. How would you manage this situation?
   a. What are the arguments for and against prescribing medicine for Mr. J.?
   b. What arrangements are commonly made for making available prescribed drugs during holidays?
   c. What follow-up arrangement (if any) would you make for Mr. J.?

J. D. E. Knox, Dundee

312 MASTER J.R.   AGED 6   SCHOOLBOY

1. Is it possible to determine the aetiological agent of an acute upper respiratory infection on the basis of your physical examination?
   a. Do you always do a throat swab for culture and sensitivity?
   b. When do you prescribe antibiotics, and if so, which antibiotics and for how long?
   c. When do you consider infectious mononucleosis in the differential diagnosis and what steps do you take to exclude this possibility?

2. What are the indications for tonsillectomy and adenoidectomy?
   a. Should all children have their tonsils out?
   b. Should any child have his tonsils out?
   c. Does frequency of acute attacks alone dictate the need for surgery?
   d. What is chronic tonsillitis and how do you make this diagnosis?
   e. How important is adenoid hypertrophy and how does it influence ear function, airway patency and facial appearance?

3. What is the role of allergy in the hypertrophy of tonsils and adenoids?
   a. Is size alone important?
   b. Why is it important to determine allergy before considering surgery?

R. L. Perkin, Toronto

313 MASTER Y.L.   AGED 4   ATTENDS NURSERY SCHOOL

1. What do you understand by the 'problem solving method', hypothesis forming', 'hypothesis testing', 'probability diagnosis', 'testing a hypothesis by treatment' and 'time as a diagnostic tool'?
   a. What are the most likely causes of this boy's sore throat, and what was the doctor's hypothesis?
   b. What is the predictive value of pus on the tonsils for a bacteriological infection?

   c.   If a bacteriological cause is isolated, which organism is it most likely to be?

   d.   How do you think a throat swab may have helped the doctor at the first and second consultations in hypothesis checking?

   e.   In what way did the doctor use time as a diagnostic tool?

   f.   Why was he waiting 10 days to re-check his hypothesis?

2.   What are your indications for tonsillectomy?
   a.   What are the disadvantages of tonsillectomy?
   b.   Discuss the natural history/ies of tonsillitis in childhood.
   c.   What condition/s has tonsillectomy been said to precipitate and why?
   d.   How would you counsel the mother on tonsillectomy?
   e.   If the doctor reacted angrily to the mother's suggestion, could his response have been appropriate?

3.   Why did the doctor prescribe penicillin VK and for the length of time he did?
   a.   Do you think the doctor should have stopped the penicillin VK after four days?
   b.   Would he have been justified changing the antibiotic after four days with or without a throat swab?
   c.   What might have happened had the doctor prescribed ampicillin/amoxycillin in this patient?
   d.   In the highly unlikely event of this patient having diphtheria, how might the doctor's initial approach have affected the natural history of this disease?

J. H. Levenstein, Cape Town

MRS. J.A.   AGED 26   HOUSEWIFE   **314**

1.   What is the likely nature of Dawn's problems?
   a.   What do you understand by the catarrhal child syndrome?
   b.   How would you treat frequent upper respiratory tract infections in a child?
   c.   Discuss the advantages of adopting a practice policy for common conditions.

2.   What are the indications for tonsillectomy?
   a.   What is the relationship between social class and the incidence of tonsillectomy?
   b.   What factors affect a patient's expectations of medical care?
   c.   What resources are available to you to improve health education amongst your patients?

3.   What are the possible reasons for aggression in a patient?

   a.   How do you deal with patient aggression directed against you?

   b.   What instructions do you give your receptionist about dealing with difficult patients?

   c.   What measures might you take if an irretrievable breakdown occurs in the doctor–patient relationship?

4.   What ethical principles govern relationships between medical practitioners?

   a.   What is your reaction when a patient criticises one of your partners?

   b.   How do you react when you feel that another doctor has undermined your relationship with a patient?

   c.   What steps can you take in your own area to avoid clashes over patient care?

T. A. I. Bouchier Hayes, Camberley, UK

315 MRS. FLORENCE A.   AGED 71   HOUSEWIFE

1.   How would you assess this patient?

   a.   What are the common sites for bones to lodge in the throat or oesophagus?

   b.   What importance has the history in impacted foreign body in the throat or oesophagus?

   c.   What are the usual features of foreign body in the upper oesophagus?

2.   How do you examine a patient with suspected foreign body in the throat?

   a.   How do you detect a bone in the pryiform fossa?

   b.   If you see no sign of the bone, what would lead you to refer the patient to an ENT surgeon?

   c.   How would he examine the patient for a possible foreign body in the oesophagus?

   d.   What radiological examination could be helpful?

3.   If the symptoms suggest a foreign body in the throat, but none can be detected, what would you do?

   a.   Could a minor laceration caused by the bone give similar symptoms?

   b.   If you decide to send the patient home, what advice would you give?

   c.   What follow up would you organize?

W. E. Fabb, Melbourne

KUMBURAI M.   AGED ?   TODDLER

316

1. What treatment should Kumburai have?
   a. What arguments are there for and against the treatment of acute upper respiratory tract infections with antibiotics?
   b. Should the mother's request for an injection be acceded to?
   c. What would she do if you said oral medication would be better?
   d. What good would a cough mixture do
      - for Kumburai?
      - for anyone with a cough?

2. Is Kumburai suffering from anything of extreme danger to him?
   a. What would happen to him if he should get gastro-enteritis, a lower respiratory infection or measles?
   b. If he had been breast fed, when would this have come to a sudden stop?
   c. What would Mrs. M. feel about future pregnancies if Kumburai should die?

3. What should Mrs. M. be told?
   a. On finding herself pregnant again, and believing that her milk was now poisonous to Kumburai what dangerous action might she take besides stopping the breast feeding?
   b. What beliefs might she hold about weaning foods?
   c. If Kumburai had been given an injection of procaine penicillin would her belief in injections as the only valuable therapy have been strengthened?

R. T. Mossop, Harare, Zimbabwe

JOHN W.   AGED 5   SCHOOLBOY

317

1. What are the likely causes of his condition?
   a. How would you distinguish between upper and lower respiratory tract infection?
   b. If there were no signs of respiratory tract infection and the rest of the examination was normal, what conditions might you suspect? What would you tell the parents when they ask, 'What's wrong with John?'?
   c. If in two days' time the child continues to have a high fever, but without additional physical signs, what conditions might you suspect?

2. How would you assess this child?
   a. What further history would you seek?
   b. What physical examination would you carry out, and in what sequence?
   c. What investigations may help in assessment?

3. What general advice would you give mother?
   a. If the child has signs of an upper respiratory infection, what advice would you give mother?
   b. What would you tell mother about fluid intake, food, rest and the use of antipyretics and tepid sponging?
   c. What follow up arrangements would you make?

W. E. Fabb, Melbourne

318 WILLIAM ANDREWS   AGED 2

1. What possible diagnoses are you considering?
   a. Could this be a case of family problems presenting as sleep disturbance in the child?
   b. How does whooping cough present?
   c. What about nocturnal asthma?

2. What investigations would you do?
   a. What findings would you expect on chest X-ray?
   b. Would pulmonary function tests help?
   c. Is it worth allergy testing this patient?
   d. How about some blood tests?

3. How would you manage this problem?
   a. Is the mother's attitude relevant in management?
   b. What antibiotics are indicated?
   c. Which bronchodilator would you give and by what route?
   d. Would antihistamines help?

R. P. Strasser, Melbourne

319 MRS. O.R.   AGED 46   HOUSEWIFE

1. What is the diagnosis?
   a. Is 'acute chest infection with local moist sounds' specific enough?
   b. Would a patholological or aetiological classification of chest infection be of much practical value?

2. Is it either desirable or possible to determine the actual infecting agent?
   a. As *Streptococcus pneumoniae*, a virus or *Mycoplasma pneumoniae* are the likely causes and psittacosis, Legionnaire's disease and Q fever the unlikely ones, does sputum culture have anything to offer?

    b.   Will a pre-treatment chest X-ray be of value in diagnosis or in deciding therapy?

    c.   Is initial management the same whatever the cause?

3. Which, if any, antibiotic is indicated?
    a.   What is the antibiotic of choice for a *Streptococcus pneumoniae* infection?
    b.   What two antibiotics could be used for a non-bacterial infection?
    c.   Should a broad spectrum antibiotic be used initially?

A. J. Moulds, Basilton, UK

E.P.   4 YEAR OLD GIRL   320

1. What diagnostic hypotheses would be in your mind?
    a.   Could measles be a possibility?
    b.   Could the child be incubating measles having been immunized?
    c.   What other possibilities are there?

2. How would you test your hypotheses?
    a.   What specific signs would make a diagnosis of morbilli?

3. How would you manage the situation?
    a.   Is there any advantage in using antibiotics at the outset?
    b.   What are the common complications?
    c.   What are the less common complications?

4. E.P. has a sister, aged eight months. Mother asks if you can prevent her getting the same condition. What would be your reply?
    a.   Is active immunization any use at this stage?
    b.   What is passive immunization?
    c.   Would it help in this case?
    d.   If so, when should it be given?
    e.   Will you need to actively immunize the baby later?

A. Himmelhoch, Sydney

MR. D.E.   AGED 18   COLLEGE STUDENT   321

1. Is your first diagnosis correct?
    a.   What is the normal course of influenza?
    b.   Is there any advantage in using antibiotics at the first visit?

2. On the second visit, what do you think has happened?
    a.   Could he die? If so, from what?

b. Before using antibiotics, should you consider doing any pathology tests?
c. Does the fact that he played football have any bearing on the course this illness may take?
d. What is the most lethal bacterium which can colonize as secondary infection in influenza?
e. Can the influenza virus cause death without secondary bacterial infection?

A. Himmelhoch, Sydney

322 DEREK B.   AGED 40   CIVIL SERVANT

1. What are the main diagnoses that you would consider for this pyrexial episode?
   a. How significant is a holiday in the Mediterranean?
   b. Is the general practitioner's list of differential diagnoses likely to be different from the specialist's?

2. What investigations might you order?
   a. What investigations are likely to give you the biggest yield?
   b. What factors influence the point at which the general practitioner starts to order investigations?
   c. What are the chances all your investigations will be negative?

3. How does a patient's past history influence the doctor's approach and management?
   a. Is a doctor prejudiced in his approach and management to a patient with frequent psychological and emotional problems?
   b. What effect might anxiety have on the presentation of physical illness?

J. C. Hasler, Oxford

323 MR. D.C.   AGED 40   COMPANY EXECUTIVE

1. Should you discuss his obvious embarrassment?
   a. Should you tell him to 'be a man' and ignore minor inconveniences?
   b. Should you tell him to 'stand up to his wife'?
   c. Should you concentrate on his physical symptom?

2. What are the likely physical findings in this case?
   a. Which systems in particular would be examined?
   b. Is a physical examination necessary?

3. If the physical findings are negative, should a chest X-ray be performed?
   a. What other investigations are mandatory?

4. Should the management include a cough suppressant?
   a. Should management of this problem include anything other than pharmaceutical prescriptions?

D. U. Shepherd, Melbourne

MR. A.C.   AGED 32   STOREMAN

32

1. If your physical examination indicates no specific abnormal findings, with the exception of possible weight loss, what are the most likely diagnoses?

2. What investigations are indicated in this case?
   a. What would you be looking for in a chest X-ray?
   b. Should the pharynx be carefully examined?
   c. Would X-ray of the nasal sinuses be of help in this case?
   d. Could examination of sputum be of help?
   e. Is bronchoscopy indicated?

3. What would you prescribe for this cough?
   a. If no carcinoma of the lung is found?
   b. If a carcinoma is found?

4. If the cough proves to be simply related to excessive smoking, how would you handle this problem?

D. U. Shepherd, Melbourne

MR. JOHN J.   AGED 75

325

1. Why should the doctor arrange a chest X-ray?
   a. What are the likely differential diagnoses?
   b. Do any of them matter at the age of 75?

2. The chest X-ray showed a carcinoma of the bronchus. What would be the doctor's immedite course of action?
   a. What treatment is available?
   b. Is it effective?

3. The chest specialist recommended no treatment. How would the doctor manage the case now?
   a. What would he say to the patient?
   b. What would he say to his wife?

J. C. Hasler, Oxford

326 THOMAS R. AGED 62

1. What are the long term complications of partial gastrectomy?
   a. What follow-up would you organize for such patients in your practice?
   b. How would you check on non-compliers?
   c. What investigations would you arrange, why and how often?

2. Give your assessment of his new symptoms.
   a. What would you do at this consultation?
   b. What explanation would you give T.R.?

3. How would you manage the likely conditions that you discover?
   a. How do you treat post-gastrectomy anaemia?
   b. What is the prognosis of the angina in T.R.?

J. Fry, Beckenham, UK

327 MR. & MRS. S. AGED 64 AND 62 PENSIONERS

1. What was the best way of managing Mrs. S.?
   a. Was the GP justified in regarding her symptoms as psychosomatic?
   b. Were investigations necessary to establish the psychogenicity of her symptoms?
   c. Why do patients sometimes persist with irrational fears about their physical health?
   d. Can phobias about illness sometimes mask other problems in the patient's life?
   e. How should the GP go about trying to discover what might be troubling Mrs. S.?
   f. What approach should he adopt if she persists in saying that there is nothing troubling her?
   g. Should psychotropic drugs have been used on Mrs. S.?
   h. Should further investigations have been performed if Mrs. S. had refused to accept the negative findings of the tests the GP had arranged?
   i. Should Mrs. S. have been offered specialist referral if she had refused to accept the GP's assurance about her physical health?

2. What was the cause of Mr. S.'s symptoms?
   a. What is the likeliest cause of gastro-intestinal bleeding in this patient?
   b. How great are the chances of a malignancy being found?

3. Was there any connection between Mrs. S.'s symptoms and those of her husband?

a. To what extent can marital difficulties cause psychosomatic symptoms?
b. To what extent could Mrs. S.'s mental state have contributed to the development of an ulcer in her husband?
c. What role do psychogenic factors play in the development and activity of peptic ulcers?
d. If the ulcer is found to be malignant, would this lead you to think that psychogenic factors did not play a significant part in its causation?

4. How are Mr. and Mrs. S. likely to present in the future?
   a. Can an increase in Mrs. S.'s symptoms be expected?
   b. How is the relationship between Mr. and Mrs. S. likely to be affected by his illness?
   c. How should the GP manage the medical and psychological problems which can be expected to arise in this couple?

S. Levenstein, Cape Town

MR. J.G.   AGED 76   328

1. Should surgery be performed?
   a. Is it reasonable to think of withholding surgery?
   b. Do you have a right to withhold it?
   c. What sort of surgery might be done?

2. Would you discuss the whole problem with the patient?
   a. What might your reasons be for frankly discussing the situation with your patient?
   b. How do you handle his son's request not to tell Dad the diagnosis?
   c. How can you proffer options to this man?

3. How could he be offered the best hope for successful surgery if that is the chosen option?
   a. What preparation will be required remembering that he has been taking aminophylline, prednisolone, and a diuretic?
   b. Would you avoid any particular drugs – why?
   c. Any particular dangers in the postoperative period?

W. D. Jackson, Launceston, Australia

MRS. I.S.   AGED 45   329

1. What is the most likely diagnosis and the initial management?
   a. What tests might you order yourself before prescribing any treatment?

    b.   Do you initiate pharmacotherapy before a cardiological consultation?

    c.   Is dietary manipulation indicated?

    d.   Is her lifestyle a problem for you?

2. Extensive cardiological investigation later establishes a diagnosis: idiopathic congestive cardiomyopathy. Now what is the management?

    a.   What is the long term prognosis?

    b.   What are the complications of long term therapy for this condition?

    c.   Can she be managed at home or will hospital be necessary?

3. You and the patient here face a rare and fatal illness, of unknown cause, with an uncertain natural history. What general principles of management do you establish?

    a.   How do you describe the prognosis to the patient?

    b.   Should you discuss the expected course and prognosis with her husband?

    c.   When and how do you approach terminal parental illness with children?

P. R. Grantham, Vancouver

330 MR. CHARLES B.   AGED 48   FARMER

1. On this evidence, what diagnostic hypotheses would you be entertaining?

    a.   What are the clinical characteristics of chronic obstructive lung disease?

    b.   What is the distinction between the so called 'pink puffer' and the 'blue bloater'?

    c.   What are the pathological elements which constitute chronic obstructive lung disease?

2. What further information would you seek?

    a.   What past history is important?

    b.   What features would you look for on physical examination?

    c.   What investigations would give useful information?

3. What plan of action would you develop if your most probable hypothesis is verified?

    a.   What regime would you initiate for this case of chronic obstructive lung disease in a self-employed farmer?

    b.   What preventive measures would you advise?

    c.   How would you help Mr. B. to use health care resources more appropriately in the future?

d. What would you tell Mr. B. about his condition, what you intend to do about it, what he should do about it, and his long-term outlook?

W. E. Fabb, Melbourne

MISS D.R.   AGED 70   RETIRED SECRETARY   **331**

1. How would you adjust her steroid dosage?
   a. Alternate day dosage or continuous?
   b. Outline a suitable dose reduction regime.

2. How would you treat her osteoporosis?
   a. Would you recommend oestrogen therapy?
   b. What other medications or supplements? What dosage?

3. What other measures would be indicated in her rehabilitation programme?
   a. Portable oxygen?
   b. Physiotherapy?
   c. Other measures?

C. T. Lamont, Ottawa

MR. J.A.   AGED 28   PLUMBER   **332**

1. What disease process is occurring?
   a. What tests would you perform in the home to possibly diagnose this case?
   b. His urine test had heavy proteinuria and showed traces of blood – Why?
   c. What further tests might be undertaken?
   d. What are the causes of CCF?
   e. What other information should be sought?

2. How would you manage the patient?
   a. In the short term?
   b. In the long term?

3. What is the prognosis?
   a. Is it likely to recur?
   b. Is long term therapy of use?
   c. How long should this be undertaken?

E. J. H. North, Melbourne

333 MR. W.G.   AGED 72   RETIRED SHOPKEEPER

1. What is the treatment of acute pulmonary oedema?
    a. Is there any useful advice that can be given on the phone before the doctor sets out to see the patient?
    b. Is oxygen essential, desirable or not necessary at home?
    c. What drugs/dosages/routes of administration should be used?

2. Was the decision to admit the patient a correct one?
    a. Has a 'silent' infarct been excluded?
    b. Will cardiac monitoring improve his chances of survival?
    c. If the GP had an ECG machine and/or a portable defibrillator would that make home care more feasible?
    d. Can the relatives realistically be expected to cope?
    e. Can the GP realistically be expected to cope?

3. What consequences are likely to flow from the refusal to admit and how can they best be coped with?
    a. Will the relatives now think the GP does not know what he is doing?
    b. Should the GP call an ambulance and send the patient anyway?
    c. If he decides to treat the patient at home what instructions should be given to the relatives?
    d. If the patient dies during the night who is going to look silly – the GP or the hospital physician?

A. J. Moulds, Basildon, UK

334 MRS. N.   AGED 72   WIDOW

1. What causes of congestive heart failure must be ruled out in this woman?
    a. What are the most common causes of congestive heart failure?
    b. What role could this woman's social circumstances play in the development of congestive heart failure?
    c. Could the drug change have had any impact?

2. Are different brands of drugs interchangeable?
    a. What factors influence the bioavailability of the drug?
    b. Can bioavailability be accurately tested?
    c. Is bioavailability of drugs more important in some drugs than others?

3. What steps may be necessary because of variable bioavailability of drugs?
    a. Name drugs in which there is variable bioavailability.

b. How may physicians avoid the above situation?
c. What role does the patient's health play in bioavailability?

W. W. Rosser, Ottawa

TIMOTHY S.   AGED 9
335

1. What is the diagnosis?
   a. Is this an acute allergic reaction due to an unknown allergen?
   b. How dangerous is the outcome if left untreated?
   c. How certain can you be of your diagnosis?

2. What therapy was instituted?
   a. Is the use of cortisone indicated?
   b. Should we use adrenaline subcutaneously?
   c. Are antihistamines of value?
   d. Is hospitalization necessary?

3. What advice should be given to the parents?
   a. What tests are available to discover the allergen?
   b. Is desensitizing of benefit to the child?
   c. Should parents be informed in the use of an emergency kit of cortisone and antihistamines and adrenaline?
   d. What dangers can possibly occur with the child?

B. M. Fehler, Johannesburg

MADAM P.L.H.   AGED 57
336

1. To what extent has the house call helped you reappraise the diagnosis of your patient's complaints?
   a. Discuss the differential diagnosis of dysphagia?
   b. What is 'globus hystericus'? To what extent are you now able to label your patient's complaints as functional?
   c. What is the place of endoscopy in this patient?

2. How would you now manage your patient?
   a. Define 'empathy'. How would this attitude assist your patient?
   b. If you inform the patient that her symptoms are functional, do you then discharge her from your care?
   c. What is the most likely prognosis for your patient?

3. How could your management of her mother's problems assist your patient?
   a. What are the clinical features of cataract?
   b. How would you rule out the possibility of diabetes in her mother?

   c.   How could you mobilize help from members of the family to assist your patient?

4.   What resources are available for the care of the elderly in your community?
   a.   Discuss the 'pros' and 'cons' of admitting your patient's mother to an institution.

F. E. H. Tan, Kuala Lumpur

337   MRS. F.B.   AGED 59   WIDOWED OFFICE WORKER

1.   What is your approach when there is a need to distinguish between the emotional and organic origin of symptoms?
   a.   Would the probabilities of differential diagnoses be changed if Mrs. F.B. was a male?
   b.   What do you understand patients to mean when they say they have palpitations? How do you clarify their meaning with them?

2.   If these symptoms prove to be emotional in origin what methods are available for Mrs. F.B.'s treatment?
   a.   What are the differences between 'operant' and 'Pavlovian' conditioning?
   b.   What are the associated symptoms of hyperventilation and what is their physical explanation?
   c.   On what other occasions may people voluntarily hyperventilate? Are there risks in doing so?

3.   What are your views on the label, sometimes given to patients, of 'suffering from mixed anxiety and depression'?
   a.   What are the pros and cons of giving benzodiazepines for symptoms of anxiety apparently produced by recent stress?
   b.   Are there any effects on mortality of the recent loss of a spouse? If there are, are they uniform for both genders? How might they be explained?

P. Freeling, London

338   MARION B.   AGED 15   SCHOLAR

1.   What questions do you ask her?
   a.   What conditions do you consider in order of frequency?
   b.   What do you expect to find on examining her?

2.   How do you manage the situation?
   a.   What do you tell Marion?

b. What treatment do you give her?

c. What is the prognosis of the syndrome?

J. Fry, Beckenham, UK

ROBERT S.   AGED 18 MONTHS

339

1. What diagnostic possibilities would you consider?
   a. What signs would suggest a diagnosis of asthma?
   b. What would make you consider a foreign body?
   c. Could he have bronchiolitis?
   d. What other diagnostic possibilities should be considered?

2. What physical signs would suggest he had a serious disorder?
   a. Colour?
   b. Respiratory rate?
   c. Pulse rate and character?
   d. Ability to take fluids?

3. What treatment would you give him?
   a. Are any medications effective for asthma in a child this age?
   b. Is inability to drink fluids a serious sign? Why?

4. If he were not ill enough to require hospitalization, what advice would you give to the family?
   a. What signs should alert them to seek review?
   b. How much fluid should he take?
   c. Would you tell the parents he had 'asthma'?
   d. What possible allergic factors should be considered?

5. How do you manage atopic eczema?
   a. What local therapy?
   b. Do oral medications help?
   c. Does diet have a role in aggravating eczema?

H. C. Watts, Perth, Australia

S.B.   AGED 3

340

1. What is the probable basis of Simon's condition?
   a. Discuss the allergic diathesis.
   b. How much does infection have a role?
   c. Is it usual to find a specific allergen in such a case?

2. What additional history might be of value?
   a. Would you expect a history of skin problems or food allergies in infancy?

    b.   What related conditions could occur in his family history?

    c.   What specific enquiries about Simon's environment would you make?

3.   What tests could be of value in diagnosis and treatment?
    a.   Discuss the role of skin testing and the RAST test for allergies.
    b.   Is there a place for empiric testing – e.g., a trial of removal of all milk products for a short period?

4.   What would you tell the anxious parents?
    a.   Explain the allergic process in lay terms?
    b.   What changes in environment would you recommend, if any?
    c.   Would you advise a normal life-style for Simon?

5.   How is treatment going to influence his condition?
    a.   How and when would antibiotics be used?
    b.   What other therapies are useful?
    c.   Would you consider Simon a candidate for 'Interval Therapy'?
    d.   Which activities should be specifically encouraged?

6.   What is the long-term prognosis and what is your long-term advice?
    a.   Is the condition likely to persist into adolescence?
    b.   What would you advise the parents about Simon's activities?
    c.   The parents are worried about the same problem developing in any other children they might have. How would you counsel them?

K. C. Nyman, Perth, Australia

341   MEHMET G.   AGED 10

1.   What does the word 'asthma' mean to patient, mother and doctor?
    a.   What is the difference between asthma and bronchitis in children?
    b.   How can you establish the reversibility of airways obstruction?
    c.   What signs and tests give a good idea of the progress of the disease?

2.   How can further attacks be prevented?
    a.   What roles do infection, allergy, exercise and stress play?
    b.   What prophylactic measures can be used?
    c.   What prognosis can you give mother?
    d.   What forms of exercise are beneficial?

3.   Should this case be managed at home, or referred?
    a.   When is asthma dangerous?

b. What emergency treatment can be given in a severe attack?

c. When, if ever, should the patient be separated from his parents?

J. Grabinar, Bromley, UK

MARK A. AGED 19 STUDENT

342

1. What is the probable diagnosis?
   a. What pointers might there be in Mark's past history?
   b. Could the family history be helpful?

2. What diagnostic tests could be helpful?
   a. Discuss the use of ventilatory function tests for such patients.
   b. What is the place of blood tests and chest X-ray in Mark's case?
   c. Would you consider a trial of empirical therapy?

3. Having established your diagnosis, how would you treat Mark?
   a. What is the place of cromoglycate?
   b. How would you use bronchodilators in this case?
   c. Would you use allergy testing, and if so what would you expect to achieve?

4. What are Mark's chances of eventual cure?
   a. Is his condition likely to be life-long?
   b. Would you advise against sport?
   c. Is his condition likely to worsen?

K. C. Nyman, Perth, Australia

KATHERINE J. AGED 10 SCHOOLGIRL

343

1. What are the possible causes of the child's condition?
   a. Could Katherine's condition be due to inadequate or incorrect use of her medication?
   b. What role does respiratory infection play in resistant asthma?
   c. What emotional factors operate in such cases?

2. What action would you take first?
   a. How would you assess the child's condition?
   b. Does chest radiology provide useful additional information in such cases?
   c. What value are respiratory function tests under these circumstances?

3. What therapy would you consider? What are the indications for each form of therapy?
   a. With what specific therapy would you begin, and why?

    b. What would be your second line of treatment if the first failed, and why?

    c. Under what circumstances would you consider hospital admission?

    d. If you send the patient home, what advice would you give the parents?

    e. What opportunity does this situation present for preventive care and health promotion?

    f. What follow up would you arrange?

W. E. Fabb, Melbourne

344   MISS S.G.   AGED 14   PENSIONER

1. What are the possible aetiological factors in this attack?
    a. What is the significance of the family situation?
    b. What is the significance of the time of the year?
    c. What would you expect to be the compliance of this girl with her current therapy?

2. What would be your short and long term management of this problem?
    a. What is the role of nebulized Ventolin?
    b. What is the value of Intal in an acute attack?
    c. Does the occurrence of this attack alter your long term management?

3. What is the significance of your examination findings?
    a. The lack of an obvious precipitating cause?
    b. The pallor?
    c. What effect does a chronic disease have on growth?
    d. In the presence of markedly decreased air entry, how accurate an assessment of lung function can you obtain with a stethoscope?

D. S. Pedler, Adelaide

345   MRS. F.   AGED 40   HOUSEWIFE

1. In contacts with patients, family doctors usually accord some kind of priority in grading their responses: why do they do this?
    a. What questions might the doctor ask Mr. F. to clarify the issue of degree or urgency?

2. What clinical phenomena constitute 'status asthmaticus'?
    a. If the doctor finds Mrs. F. in status, does the fact that she is already taking prednisolone by mouth influence management?

3. What might the doctor carry in his emergency bag to be ready to deal with this situation?
   a. How do doctors cope with the need to comply with security regulations and also ensure ready availability of potent drugs?

J. D. E. Knox, Dundee

JAMES P.   AGED 15   346

1. What would be the best way of assessing James' asthma?
   a. What are the common patterns of asthma in relation to triggering factors and time of day?
   b. Why can patients have quite severe asthma and yet produce normal peak expiratory flow rates in the middle of the morning?
   c. What place does a peak flow meter have in the assessment of asthma?

2. How might the doctor handle the apparent unwillingness to take the asthma seriously?
   a. What are the likely reasons for this attitude?
   b. What specific approaches in the consultation are likely to be productive or otherwise?

3. What drug therapy might be considered for this patient?
   a. What are the advantages and disadvantages of aerosols versus oral medication?

J. C. Hasler, Oxford

MICHELLE V.   AGED 16   SCHOOLGIRL   347

1. What are the factors critical to the clinical assessment of this patient?
   a. What information should be sought in taking the history?
   b. What information should be sought in the physical examination?
   c. What investigation should be performed in order to define the nature and severity of Michelle's disability?

2. What factors will influence the doctor's management plan?
   a. What is the value of skin tests for allergens?
   b. What tests can or should be performed in the consulting room to assess Michelle's response to bronchodilators?
   c. How might beta stimulator aerosols be used more effectively with this patient?
   d. What other drug therapies are likely to be beneficial and how is this best evaluated?

3. What are the important issues to be addressed in the education of this patient regarding long term management of her asthma?
    a. What special advice should be given concerning respiratory tract infection?
    b. What special advice should be given regarding the use of aerosols?
    c. How can the doctor and the patient ensure that continuity of medical care is guaranteed despite the problems of holidays, travel and communications?

W. L. Ogborne, Sydney

348   MRS. S.   AGED 70   PENSIONER

1. What are the pro's and con's of issuing prescriptions to patients without seeing them at the time of issue?
    a. What systems exist for regulating 'repeat prescriptions'?
    b. What are the basic features of a repeat prescription card, which many practices now use?

2. What is the role of antibiotics in 'secondary prevention', i.e. preventing exacerbations of chronic bronchitis?
    a. Would you comply with Mrs. S.'s request for the 'major breakthrough' penicillin?

3. Patients' needs are not synonymous with patients' demands. What factors govern the creation of patient expectations?
    a. If a doctor wishes to modify a patient's demands in the light of his professional assessment of the situation, what techniques are likely to achieve his objective?
    b. How would you cope with Mrs. S.'s demand?

J. D. E. Knox, Dundee

349   MR. C.C.E.   AGED 28   UNEMPLOYED

1. What determines someone's personality?
    a. Is personality purely inherited?
    b. Can low self esteem result from a physical disorder such as asthma? If so, how?
    c. Does personality often contribute to associations between unlikely diseases (such as asthma with urethritis)?
    d. What suggestions could be used to boost this patient's ego?

2. What constitutes patient compliance?
    a. Do GP's tend to think of compliance simply in terms of drug therapy?

b. What factors would have made this patient accept the use of fenoterol but not accept the use of beclomethasone and sodium cromoglycate?

c. Having been advised by a consultant to use both beclomethosone and sodium cromoglycate, how is the patient's compliance likely to be affected by the warning (printed in the GP's prescribing schedule) that the simultaneous use of beclomethasone and sodium cromoglycate is not recommended?

d. Have doctors any moral or ethical right to expect patients not to be promiscuous?

e. Have doctors any right to expect promiscuous patients to wear a condom?

f. Where alcohol abuse is controlled how much credit can the doctor claim in achieving compliance?

g. Where fenoterol abuse exists should compliance be achieved by refusing to prescribe the drug?

3. What prognostic factors are evident in this case?
   a. What are the prospects of changing a person's personality?
   b. Once an alcohol abuser, always an alcohol abuser?
   c. What is the relationship between compliance and prognosis in asthma?
   d. What is the likely outcome of a prescription supplied for amoxy-cillin 250 mg 8 hourly for a week?

D. Levet, Hobart

MR. H.D.   AGED 49   BUSINESS EXECUTIVE

350

1. What salient physical findings should be sought?
   a. Is the fact that the patient appears acutely ill of diagnostic significance?
   b. What diagnostic possibilities are entertained by finding dullness to percussion of the left base of the lung with bronchial breath sounds, both associated with increased vocal and tactile fremitus and rales in the left base?
   c. What positive diagnostic and prognostic considerations are suggested by the finding of generalized wheezing throughout both lungs with a prolonged expiratory phase?

2. What laboratory aids might be expected to offer positive diagnostic information?
   a. What is the significance of the blood culture revealing a Gram negative organism grown two days after plating?
   b. What is the significance of serum obtained on admission showing group B *Haemophilus influenzae* antigen on counter immunoelectrophoresis (CIE)? Is this helpful?

    c.   What are the differential diagnostic possibilities when the chest X-ray report reveals infiltration of the left lower lobe with some fluid in the left pleural cavity?

    d.   Does a Gram stain of the sputum help in determining immediate appropriate therapy?

3.   What are the most likely aetiological causes for secondary or post-influenzal pneumonia, more likely with underlying pulmonary disease such as asthma?

    a.   What changes are likely because of damage to the bronchial epithelium and transient impairment of normal pulmonary clearing mechanisms, such as cilia and mucus flow following influenza?

    b.   What factors make *Mycoplasma* infection unlikely as an aetiological agent in this patient?

    c.   What historical factors and diagnostic procedures would be helpful in ruling out pulmonary embolism in this case?

    d.   What further considerations are important, knowing that this patient has been on prednisone for five years as part of the therapy for asthma?

L. H. Amundson, Sioux Falls, SD, USA

351   MR. L.S.   AGED 62

1.   Does this patient suffer from bronchitis or asthma?

    a.   What investigations are available to help determine this?

    b.   Is a therapeutic trial of steroids justifiable even though reversible airways obstruction cannot be demonstrated?

2.   Discuss the management of late onset (intrinsic) asthma.

    a.   Could his occupation be relevant?

    b.   What drugs are available to combat bronchospasm: are these best delivered orally or by aerosol?

    c.   Discuss inhalation techniques and the various types of inhaler.

A. G. Strube, Crawley, UK

352   MRS. T.   AGED 23   BANK CLERK

1.   Why was the patient's illness initially refractory to treatment?

    a.   What is the medical management of bronchitis with bronchospasm?

    b.   Could allergy play a role in the response to treatment?

    c.   Could psychogenic factors play a role in the response to treatment?

    d.   What role does the severity of symptoms play in the response to treatment?

    e.   Is a change of antibiotic justified if there is an initial failure of response to treatment?

2.   How would you manage this patient further?

    a.   What role could the patient's smoking habits play in perpetuating her respiratory problems?

    b.   How can the GP help the patient to reduce her cigarette smoking while also giving attention to her emotional state?

    c.   To what extent, if any, should the GP give advice?

    d.   What attitude should the GP adopt if the patient continues smoking?

    e.   What is meant by non-judgmental acceptance?

    f.   Of what value is the peak flow meter in assessing the patient's respiratory status?

S. Levenstein, Cape Town

MR. L.B.   AGED 52   **353**

1.   How could the diagnosis have been made earlier?

    a.   Would earlier intervention have influenced the final outcome?

    b.   Could he have been treated at home?

    c.   Does the involvement of three different doctors make management less effective?

    d.   How can this be avoided?

2.   What is meant by the term 'congestion'?

    a.   Describe the signs in the lungs and heart which may occur in left ventricular failure.

    b.   How may this be distinguished from asthmatic bronchitis?

A. G. Strube, Crawley, UK

MR. G.   AGED 32   FARMER   **354**

1.   What further historical information is necessary to confirm the diagnosis?

    a.   What details of style of farming are important in this man's history?

    b.   What season of the year was this man likely to present in?

    c.   What characteristic of the climate is this problem related to?

2.   What further investigations would be helpful at this point in time? Even though a chest X-ray was done one month previously would a repeat chest X-ray be of benefit?

   a. Would a complete blood count and differential be helpful in confirming the diagnosis?
   b. Are there very specific blood tests that might be helpful in confirming this diagnosis in this situation?
   c. What X-ray findings are most likely with the history?

3. Why have previous efforts to treat this man failed?
   a. Why do antibiotics not help in this situation?
   b. What is the treatment of choice in this situation?
   c. How rapidly would you expect a response to the treatment of choice?

W. W. Rosser, Ottawa

355   MR. PETER Z.   AGED 57   STOREMAN

1. What investigations would assist in diagnosis?
   a. Are you worried by the sudden onset of pneumonia, with no previous respiratory history?
   b. Is iron deficiency anaemia a contributory cause to pneumonia?
   c. Is further investigation of the respiratory tract necessary?
   d. Are further investigations of the anaemia necessary?

2. If all your investigations regarding the cause of the anaemia were negative, how would you manage the patient in the future?
   a. If expense were a problem in repeated investigation what would your priority be over the next 6 months?

R. M. Meyer, Johannesburg

356   MRS. BETINA A. & MR. HARRY A.   AGES: BETINA 42, HARRY 44
BETINA: HOUSEWIFE   HARRY: PANEL BEATER

1. What are some common causes of accelerated biological ageing?
   a. Is the comparison of chronological age and biological age a significant diagnostic process?
   b. How often do visual 'clues' play a role in clinical decision making?
   c. Are medical graduates trained to think of industrial toxins as a cause of ill-health?
   d. What industrial toxins can cause or aggravate obstructive lung disease?

2. What diagnoses are you considering at this stage?
   a. What cues triggered off the thoughts leading to your diagnostic postulates?

    b.   What conditions can you think of that can be diagnosed by simple observation?

    c.   How often do you need special investigations to confirm diagnoses made by observation?

3.   Given that you have limited time available, how will you manage the consultation from this point onwards?

    a.   How do you manage a patient consultation where there is:
- a mixture of organic and psychological problems?
- more than one problem?

    b.   What is the significance of a spouse attending during a consultation with the other member of a marriage?

    c.   In your experience, how often would illness in a spouse produce this kind of domestic relationship?

    d.   What kind of illness in a spouse is commonly associated with this kind of husband–wife interaction?

M. W. Heffernan, Melbourne

MR. R.S.   AGED 38   TRUCK DRIVER   357

1.   What does the family physician suspect as the aetiology at the first visit?

    a.   What clinical signs and symptoms support this?

    b.   Do you think he suspects a bacterial or viral aetiology?

    c.   If viral, do you think he would/should prescribe antibiotics?

    d.   How often do physicians prescribe antibiotics for chest infections which are suspected to be viral in origin?

    e.   Why do they do this; do you agree?

    f.   From what disease entity was this man suffering?

2.   How commonly do patients suffer from occupational related diseases?

    a.   Are they usually, sometimes, or seldom recognized by family physicians?

    b.   Are physicians usually trained to recognize occupationally related diseases?

    c.   What resources are available to physicians with questions related to occupational health?

    d.   Do you believe pre-employment physicals are useful?

    e.   What is the role of an occupational hygienist?

3.   What are the issues – ethical, moral and legal, relating to this man's concerns about reporting his disease?

    a.   Is it the doctor's moral responsibility to protect this man's job, or the other employees who may be similarly exposed?

b. Does the physician have a legal responsibility to override his patient's concerns and report this hazard?
c. What are the ethical implications to the physician in view of the source of his information, his patient being reluctant to have it revealed?
d. How should employees be protected from health risks in the workplace?

C. A. Moore, Hamilton, Canada

358 MR. B.P.   AGED 18   FARM LABOURER

1. What additional information is required to reach a diagnosis?
   a. Would the taking of a complete family history be justified at this first urgent consultation?
   b. Should a traumatic cause be seriously considered?
   c. Is it important to know his state of health immediately prior to the football match?

2. What possible causes should be considered?
   a. What are the probabilities of this condition being skeletal in origin?
   b. Does the age of the patient exclude serious myocardial vascular disease?
   c. To establish early diagnosis in this case, which would be more important, the history, the examination, or any immediate investigations?

3. How should this patient be managed?
   a. Would an immediate ECG be likely to elucidate the problem?
   b. Should the patient be kept in the small hospital for observation or should he be transported to a larger base hospital?
   c. If there are ECG changes apparent suggesting myocardial vascular disease, what further investigations should be advised?
   d. How would you describe the prognosis to the patient?
   e. What preventive advice should be given?

T. D. Manthorpe, Port Lincoln, Australia

359 JOE SMITH   AGED 33   ELECTRICIAN

1. What are the possible causes of his chest pain?
   a. Could this be cardiac ischaemia?
   b. What features suggest pulmonary chest pain?
   c. What other possible causes of this pain are there?

2. What investigations are indicated?

    a.   What information would an ECG give you?
    b.   How would X-rays help you?
    c.   Would any blood tests contribute anything?
    d.   Which tests are 'cost effective' on a Sunday afternoon?

3. What is this patient's main problem?
    a.   What is a workaholic?
    b.   Is this his only problem?
    c.   How are others affected?

4. How would you manage this problem?
    a.   How would specialist referral help?
    b.   How might changes in life style be achieved?
    c.   In what way should his wife and family be involved?
    d.   What opportunities are there for health promotion?

R. P. Strasser, Melbourne

MR. M.T.   AGED 31   CLERK   360

1. What diagnostic possibilities would you consider whilst driving to the patient's home?
    a.   Which of these conditions is life-threatening?
    b.   What action would you take?
    c.   What is the place of a mobile resuscitation unit (coronary ambulance) in the management of acute chest pain outside of the hospital?

2. Why might he be hyperventilating?
    a.   What are the effects of hyperventilation?
    b.   Why should he have incipient tetany?
    c.   How would you demonstrate this?
    d.   How would you manage the situation?

3. What factors tend to make relatives particularly anxious about a patient's condition?
    a.   How would you explore the underlying problems in this case?
    b.   How can you be sure that you are 'reassuring' the patient and family rather than yourself?

E. C. Gambrill, Crawley, UK

JOHN ROBERTS   AGED 48   COMPANY MANAGER   361

1. What is the problem in this case?
    a.   Despite the normal ECG, could this be cardiac ischaemia?
    b.   Describe the features of an acute anxiety attack?
    c.   What is 'cardiac neurosis'?

2. Are any further investigations indicated?
   a. How would any further tests help you?
   b. Would further investigations help the patient?
   c. Would specialist referral help at this stage?

3. How would you manage this problem?
   a. What medications are indicated?
   b. Will the problem be resolved with just one consultation?
   c. Who else might you involve in managing this case?
   d. What opportunity does this event present for health promotion and preventive care?

R. P. Strasser, Melbourne

362 MRS. S.S.   AGED 45   CLERICAL WORKER

1. What is your differential diagnosis for the emergency consultation?
   a. What are the advantages and disadvantages of hospital admission for myocardial infarction in patients without shock or cardiac arrhythmia?
   b. What do you know about costochrondrosis and its management?
   c. What are the possible clinical findings when a patient complains of palpitations?

2. What is your problem list for Mrs. S.S.?
   a. What do you know about associations between hysterectomy and emotional state?
   b. What are your criteria for the diagnosis of spastic colon?
   c. What do you understand by the term 'random association' and give clinical examples of it?

3. What are your criteria for giving anti-depressant medication?
   a. What are the common stages of bereavement experience and their duration?
   b. Is anti-depressant medication ever justified for recently bereaved people?
   c. What are the side-effects of the commonly used anti-depressants? Do these side-effects alter with dosage or duration of treatment?

P. Freeling, London

363 MR. M.F.   AGED 59   RETIRED CLERK

1. What are the aetiological factors in this man's myocardial infarction?
   a. What are the risk factors for myocardial infarction?

    b.   What is the role of the beta-blocker in the prevention/diminution of the size of a myocardial infarct?

2.   What is your management of this situation?
    a.   How would you provide pain relief to this man?
    b.   Does an anti-arrhythmic have a place in this situation?
    c.   How do you organize the transfer of this man to hospital (if that is your plan of management)?
    d.   What would you include in your explanation to this man's wife?

D. S. Pedler, Adelaide

HAROLD O'HALLORAN   AGED 85   PENSIONER   **364**

1.   How do you explain the episode of agitation and confusion three years ago?
    a.   Could pneumonia alone cause such an episode?
    b.   How does senile dementia affect people?
    c.   Might hospital admission itself have contributed?
    d.   What is 'acute brain syndrome'?

2.   Is hospital admission indicated this time?
    a.   Would you (cardiac) monitor this patient?
    b.   What are the advantages of hospital treatment?
    c.   What disadvantage might there be with hospital treatment?

3.   Could you manage this patient at home?
    a.   Is family support sufficient to manage his medications and recognize any sudden change in his condition?
    b.   How could the district nurse help?
    c.   With frequent home visits by you, how would his medical care differ at home from that in hospital?
    d.   Who else in the community might you involve?

R. P. Strasser, Melbourne

MR. M.S.   AGED 42   **365**

1.   What are the diagnostic possibilities you would consider?
    a.   How can you exclude the more serious causes?

2.   What other information would you wish to obtain to arrive at a more precise diagnosis?
    a.   What other factors in the history would you enquire about?
    b.   What investigations, if any, would you perform?
    c.   What physical signs would you look for?

3. How do you exclude a diagnosis of ischaemic disease in a young man?
   a. What features in the history enable you to arrive at a diagnosis?
   b. What physical signs would support such a diagnosis?
   c. What investigations can you perform? What are the indications and risks?
   d. What else can help you to confirm a diagnosis of angina? Would a trial of a drug for angina help?

4. In a patient with proven ischaemic heart disease, when do you refer him to a consultant?
   a. What are the indications for surgery in ischaemic heart disease?

H. C. Watts, Perth, Australia

366 MR. K.W. AGED 38 BUSINESSMAN

1. What is the significance of his chest pain?
   a. Is there anything else you should do to elicit the cause?
   b. If it is not cardiac in origin what might it be?
   c. How can the physician take advantage of his present symptoms to his benefit?

2. What are the most important risk factors in cardiovascular disease?
   a. Should you treat his blood pressure?
   b. Does lowering the BP improve the prognosis in cardiovascular disease?
   c. What should you do about his hypercholesterolaemia?
   d. What should you do about his smoking and alcohol intake?

3. What should you do about his other risk factors?
   a. What are the effects of stress on cardiovascular disease?
   b. What are the signs of stress?
   c. Would a change of lifestyle alter this man's chances of developing cardiovascular disease?

W. F. Glastonbury, Adelaide

367 MR. L.P. AGED 54 CLERGYMAN

1. How do you decide if chest pain is serious?
   a. Is the history or physical examination more important?
   b. Does a normal physical examination exclude serious disease?
   c. Is it safe to make a diagnosis of benign chest wall pain by exclusion only?

2. What diagnostic tests help?
   a. Is the ECG always abnormal?
   b. Does a chest X-ray often give helpful information?
   c. What is the timing of cardiac enzyme changes?
   d. What about a therapeutic trial of nitroglycerine?
   e. What other tests do you order if the cardiac investigation is negative?
   f. When would you perform an exercise ECG?

3. What counselling do you give to the patient with coronary artery disease and to his family?
   a. What is the appropriate timing of such advice?
   b. Do you always say the same thing to the patient and to the family?
   c. How important is diet?
   d. How do you prescribe an exercise program?
   e. How soon can a 'heart' patient resume sexual activity?
   f. What psychological problems may you encounter after the patient returns home?
   g. How do you decide when the patient can resume work?

R. L. Perkin, Toronto

MRS. C.D.   AGED 55   HOUSEWIFE   368

1. What is the cause of the pain?
   a. What other physical sign might develop in the next 48 hours to help clarify the diagnosis?
   b. Does the diagnosis depend on this sign?
   c. If this sign develops, will it be possible to make an exact diagnosis?

2. What place have corticosteroids in the treatment of this patient?
   a. Will corticosteroids ease the pain?
   b. Will corticosteroids interfere with the patient's immune response in relation to the malignancy or the cause of the pain?
   c. How often should this patient be reviewed?

3. How much of this patient's illness has been due to cigarette smoking?
   a. In what way would the course of her illnesses be altered by the immediate cessation of smoking?
   b. Would reduction but not cessation of smoking be beneficial?
   c. How can a general practitioner assist a person who wants to stop smoking?

B. H. Connor, Armidale, Australia

369   MR. A.W.   AGED 31   CLERK

1. How would you manage his clinical problem?
   a. How would you treat him medically?
   b. What are the risks in coronary arteriography?
   c. What are the indications for a coronary bypass operation?

2. How do you prevent the patient from becoming a cardiac invalid?
   a. How would you advise him regarding exercise and sexual relations?
   b. What is his prognosis?

3. How would his problem affect his family and his community?
   a. What is your approach in informing his wife of his condition?
   b. What are the community resources available for such a cardiac patient in your community?

F. E. H. Tan, Kuala Lumpur

370   WALTER M.   AGED 45   STOREMAN

1. What diagnostic suspicions should these findings arouse in the doctor's mind?
   a. What special information could the radiologist be expected to provide in his report on the fractured ribs?
   b. What particular physical findings should be sought by the doctor in the light of the patient's presentation?
   c. What tests should the doctor now select in order to make the diagnosis?

2. What is the most likely cause of Walter M.'s rib fracture?
   a. Apart from X-raying the ribs what other X-ray could be ordered that would clinch the diagnosis?
   b. What would be the significance of a raised blood urea?
   c. What would be the value of a protein electrophoretogram (EPG)?
   d. Would an EPG be of diagnostic value on any other body fluids?
   e. What, if any, diagnostic findings would the pathologist expect from bone marrow biopsy?

3. What matters should the family doctor discuss with the patient and his family?
   a. Who should be present at these discussions?
   b. How should the doctor respond if asked the question – 'Is it cancer?'
   c. How should the doctor respond if asked the question – 'Am I going to die?'

W. L. Ogborne, Sydney

MR. T.S.   AGED 45   BUSINESS EXECUTIVE   **371**

1. What is your differential diagnosis?
   a. What are the possible presenting features of carcinoma of the bronchus?
   b. What are your criteria for the diagnosis of chronic bronchitis?
   c. What features of a patient's history might lead you to suspect alcohol abuse?
   d. What disorders might present with bruising?

2. Which one diagnosis would most logically explain all the features of this patient's history and examination?
   a. What blood tests would help to substantiate a diagnosis of chronic alcohol abuse?
   b. Describe the progression of the alcoholic from social drinking to chronic alcohol dependence.
   c. What methods and agencies are available to help the chronic alcoholic?
   d. What are the features of the alcohol withdrawal syndrome?

3. To what aspects of the history and examination would you pay particular attention in carrying out a routine check-up on a 45 year old man?
   a. With what conditions is cigarette smoking associated?
   b. How would you advise a patient who wished to give up smoking?
   c. Devise an exercise plan for a middle-aged man who has led a sedentary life for the past ten years.
   d. What measures would you take if you found a 45 year old man to have a BP of 160/105?

T. A. I. Bouchier Hayes, Camberley, UK

MISS P.C.   AGED 25   OFFICE CLEANER   **372**

1. What are the likely diagnoses here?
   a. Is the infection likely to be viral or bacterial?

2. What investigations would you undertake?
   a. What would you expect on chest X-ray?
   b. What would you expect on blood film examination?

3. Does a negative chest X-ray alter your diagnosis?

4. What is the significance of her statement that her father died from lung cancer?

    a.   How would you help her anxiety in relation to her present illness?

    b.   How would you help her anxiety in relation to her father's death from lung cancer?

D. U. Shepherd, Melbourne

373   MRS. J.P.   AGED 51   HOUSEWIFE

1. What is the pathogen?
    a.   How many types of *Pneumococcus* are identified?
    b.   How are they distinguished from each other?
    c.   What is the quickest method of making the diagnosis?
    d.   What will the chest X-ray show at the beginning, and later on?
    e.   What pre-existing conditions are often present in patients with pneumococcal infection?

2. How would you treat the patient?
    a.   What dose of penicillin is appropriate?
    b.   What alternative drugs can you use if the patient is allergic to penicillin?
    c.   How long would you treat the patient?
    d.   Is type specific pneumococcal antiserum ever used? If so, in what circumstances?

3. What preventive measures would you advise for the future?
    a.   Is it important for the patient to stop smoking?
    b.   Does one bout of pneumococcal pneumonia confer lifelong immunity?
    c.   Would you give the patient pneumococcal vaccine (Pneumovax)?
    d.   How often does the patient need booster doses of Pneumovax?

R. L. Perkin, Toronto

374   MR. B.F.   AGED 44   PLANT WORKER

1. What are the essential problems and their differential diagnosis?
    a.   Chest pain?
    b.   Dyspnoea?
    c.   Hypertension?
    d.   Past history of thrombophlebitis?

2. What are the possible risk factors to be considered in this case?
    a.   Would a history of moderate smoking be significant?
    b.   What specific family history should be obtained?

c. Would a history of previous response to anti-hypertensive medication have any bearing on the differential diagnosis of hypertension?

d. Would it be important to obtain a history of any trauma, immobilization or surgery, as well as the work habits of this plant worker?

e. What drug related complications might be expected during the therapy of this patient?

    a. What are the main complications of heparin and coumarin?

    b. What side effects might be observed from the use of diuretics and digitalis?

    c. What complications might be expected from the diagnostic use of lymphangiography, venography, and Doppler ultrasound?

f. What chronic changes can occur in the leg from repeated thrombophlebitis?

g. How might his diagnosis and therapy influence his job description upon return to work?

L. H. Amundson, Sioux Falls, SD, USA

MR. K.   AGED 45   BANK CLERK   375

1. What was the first GP's diagnosis?

    a. How can one distinguish between chest pain of cardiac and non-cardiac origin?

    b. What are the commoner non-cardiac causes of chest pain in general practice?

    c. To what extent may the patient's previous cardiovascular status have influenced the GP's initial assessment?

2. Why was the patient so anxious at the consultation with the 'locum' GP?

    a. Was the effect of the first GP's 'reassurance' cancelled out by the 'double-message' of being told to go to bed for 3 days?

    b. How effective is reassurance in allaying patients' anxieties?

    c. To what extent may the patient's anxiety have been due to his regular GP having gone on leave at that time?

    d. To what extent may the patient's anxiety have been unrelated to his present symptoms?

3. Why was the patient relieved after the consultation with the 'locum' GP?

    a. To what extent is the use of an ECG to reassure a patient justified?

    b. Was the patient reassured by being told he could return to work the next day?

   c.   Was the GP justified in telling the patient he could return to work the next day?

   d.   Is the patient likely to remain 'reassured' for long?

   e.   Is the patient likely to develop chest pain again?

   f.   If the patient does develop chest pain and/or anxiety symptoms again, how should the GP manage the situation?

S. Levenstein, Cape Town

376   MR. C.H.   AGED 57   LABOURER

1.   What syndrome does Mr. H.'s story illustrate?

   a.   What are the characteristics of angina?

   b.   What investigations would you undertake if you suspected ischaemic heart disease? How would you advise a patient who displays cardiac neurosis?

   d.   Design a protocol for the differential diagnosis of chest pain.

2.   What are the reasons for frequent office attendance by a patient with no evidence of physical disease?

   a.   What do you understand by the concept of 'the doctor as treatment'?

   b.   What strategies might you use to end a consultation when useful communication has finished?

   c.   What do you feel about the doctor's role as counsellor?

   d.   Of what significance is physical contact between doctor and patient?

3.   What resources are available for the health education of patients?

   a.   How can the various members of the primary care team contribute towards health education in the practice?

   b.   What problems may be caused by media coverage of medical topics?

   c.   What subjects would you cover if asked to speak to a lay audience on the topic of ischaemic heart disease?

T. A. I. Bouchier Hayes, Camberley, UK

377   MRS. S.H.   AGED 40   HOUSEWIFE/SOCIAL WORKER

1.   What investigations might be indicated at this most recent visit?

   a.   Is it possible that repeated investigations might be 'reinforcing the illness' in the mind of the patient?

   b.   What new historical or objective data might cause you to reinvestigate the symptoms?

2. What referral(s) might be indicated at this most recent visit?
   a. Is it possible that repeated referrals might be 'reinforcing the illness' in the mind of the patient?
   b. What new historical or objective data might cause you to again refer this patient to a consultant physician?
   c. Is it likely that referral to a psychiatrist would be useful?

3. What is the most likely cause of this patient's symptoms?
   a. What are some of the clinical features of angina pectoris?
   b. What are some of the clinical features of hyperventilation related to anxiety?
   c. What are some of the clinical features of cardiac neurosis?

G. G. Beazley, Winnipeg

MR. J.P.   AGED 53   EXECUTIVE   378

1. What would be your strategies for dealing with such an obviously complex problem in a busy consulting session?
   a. Given plenty of time how would you proceed from the initial history above?

2. How can you distinguish between the various causes of retrosternal and epigastric pain?
   a. What characteristics of history do you recognize?
   b. What physical signs may help in your differential diagnosis?
   c. What tests may help?

3. What would you do if you're not sure of the diagnosis even if you have sought another opinion?

F. Mansfield, Perth, Australia

LES B.   AGED 32   SALESMAN   379

1. What is the single most likely process by which Les B.'s symptoms will be diagnosed?
   a. What fundamentals of history taking must be observed if the diagnostic clues are to be recognized?
   b. What anatomical considerations should govern the clinician's approach to chest pain around the left breast?
   c. What simple diagnostic manoeuvres can be employed in the consulting room in order to identify the cause of Les B.'s chest pain?

2. Why have so many doctors failed to diagnose the cause of Les B.'s chest pain?
    a. What factors inherent in the medical consultation hinder the diagnostic process?
    b. How does the doctor's perception of his professional role influence the diagnostic process?

3. During physical examination the spinous processes of T3 and T4 are very tender when firm pressure is applied with the thumb. What relationship, if any, does this finding have to Les B.'s chest pain?
    a. Is the tenderness to pressure on the spinous processes T3 and T4 compatible with any elements of Les B.'s history?
    b. What simple procedure can be performed in the consulting room to relieve Les B. of his chest pain?
    c. How is this procedure performed?
    d. What advice should be given to Les B. regarding recurrence of his chest pain?
    e. What factors will determine whether or not such recurrences will occur?

W. L. Ogborne, Sydney

380   DESMOND K.   AGED 58   FACTORY MANAGER

1. What are the characteristics of the pain of angina pectoris?
    a. What instructions and explanation should be given at the time the glyceryl trinitrate was prescribed?
    b. What other drug therapy might have been given in this case?
    c. What other causes of retrosternal pain must be considered in the differential diagnosis?
    d. What general advice should this patient have been given at the initial consultation?

2. What action should the general practitioner take in relation to the patient's complaints at the most recent consultation?
    a. What are the possible advantages and disadvantages of a conservative approach?
    b. How important is the general practitioner in improving the statistics dealing with morbidity and mortality from common diseases?
    c. What further treatments may be available to this patient, what success has been achieved, and what are the social and economic implications of making these treatments increasingly available?

J. G. P. Ryan, Brisbane

MR. M.N.　　AGED 41　　FORK HOIST DRIVER

381

1. How should Dr. Y. advise the patient?
   a. What are his responsibilities for making sure that the patient is handed back to his family doctor?
   b. How does he make it clear that it is Dr. Y.'s duty to inform the locum tenens of his interest in the patient's ability to work and any proposed treatment which may affect his working performance?

2. How should Dr. Y. advise the employer?
   a. What is the nature of the relationship between an industrial medical officer and the company for whom he works?
   b. Is there any change in the nature of the doctor's duty towards the patient?
   c. If this patient refuses to allow the doctor to discuss his medical condition with officials of the firm, what does the doctor do next?

3. What should Dr. Y. do with regard to the patient's own doctor's locum?
   a. What do you know about established rules for ethical practice of medicine by industrial medical officers?

P. L. Gibson, Auckland

THOMAS D.　　AGED 52　　COMPANY EXECUTIVE

382

1. How would you manage the continuing care of his angina and transient ischaemic attacks?
   a. What drugs are useful in these conditions?
   b. What should the patient be told about his prognosis?

2. How would you react to the decision preventing him from driving a car?
   a. What kind of feelings might it arouse in the patient?
   b. What role should the doctor adopt?

3. What responsibility does the general practitioner have in the prevention of arterial disease?
   a. What are the main predisposing factors for ischaemic heart disease and stroke?
   b. Can the doctor influence any of these factors?
   c. Should he attempt to do so?
   d. What would be the implications in terms of time and resources?

J. C. Hasler, Oxford

383   MR. W.R.   AGED 65

1. Are coronary heart disease and peripheral vascular disease related?
   a. What are the predisposing factors?
   b. What actual pathological features are involved?
   c. Why does propranolol help angina but aggravate peripheral disease?
   d. Why does glyceryl trinitrate help angina but not peripheral disease?

2. What is the basis for this patient's hypertension?
   a. If a patient has rigid blood vessels and an ischaemic myocardium, what treatment is rational for the blood pressure?
   b. What are the fundamental effects of beta-blocking drugs in hypertension?
   c. What is the rationale for trying a cardio-selective beta-blocking agent in this case?
   d. How does prazosin work in hypertension? Is it more suitable than beta-blockers?

3. Is it rational to treat this patient's blood pressure?
   a. What is the risk of stroke if blood pressure is treated or untreated?
   b. How does one explain to the patient that one is treating the blood pressure and not the ischaemic heart disease. Does this distinction matter?

A. L. A. Reid, Newcastle, Australia

384   MRS. P.M.   AGED 65   HOUSEWIFE

1. What are possible causes of her problem?
   a. Is there likely to be a significant functional element?
   b. Can ischaemic heart disease be confused with gastrointestinal problems?
   c. Could anaemia be responsible for her symptoms?
   d. Could incipient cardiac failure be responsible for her symptoms?

2. What are the next steps in the management of this patient?
   a. What blood tests should be ordered?
   b. If she had iron deficiency anaemia what would be the likely cause?
   c. To whom should she be referred?

3. What principles in overall management are embodied in the management of this patient?
   a. Should general practitioners care for members of their own family?

b. What common illnesses can act as 'masquerades' in day to day medical problems?

c. How can one clinically separate symptoms caused by ischaemic heart disease and gastro-intestinal disease?

d. Does familiarity with problems lead to 'missed' diagnosis?

e. Do positive investigatory findings serve as a 'smoke screen' for other unrelated co-existing problems?

f. Do relatives of the medical profession receive inappropriate management – either under or over investigation/treatment?

g. Should the patient be counselled that she is unlikely to harbour malignant disease?

J. E. Murtagh, Melbourne

MR. A.P.   AGED 27   DEPARTMENT STORE SUPERVISOR   385

1. What further information would you elicit in relation to food?
   a. What types of food ease the pain?
   b. What medication helps?
   c. What food precipitates or aggravates the pain?
   d. Are meals regular and adequate?

2. What further information would you elicit in relation to habits?
   a. Does Mr. A.P. smoke cigarettes?
   b. Does he drink alcohol?
   c. Does posture precipitate the pain?
   d. Is any stress involved in his work?

3. What family history would be of help?
   a. Is there a family history of gall bladder problems, peptic ulcer or other pancreatic, gastro-intestinal and/or liver disease?

4. What investigations are indicated in this patient?
   a. Is barium meal and/or gastroscopy required?
   b. Is a cholecystogram also indicated?

5. What advice would you give to this patient?
   a. In relation to food and habits?
   b. Medication?

6. Is surgery preferable to medical management in this case?

D. U. Shepherd, Melbourne

MR. A.H.   AGED 55   386

1. Could these long-standing symptoms of 'indigestion' have been due to cardiac pain?

    a. Discuss the differential diagnosis of the pain of reflux oesophagitis from cardiac pain.

    b. How would you have modified management of this patient if you had considered the possibility of cardiac pain?

A. G. Strube, Crawley, UK

387   MR. A.R.   AGED 22   UNEMPLOYED LABOURER

1. What are the possible sources of Mr. A.R.'s indigestion?
    a. Do you use any classification of drinking habits?
    b. Do you have any explanations in psychological and social terms of the motivations of people to self-abuse with drink or drugs?
    c. What objective criteria might there be to determine whether or not Mr. A.R. self-abuses with drugs and/or drink?

2. What is your approach to the management of asthma in young people?
    a. How would you set up a recall system in your practice to check on the control of asthma?
    b. What psychological defence mechanisms may be reflected in a young person's refusal to have their asthma monitored?

3. What is your response to the information that a patient has a criminal record?
    a. Is deviance an illness?
    b. What problems would exist for you if the police called you to give evidence in court concerning Mr. A.R.'s health record?
    c. Is crime a symptom of illness?

P. Freeling, London

388   TONY C.P.W.   AGED 15   HIGH SCHOOL STUDENT

1. What is the treatment of peptic ulcer?
    a. What are the indications for surgery?
    b. What type of surgery is being contemplated?
    c. What pathological and psychological effects will surgery have on a 15 year old boy?

2. Why is Tony suffering from this condition?
    a. Why has medical treatment failed?
    b. What factors may be involved in the aetiology?

3. What is child abuse?
    a. Are there such things as mental abuse or social abuse?

b. Are there similar cultural and social pressures in your society which lead to serious psychosomatic illnesses among school children?

N. C. L. Yuen, Hong Kong

MRS. M.   AGED 63   WIDOW

389

1. How much can a doctor rely on previous experience and pattern of behaviour in a patient?
   a. How does one decide which new or old symptoms can be ignored?
   b. Can symptomatic treatment ever be justified ethically?
   c. Can one rely on response to symptomatic treatment as an index of correct management?
   d. Is symptomatic treatment a justifiable diagnostic procedure?

2. Why is this woman a kleptomaniac?
   a. Is it due to the drug therapy?
   b. Is it due to wrong therapy?
   c. Is it reasonable to accept the view that inadequate coping mechanisms which produce anti-social behaviour must be tolerated by the community?
   d. Why does she reject help from the family and social agencies?

3. Should this patient's medical problem be given priority over her psychiatric condition?
   a. Would surgery ever be a real option?
   b. If home treatment for the ulcer is agreed between patient and doctor, what medical and social agencies should the doctor insist be involved?
   c. With the risk that invasive investigation e.g. gastroscopy could produce a further episode of kleptomania, is it justifiable to discuss this investigation?

P. F. Gill, Hobart

MR. G.P.   AGED 29   SCHOOLTEACHER

390

1. How significant are the negative physical findings?
   a. Could he have an ulcer?
   b. If not, what is the cause of his pain?
   c. How extensively should you investigate this man's pain?

2. What role could tension play in producing his pain?
   a. Is there a place for tranquillizers in the treatment of his pain?
   b. How do you get him to recognize the cause of his pain?
   c. What can you do to relieve his symptoms?

3. What does the future hold for him with his current alcohol and cigarette consumption?
    a. What alcohol intake would you consider normal for his age?
    b. Is he an alcoholic? How do you define alcoholism?
    c. In the absence of a family history of cardiovascular disease, what level of risk exists in this man?

4. Where do you begin with counselling this man?
    a. Bearing in mind ethics regarding secrecy, should you discuss the situation with his wife at this time?
    b. What can she do to help?
    c. Should he consider a change of occupation?

W. F. Glastonbury, Adelaide

391 THE D. FAMILY

1. What are the most likely causes of B.'s abdominal pain?
    a. What is the evidence to support these possibilities?
    b. Which is the most likely?
    c. Were further examinations or tests indicated at the initial visit?
    d. If not, why not?
    e. Should she have been reviewed later?

2. How should the general practitioner manage inconsiderate patients?
    a. Are doctors justified in classifying some patients as inconsiderate?
    b. What are the dangers, if any, in making this judgement?
    c. What is meant by 'availability' of the general practitioner to his patients?
    d. Would he have been justified in deferring the visit to B. and await the outcome of advice of symptomatic treatment given over the phone?
    e. How could you modify this family's help-seeking behaviour?

3. What are the possible reasons for Mr. D.'s request for medical advice for 'hayfever and sinusitis'?
    a. Should the general practitioner have taken the opportunity to pursue this at the time of Mr. D.'s proffered symptoms?
    b. What, if any, is the role of the 'family' in either or both of these episodes of illness?

D. A. Game, Adelaide

392 MARY L.   AGED 11

1. What do you consider the significance of the pains having been present for 2 years?

   a. What is the usual time sequence in appendicitis?

   b. Differentiate between the signs and symptoms of appendicitis and appendicular colic?

   c. What is the periodic syndrome?

2. What pressures face the mother?

   a. What further information would you like about Mary's family?

3. What examination and investigation would you perform?

4. What is your management of abdominal pain in children which seems almost certainly 'benign'?

   a. In this instance would you consider any of the following: *Giardia lamblia*, peptic ulcer, Meckel's diverticulum, abdominal migraine, urinary tract infection, irritable colon, sore throat?

F. Mansfield, Perth, Australia

MRS. S.T.   AGED 30   HOUSEWIFE   393

1. What things are in your mind before you proceed to examination and investigation?

   a. What are the social factors in modern life which make alcohol and tobacco abuse such attractive activities?

2. If examination was to reveal only a slightly elevated blood pressure (135/90), how would you describe your assessment to the patient?

   a. Should mild hypertension be treated by weight loss alone initially or should drug treatment be instituted also?

3. How would you reply to the question: 'I haven't got cancer, have I, doctor?'

   a. What do you know of the incidence of carcinoma of the lung in a patient of this age?

   b. What do you know about the incidence of gastrointestinal malignancy in such a patient?

P. L. Gibson, Auckland

MRS. P.S.   AGED 43   394

1. What do you say to this woman when she has recovered from the anaesthetic?

   a. Would earlier, more extensive investigation or better record keeping have altered the outcome?

   b. Are there any known predisposing factors you might consider?

   c. What is the natural history of reticulum cell sarcoma?

2. What happens next?
   a. What are the common side effects of radiotherapy, chemotherapy, immunotherapy?
   b. What will be your role as her family doctor in her ongoing treatment?
   c. Are there family factors to consider?
   d. Can she return to work?

3. How do you respond to questions about the prognosis?
   a. Do you differ the presentation of information given to (i) the patient, (ii) her husband, (iii) her children, (iv) her parents, (v) her lawyer who threatens a malpractice suit based on failure to diagnose in time.
   b. Do high achievers pose any special problems?

P. R. Grantham, Vancouver

395 CHERYL C.   AGED 10

1. What are the most likely diagnoses you would consider?
   a. Upper respiratory infection?
   b. Urinary tract infection?
   c. Appendicitis?
   d. Mesenteric adenitis?

2. How will the history you take influence your thoughts?
   a. Nature of pain?
   b. Frequency and distribution?
   c. Associated symptoms?

3. What examination will you perform?
   a. ENT?
   b. Respiratory system?
   c. Abdomen?
   d. Urine?
   e. Will you perform a rectal examination?

4. What will your advice be if the examination is negative apart from some general abdominal tenderness?
   a. What investigations, if any?
   b. What discussion with the mother in relation to possible outcomes?
   c. What follow-up will you arrange?

J. R. Marshall, Adelaide

MR. J. McN.   AGED 65

1. What might have alerted the doctor to the seriousness of the illness?
   a. What test would have lead to the correct diagnosis?
   b. How much emphasis can one place on altered behaviour for an individual patient?
   c. How can one tell when a patient is not complaining enough?

2. How could delayed care have been avoided?
   a. How can one select those patients who should be investigated, without over-investigating those with a similar history during an epidemic.
   b. How can one guard against wrong diagnosis because of epidemic similarity?
   c. How can more effective communication between partners be achieved?
   d. How can one avoid having patients who do not observe instructions given?

G. M. Dick, Hobart

MRS. S.   AGED 58   HOUSEWIFE

1. What diagnosis was made?
   a. How significant is the history in diagnosing appendicitis?
   b. Was the diagnosis justified in these circumstances?
   c. Were further investigations or referral indicated?
   d. If the diagnosis is made is there justification in deferring operative treatment in a patient aged 55?
   e. What effect does age make in the assessment of the condition and the subsequent treatment?

2. Was the general practitioner justified in performing the operation?
   a. Should he have planned the operation in the first instance?
   b. Should he have removed an appendix which was not acutely inflamed?
   c. What was the significance of the histo-pathological report of the appendix?
   d. Is there any justification in letting social conditions influence what should be a scientifically based decision?

D. A. Game, Adelaide

JOANNE W.   AGED 11

1. Is it advisable to seek another opinion at this time?
   a. What is the most likely diagnosis?

    b.   What are the chances of this being appendicitis?

    c.   How significant is the normal throat and cervical glands?

    d.   Can you be sure of the diagnosis?

2.   How significant was the consultation 4 days ago?
    a.   Has this any bearing on her present abdominal pain?
    b.   Do these relate to Mrs. W.'s impending absence?
    c.   In what other ways can this condition present in children?

3.   What is the management of this situation?
    a.   Do you hospitalize Joanne?
    b.   What do you expect to find when you visit her again in two hours?
    c.   How do you explain these abdominal pains to Joanne and to her mother?
    d.   How can you help Mrs. W. to cope with this situation?

W. F. Glastonbury, Adelaide

399   MISS D.W.   AGED 12   SCHOOLGIRL

1.   What would be your immediate management of this problem?
    a.   Is there an urgent necessity to arrive at a specific diagnosis with this problem?
    b.   What are the chances of the cause of the abdominal pain being functional?
    c.   Would you treat the patient at home or would you admit her to the small village hospital?

2.   What additional information should be sought?
    a.   What other specific information would you obtain from her history?
    b.   Who else may help in elucidating the problem?
    c.   What simple clinical tests would you perform within the first 24 hours?

3.   How would you undertake the long term management of this problem in order to prevent further attacks?
    a.   If no organic condition is found, what preventive advice can be given to the patient?
    b.   How can other members of the family help in the management of this problem?
    c.   Is medication indicated or are there alternative methods of treatment?

T. D. Manthorpe, Port Lincoln, Australia

MISS B.S.   AGED 3

400

1. What is your diagnosis?
   a. How would you convey your thoughts to her parents?
   b. Would you expect dysuria in a urinary tract infection in this age group?

2. What investigations would you arrange?
   a. Is microscopy of urine a useful and necessary side-room skill?
   b. What value is there in a white cell count in such a situation?
   c. At what stage would you ask for a chest X-ray?

R. W. Roberts, Ravensthorpe, Australia

JENNIFER E.   AGED 8   SCHOOLGIRL

401

1. What diagnostic hypotheses would you entertain?
   a. What features in this case would suggest urinary tract infection?
   b. What features would make a diagnosis of appendicitis unlikely?
   c. What other diagnoses are possible?

2. How would you assess this patient?
   a. What further history and physical examination would you carry out?
   b. What investigations would you consider essential?
   c. What role does time play in the diagnosis of abdominal pain?

3. What follow up might be required?
   a. If urinary tract infection was established by culture, what further investigations would be needed?
   b. What advice would you give the mother about the immediate management of the urinary tract infection?
   c. If no anatomical abnormality was demonstrated by further investigation, what advice would you give mother about preventing recurrences?

W. E. Fabb, Melbourne

MR. E.   AGED 38   BANK CLERK

402

1. What conditions should be considered in the differential diagnosis?
   a. Does the absence of waxing and waning of intensity of pain rule out the diagnosis of renal or gall bladder colic?

2. What should be done to help Mr. E?
   a. If a diagnosis of acute renal colic is considered most probable, should he be admitted to hospital as an emergency?

    b.   In the absence of definitive evidence of a specific pathology, what should the general practitioner do to ease Mr. E's intense pain?

    c.   What potent analgesics are carried by family doctors?

    d.   If emergency hospital admission is indicated, what considerations influence the choice of hospital, department or ward by the family doctor?

    e.   How is emergency admission arranged in your district?

J. D. E. Knox, Dundee

403   MRS. J.S.   AGED 54   HOUSEWIFE

1.   What is the most likely cause of Mrs. S.'s abdominal pain?

    a.   Are any investigations necessary to reach a diagnosis?

    b.   If so, what investigations would you perform?

    c.   How do you convince Mrs. S. that you are correct in your diagnosis?

2.   How would you manage this problem?

    a.   How do you approach the subject of psychosomatic disease?

    b.   How do you manage the influence of the family problems on Mrs. S.?

3.   What will be the most likely course of Mrs. S.'s condition?

    a.   Apart from abdominal pain, how else may this condition present?

    b.   How successful is your treatment likely to be in modifying the course?

    c.   What is the place of antispasmodics and antacids?

    d.   Is there a place for tranquillizers?

W. F. Glastonbury, Adelaide

404   MRS. Q.   AGED 35   HOUSEWIFE

1.   What is your differential diagnosis?

    a.   What anatomical structures may be involved?

    b.   What pathological processes may be occurring?

    c.   What are your comments about the duration of symptoms?

2.   What would you say to the husband?

    a.   What are his concerns?

3.   What would be your management?

    a.   Hospital?

b. Leave home and revisit?
c. Gynaecologist opinion?
d. General surgical opinion?

F. Mansfield, Perth, Australia

MRS. Y.   AGED 24   HOUSEWIFE   **405**

1. What is the diagnosis?
   a. How does one make a differential diagnosis of dysfunctional uterine bleeding, incomplete abortion or missed abortion in the early days of amenorrhoea?
   b. In an ectopic pregnancy can the endometrium show a secretory phase and no decidual changes?
   c. Can a perforated uterus following curettage present as an acute abdomen one week later?

At operation it was found she had a ruptured endometrial cyst with widespread endometriosis and adhesions of both tubes.

2. How does one advise the patient regarding the possibility of a future pregnancy?
   a. What are the chances of a pregnancy having had one ovary and tube removed, with the other ovary showing areas of endometriosis and adhesions?
   b. Is there any effective treatment for endometriosis?
   c. Is micro-surgery likely to help?

N. C. L. Yuen, Hong Kong

MISS G.A.   AGED 17   BANK CLERK   **406**

1. What is the most likely differential diagnosis?
   a. She has been 'at risk' of pregnancy and the last of several irregular periods was 'small' and late.
   b. Is mild hyperaesthesia over the right lower abdominal region without rebound significant?
   c. If albuminuria was present and several white blood cells are seen on microscopy, what single dose therapy preceded by what question could be used while awaiting a culture report?

2. Why if the discomfort is so severe may a young girl not readily seek medical care unprompted?
   a. What, if any questions, about her sexuality would you explore?
   b. What non-interpersonal relationship diagnoses related to her sexuality would you consider?

    c.   What areas might you explore regarding her fear of retrenchment as she has had many days off over the past year?

    d.   Who would you get to follow this up if it proved to be a significant problem?

3.   Questioning reveals that she had been treated for a 'bladder infection' 3 months earlier. What might have been missed?

    a.   Why might no follow up have been undertaken after that episode?

    b.   What should have been done, when?

    c.   A different organism is found on this occasion – what should that alert you to?

    d.   Further questioning reveals six or more episodes of UTI over the past decade. What further office, laboratory and other investigations are indicated?

A. J. Radford, Adelaide

407 MISS M.B.J.   AGED 14   SCHOOLGIRL

1.   What conditions would you consider in the differential diagnosis?

    a.   What masses may arise from the pelvis in a pubertal girl?

    b.   What is the significance of retention of urine and the low grade fever in this patient?

2.   What relevant history and physical signs would you try to obtain?

    a.   Describe the physiological changes which take place during puberty?

    b.   How would a genital examination assist you in your diagnosis?

    c.   Describe the development of the vagina and how an imperforate hymen could be formed?

    d.   How would a rectal examination help?

3.   How would you manage this patient?

    a.   What is the immediate management?

    b.   What other investigations would you request at a later date?

    c.   The patient and her mother are anxious regarding her child bearing capability. How would you go about reassuring them?

F. E. H. Tan, Kuala Lumpur

408 MRS. M.W.   AGED 68   HOUSEWIFE

1.   What should the doctor tell her at this point?

    a.   How could arrangements be made for the care of her husband while she is being investigated and treated?

    b.   To whom should this patient be referred?

    c.   How urgently should this be done?

    d.   Should any further tests be done?

2. What are the available treatment modalities?

    a.   What are the indications for surgery?

    b.   What are the indications for a colostomy – temporary or permanent?

    c.   When is radiation therapy indicated?

3. Assuming she has metastatic disease and an inoperable tumour, how could she be managed?

    a.   What community resources are available?

    b.   What are the common causes of discomfort and appropriate therapies thereof?

    c.   What are the indications for and possibilities of admission to a palliative care unit?

E. Domovitch, Toronto

MRS. C.D.   AGED 36   HOUSEWIFE AND SHIFT WORKER   409

1. What questions need to follow with respect to her abdominal pain and diarrhoea?

    a.   What considerations may be important with respect to her employment regarding aetiology? Do you always enquire re the nature of employment in such presentations?

    b.   What aspects of the history would lead you to believe that a parasitological aetiology should be considered?

    c.   What are the most common aetiological agents in travellers' diarrhoea?

    d.   What sensible advice should you give the traveller regarding the minimization of bowel problems while travelling?

2. What management plan would you institute on empirical grounds if further questioning provided no significant positive findings?

    a.   What indications should encourage the use of laboratory tests in such patients?

    b.   Why is an antibacterial agent *not* indicated in the majority of *Shigella* and *Salmonella* infections?

    c.   What empirical therapy, if any, might be tried if you suspect, as distinct from know, you are treating a giardial infection?

    d.   Assuming that it is the second or third episode over weeks or months what might you see on proctoscopy (or sigmoidoscopy).

3. What line of questioning would you pursue regarding her request for vitamins?

    a.   What are the valid indications for recommending multi-vitamin combinations?

    b.   What is the presumptive and scientific validity for megavitamin therapy?

    c.   Do you have a systematic approach to taking a history from a person complaining of tiredness?

A. J. Radford, Adelaide

410 MRS. J.C.   AGED 21   STENOGRAPHER

1. What is the likely diagnosis?
    a.   List those things that help you come to the correct conclusion.
    b.   How would a faecal investigation help?
    c.   Is there any need for X-rays or sigmoidoscopy?

2. How important is further history in this situation?
    a.   Is there a need for counselling?
    b.   How would you go about this?

3. If the patient asked about the possibility of cancer what would you say?
    a.   Should cancer be a provisional diagnosis?
    b.   How would you easily exclude it?

D. S. Muecke, Adelaide

411 MRS. M.C.   AGED 23   FARMER'S WIFE

1. What is your diagnosis?
    a.   What features are suggestive of bacterial infection?
    b.   What are the common organisms associated with this picture?
    c.   What are the clinical features of a *Shigella* infection?

2. What investigations would you order?
    a.   What do you hope to find on microscopy of the stool specimen?

3. What treatment would you institute?
    a.   What intravenous fluids would you use?
    b.   Is antibiotic therapy indicated if a *Salmonella* is isolated?

R. W. Roberts, Ravensthorpe, Australia

412 GEORGE TE H.   AGED 6   MAORI SCHOOLBOY

1. What is the likely cause of the diarrhoea?
    a.   What particular organism is associated with shellfish?
    b.   Is the condition infectious?

2. What public health measures are needed?
   a. Do you notify the disease as infectious?
   b. What steps will help eradicate the problem?

3. How will you manage the diarrhoea?
   a. General measures?
   b. Preventive measures?
   c. Specific treatment?

J. G. Richards, Auckland

MR. G.L.   AGED 28   FARMHAND   **413**

1. What are the likely causes in this case?
   a. If ulcerative colitis was the cause, how long could it last?
   b. How could trauma cause this problem?
   c. What changes might occur?

2. How can the condition be treated?
   a. When would a change in treatment be undertaken?
   b. How successful are various methods of treatment?
   c. What psychological implications has the disease on the patient?
   d. How can the disease affect the family?

E. J. H. North, Melbourne

MR. GORDON B.   AGED 32   CLERK   **414**

1. What problems need to be considered in the diagnosis?
   a. In what way is the diarrhoea related to his anxiety?
   b. What has probably happened to his ulcerative colitis?
   c. Is he likely to have glaucoma?
   d. What could have produced the high pressure reading in the survey?

2. How can a diagnosis be made?
   a. What would sigmoidoscopy reveal in acute ulcerative colitis?
   b. What would a barium enema X-ray show in Mr. B?
   c. Would a therapeutic trial establish the diagnosis?

3. What is the treatment of acute ulcerative colitis?
   a. What is the place of parenteral corticosteroids?
   b. How are topical corticosteroids administered?
   c. What is the place of sulphasalazine in therapy?
   d. When is surgery required?

4. What are the pros and cons of health screening measures?

    a.   What are the dangers of using inadequately trained personnel?
    b.   How should screenings be organized so as to allay anxiety?
    c.   What screening procedures are of proven cost effectiveness?

D. G. Chambers, Clare, Australia

415   MRS. P.W.   AGED 50   CINEMA USHERETTE

1. What explanation can you offer for her complaint?
    a.   What features of a consultation alert you to a psychotic illness?
    b.   Could the patient be telling the simple truth?
    c.   How can you explain to her the origin of these 'messages'?
    d.   What should you do if the patient denies a psychiatric problem, and refuses psychiatric referral?

2. How relevant is her past medical and personal history?
    a.   In someone of this age what other causes of a paranoid psychosis, apart from schizophrenia, should be explored?
    b.   Is the marital problem cause or effect?
    c.   Should her family be consulted?
    d.   What electrolyte abnormalities may be suspected?

3. How can she be persuaded to accept treatment?
    a.   Is treatment by subterfuge ever justified?
    b.   Should she be formally admitted to a mental hospital?
    c.   Can treatment be started without consultant advice?

J. Grabinar, Bromley, UK

416   JASON L.   AGED 6 MONTHS

1. Why do people request 'trivial' calls at night?
    a.   What are the possible dynamics of this family?
    b.   How does the doctor cope with his own feelings?
    c.   What reasons make people perceive mild illness as urgent?
    d.   Should one take steps to try to reduce the number of calls such as this: if so, what steps would be appropriate?

2. Why couldn't this baby have been given some 'proper' treatment?
    a.   What is the patho-physiological basis for treatment with fluids only?
    b.   Are there any real problems with anti-emetics, anti-diarrhoeals and electrolyte rich solutions in this situation?
    c.   Are there any reliable markers of dehydration?

    d.   What are the chances of convincing Mr. P.L. that his baby has been offered proper treatment? How would one proceed?

3.   How does the doctor feel about advice as treatment?

A. L. A. Reid, Newcastle, Australia

WILLIAM P.   AGED 10 MONTHS

417

1.   What is the likely cause of the diarrhoea?
    a.   How often is diarrhoea associated with upper respiratory infection?
    b.   What organisms commonly cause diarrhoea?
    c.   Is the condition infectious?

2.   What treatment would you have prescribed initially?
    a.   General advice given?
    b.   Specific therapy?

3.   Is it possible that the treatment prescribed influenced the outcome?
    a.   Does amoxycillin cause diarrhoea?

J. G. Richards, Auckland

MADELINE P.   AGED 4 MONTHS

418

1.   What is the likely cause of the diarrhoea?
    a.   What infections cause diarrhoea at this age?
    b.   What dietary problems are present?

2.   What counselling does Mrs. Phillips need?
    a.   Developmental ranges of normality?
    b.   What basic advice is necessary related to diet?
    c.   Is counselling your responsibility or that of the district nurse?
    d.   What are common problems associated with first born children?

J. G. Richards, Auckland

MRS. DONNA M.   AGED 53

419

1.   How important is a change in bowel habit in a woman of 53?
    a.   What processes affect the size and frequency of stools?
    b.   How does bran work to improve bowel function?
    c.   How likely is malignancy in the absence of weight loss or rectal bleeding?

2. What principles govern the amount of investigation you would order to elucidate a minor complaint in an anxious person?
   a. Do you investigate anxious persons early, hoping to reassure them better, or later to spare them unnecessary worry?
   b. How much responsibility should the doctor take for such decisions without sharing them with the patient and the patient's family?
   c. How commonly would you find correctable pathology with this history?
   d. Could disease above the colon produce these symptoms?
   e. What is the epidemiology of carcinoma of the colon?
   f. In suspected cases of carcinoma of the colon, how effective are tests for occult stool blood? Barium enema? Sigmoidoscopy? Colonoscopy?
   g. If at surgery an operable carcinoma of the rectum was found, would there be any indication for oophorectomy?
   h. If at operation no carcinoma was found, but a routine survey by the surgeon showed multiple gallstones, should these be removed?

F. B. Fallis, Toronto

420 **MR. L.C.   AGED 20   4TH YEAR DENTAL STUDENT**

1. What is the differential diagnosis?
   a. Is there a single condition involving all problems?
   b. Is this ulcerative colitis or carcinoma of the large bowel?
   c. Is this a case of regional ileitis (Crohn's disease)?
   d. How certain can you be of the diagnosis?

2. What diagnostic procedures should be advised?
   a. Are barium enemas and barium meals necessary?
   b. Is sigmoidoscopy of value?
   c. What blood investigations should be performed?
   d. Is examination of stools necessary?

3. What medical treatment would be ordered?
   a. Is hospitalization necessary?
   b. Is a surgical opinion required?
   c. Should vitamin B12 and folic acid be advised?
   d. Are steroids necessary?
   e. What medication is advised?

4. What is the prognosis?
   a. Is the disease curable or controllable?
   b. How long is medication required?
   c. Is the disease life threatening?

d. Can he live a normal life?

e. Is he neurotic?

B. M. Fehler, Johannesburg

MR. C.   AGED 45   FIRE OFFICER   421

1. What are common inter-professional communication problems in 'transfer of care' in either direction across the general practice/hospital interface?
   a. Why is it especially important for the family doctor to be kept up-to-date on what is happening to his hospitalized patients?
   b. How might the family doctor's situation have been eased in the consultation with Mr. C.?

2. What is Crohn's disease?
   a. What is the likely sequence of pathological events in Mr. C.'s case?

3. What management decisions need to be taken in Mr. C.'s case?
   a. What arrangements need to be made to ensure continued professional monitoring and treatment of his sinus?
   b. What drug therapy, if any, might be considered at this stage?
   c. How long is Mr. C. likely to remain off work?

J. D. E. Knox, Dundee

MRS. A.C.   AGED 43   HOUSEWIFE/PHARMACIST   422

1. What is the differential diagnosis?
   a. How do you differentiate between an infective or obstructive jaundice?
   b. What viruses cause hepatitis and how is each disease acquired?

2. What basic diagnostic investigations would you suggest?
   a. How would you decide upon these investigations?
   b. Should a full liver survey be advised – or does the cost factor play a part?
   c. Are X-rays of any value?
   d. Would ultrasound help?
   e. Would cholecystography help?

3. What advice would you give the patient?
   a. Do you put the patient to bed?
   b. What diet do you advise?
   c. Is any medication necessary?
   d. What precautions do you advise the patient's family to take?

4. Is immunization of contacts necessary?
   a. Should the patient's own family be given gammaglobulin?
   b. Colleagues at work – should they be immunized?
   c. Should the patient's children be allowed to attend school?
   d. Are there any dangers in the use of gamma globulin?

B. M. Fehler, Johannesburg

423 MRS. A.J. AND JOHN J.   AGED 55   MANAGER

1. What is primary biliary cirrhosis?
   a. Why might it give rise to icterus?
   b. How might the disease give rise to episodes of severe abdominal pain?
   c. What sort of course does the disease usually follow?

2. What is the role of drug therapy in this disease?
   a. Why is John receiving vitamin preparations?
   b. Why is vitamin D given by injection when vitamin K is being given by mouth?
   c. What is the mode of action of cholestyramine?

3. How would you manage the consultation with Mrs. M.?
   a. What ethical considerations may arise?
   b. What additional information might be needed?
   c. Even if all the necessary information is available, what might you consider to be the most important issues in your role as family doctor?

J. D. E. Knox, Dundee

424 MR. P.   AGED 68   RETIRED PLUMBER

1. What is the differential diagnosis of painless jaundice?
   a. What steps would you take to make a diagnosis?
   b. What causes of fibrosis of the pancreas do you know?
   c. What are the clinical features of haemochromatosis?

2. Was this doctor wise in not informing the patient of the diagnosis?
   a. Was this doctor wise in informing the patient's wife of the diagnosis?
   b. What do you understand by the term 'collusion of anonymity'?
   c. What do you understand by the term 'conspiracy of silence'?
   d. What principles would you adopt in talking to patients about their prognosis?

J. G. Richards, Auckland

MISS A.S.   AGED 19

425

1. What is your management and treatment?
   a. What laboratory investigations are necessary?
   b. Is it necessary to wait for laboratory findings before commencing treatment?
   c. What other facts in the history or in the examination should be sought?
   d. What follow up care is necessary?

2. Discuss the necessity for correct laboratory diagnosis?
   a. What other organisms may be present besides the usual urinary pathogens?
   b. What is the difference in symptoms and signs between urethritis, trigonitis, vaginitis and cystitis?

3. What underlying factors should be discussed with the patient, both for primary and secondary prevention?
   a. If sexual contact has occurred, what other problems may be revealed?
   b. Why does she look worried?

G. M. Dick, Hobart

JAN H.   AGED 17

426

1. What is the correct management for a first case of cystitis at age 17?
   a. What questions are essential to manage this patient?
   b. What investigations, if any, are necessary? Are these influenced by the full history?
   c. What treatment(s) would be appropriate for the bladder problem?

2. In family medicine, how does one decide when to treat an individual and when to look at the family?
   a. How many problems are there in the case described; to whom do they belong?
   b. How many specialists would be needed to cope with the problems described if there were no generalists? Could they do it?
   c. Should one delve deeply into simple problems?

3. Is there any relationship between stiff neck and tension?
   a. What measures might help Jan's mother?
   b. Are chiropractors useful allies or charlatans?

A. L. A. Reid, Newcastle, Australia

427 **MRS. S.R.** **AGED 28** **HOUSEWIFE/UNIVERSITY GRADUATE**

1. What is your approach to the management of urinary frequency and dysuria in the long and short term?
   a. What advice would you give to a woman who has recurrent symptoms of dysuria and frequency but no underlying anatomical abnormality on further investigation?
   b. What would be your approach to a male of the same age as Mrs. S.R. with the same symptoms?

2. What, if any, may be the relationship between Mrs. S.R.'s physical problems and her failure to conceive?
   a. How long would you wait before investigating a 'case' of apparent secondary infertility?
   b. Could any organic diagnoses link together Mrs. S.R.'s complaints and physical findings?
   c. What importance would you attach to finding a cervical erosion on examining Mrs. S.R.? How would you explain to her what a cervical erosion was?

3. What is your approach to the antenatal care of women with Mrs. S.R.'s history of urinary problems?
   a. What do you know about the screening for asymptomatic bacteriuria of:
      – pre-pubertal children?
      – pregnant women?
   b. With what, if any, drugs would you treat asymptomatic bacteriuria in a pregnant woman?

P. Freeling, London

428 **SUSAN M.** **AGED 10**

1. Are the symptoms presented by Susan common in children?
   a. What is the most likely cause?
   b. How did the doctor arrive at his initial diagnosis?
   c. Can knowledge of the family sometimes hamper accurate diagnosis?
   d. What tests are helpful when symptoms are vague and nonspecific?

2. How do urinary tract infections in girls of this age usually present?
   a. How reliable are laboratory reports of MSUs as indicators of urinary tract infection?
   b. When would you ask for an IVP?
   c. What are you looking for?

3. What are the dangers of missing a diagnosis of urinary tract infection in a child?

    a.   When would you refer to a consultant?

    b.   What sort of follow up should Susan receive?

4. How would you manage this case?

    a.   What medication would you prescribe?

    b.   How long should it be continued?

G. Strube, Crawley, UK

DOROTHY A.   AGED 3   429

1. What are the common presentations of significant lower urinary infection in young children?

    a.   When are IVP and cystograms indicated? Are the indications the same for boys and girls?

2. Are there hygienic measures to be taken with a young girl with urinary tract infection to prevent recurrences?

    a.   Are proper bladder and bowel habits important?

    b.   Why should bubble baths and tight panties be avoided?

    c.   Do constipation or pinworms require treatment?

    d.   How would you advise a mother who thought her three year old daughter was masturbating?

3. How would you now treat Dorothy A. if she had a definite recurrence of symptoms?

    a.   In view of the above investigation, how many recurrences would you now accept if they were easily cleared on cotrimoxazole?

    b.   Is end stage renal failure often the result of inadequate treatment of renal infections in childhood?

    c.   How frequently and for how long would you follow Dorothy A.?

F. B. Fallis, Toronto

MRS. S.E.   AGED 85   PENSIONER   430

1. Is she likely to have a urinary infection – if not, why not?

    a.   If so, what level of the urinary tract would this affect?

    b.   Could the pernicious anaemia have a bearing?

2. Could these symptoms have a psychological basis?

    a.   What makes you think so?

    b.   Why would she produce nocturnal symptoms only?

3. List likely possibilities!

4. What investigations are necessary?

D. S. Muecke, Adelaide

431 MRS. J.F.   AGED 34   SECRETARY

1. What is the likely cause of her problem?
   a. Is the problem basically functional or organic?
   b. Is chronic infection likely to cause these symptoms?

2. What problems confront patients who directly consult specialists about their medical problems?
   a. Are patients prone to select an inappropriate consultant?
   b. Do specialists tend to approach problems with a 'tunnel vision'?
   c. Are general practitioners astute in selecting the most appropriate consultants for their patients?
   d. Do specialists fail in giving total patient care, especially on psychosocial problems?

3. What are the important aspects in total care of this patient?
   a. Why has this patient eventually consulted her general practitioner?
   b. Do patients really need a general practitioner/family doctor?
   c. Should the general practitioner act as a liaison person between the urologist and the patient?
   d. Should the patient be referred to a gynaecologist?

J. E. Murtagh, Melbourne

432 SUSAN STONE   AGED 22   STENOGRAPHER

1. What was the sequence of the diagnostic labels applied to this patient as her story unfolded?
   a. What were the possible consequences if the doctor had considered only the presenting symptom at the first consultation?
   b. Could the eventual diagnosis of a kidney malignancy be considered to have been reached 'more by luck than good management'?
   c. What is the normal process of reaching a diagnosis in the primary care situation?

2. What sequence should be followed in treating and investigating a recurrent urinary tract infection in a female?
   a. What are some of the possible causes that may lead to such infection?
   b. What drugs are most often used for the treatment of the acute infection?
   c. What general advice should be given to the patient to help her prevent further episodes if no correctable anatomical abnormality is discovered?

d. What are the social and psychological problems that could be associated with recurrent urinary tract infection?

J. G. P. Ryan, Brisbane

MISS C.L.   AGED 6

433

1. Would you feel the psychosocial aspects of this child's environment are the key issue to diagnosis and management?
    a. How would you assess the importance of psychosocial aspects?

2. What do you advise parents about 'potty training?'
    a. Is 'potty training' necessary?
    b. Can it cause difficulties with control of micturition?

3. How do you monitor and control renal tract infection in such a case?
    a. Should urine samples be regularly checked?
    b. If so how and where?
    c. When would you cease such monitoring?

W. D. Jackson, Launceston, Australia

DEBBIE   AGED 12   SCHOOLGIRL

434

1. What steps should one take to deal with Debbie's enuresis?
    a. Is a physical cause likely?

2. How might the question of her school work be investigated?
    a. What kind of professional assessment of her educational abilities can be made?
    b. Do the school teachers have any part to play?

3. How might Debbie's emotional problems be further explored?

J. C. Hasler, Oxford

N.L.   AGED 15   SCHOOLBOY

435

1. What would you do in these circumstances?
    a. What advice would you give?
    b. What treatment would you offer?
    c. What investigations might you undertake?
    d. What other help might you seek?
    e. When would you prefer to commence treatment of an enuretic?

2. What other course might the parent/s take?
    a. If they had done nothing what would the outcome have been?

    b.   What are the chances of success in these cases?

    c.   What advice would you give to the parent/s on the role they should play?

    d.   How can the parents help?

    e.   What common mistakes are likely to aggravate the problem?

3.   What is the incidence of this condition?

    a.   Is it more common in certain social classes?

    b.   What differences are found between the male and female bed wetter?

E. J. H. North, Melbourne

436   MRS. M.P.   AGED 38   HOUSEWIFE

1.   Is the symptom likely to be physical or psychogenic?

    a.   What may she be trying to tell you about her marriage?

    b.   What investigations are warranted?

    c.   Is a trial of drug therapy justifiable? If so, what drug?

2.   What are the possible organic causes?

    a.   What neurological signs would you look for?

    b.   Could her obstetric history have produced the present problem? How?

3.   What specialist advice would you request, if any?

    a.   On neurological referral, multiple sclerosis is diagnosed; what do you tell the patient?

    b.   What other symptoms do you inquire about?

    c.   What are her long-term prospects?

    d.   What therapy do you advise?

J. Grabinar, Bromley, UK

437   MR. A.F.   AGED 77   RETIRED FROM ARMY

1.   How do you manage this patient's incontinence?

    a.   What general measures might improve bladder control?

    b.   Do any drugs help in the treatment of neurogenic bladder?

    c.   Would control of infection help?

2.   How would you manage the bowel dysfunction?

    a.   What dietary factors are of importance?

    b.   Laxatives, stool softeners?

3.   What support will he need if he returns home?

C. T. Lamont, Ottawa

MR. K.V.   AGED 40   BUSINESS MAN

438

1. What is the **most** likely diagnosis?

2. What important question should be asked in the history?
   a. What family history is there of gout, renal calculi or renal disease, other metabolic disorders?
   b. What history of previous illness or similar episodes does this patient have?
   c. What medication is this patient taking?

3. What investigations should be performed?
   a. What is the likely outcome of a general physical examination?
   b. What investigation of urine could you undertake on the spot?
   c. What investigations could you also obtain within 12 hours?

4. What should be the management of this case?
   a. Is any initial management required?
   b. Should the patient be given a statement of the history and findings?
   c. Should the patient be advised to consult his own doctor if no further symptoms occur?

D. U. Shepherd, Melbourne

MRS. BETTY F.   AGED 29   CLEANER

439

1. There are two main issues here, the one of the family history of coronary artery disease and the second issue of a possiblity of renal disease. How would you proceed? What would be the value of asking the following questions:
   a. Does the patient smoke?
   b. Is she overweight?
   c. What is her diet like?
   d. What are her cholesterol, triglycerides and lipoproteins?
   e. What is the family history of renal disease?
   f. Did she have any problems of kidney disease during pregnancy?
   g. What is her analgesic consumption now and in the past?
   h. Does she have a history of easy bruising or spontaneous bleeding?

2. You discover that her serum cholesterol and triglycerides are borderline. She had a cholecystectomy in 1975 and hepatitis in 1972. She is 51 kg in weight and 155 cm tall. What advice would you give her about coronary artery disease?
   a. What advice would you give her about smoking?
   b. What are the risks of her having a heart attack?

    c.   Is it necessary for her to keep her weight down?
    d.   Is it necessary for her to reduce her cholesterol and triglycerides?
    e.   Should she remain on the pill?
    f.   Does exercise play any part in her treatment?

3.   What should you do about the renal disease?
    a.   What value are the serum electrolytes and renal function tests?
    b.   Does she need any further investigations, e.g. intravenous pyelogram or a renal scan?
    c.   What should you do about the blood in her urine?

M. D. Mahoney, Brisbane

440   MR. F.R.   AGED 62   STOREMAN

1.   Was it reasonable for the other practitioner to accept negative results as indicative of no serious disease?
    a.   How often does blood loss occur from a benign disease process?
    b.   What are the causes of painless haematuria?
    c.   What are the causes of painful haematuria?

2.   How would you set about investigating this man?
    a.   How reliable is urinary cytology?
    b.   Is there a place for ultrasonography in this man?
    c.   Is a bone scan indicated?

3.   What is the likely disease process involved in a patient of this age?
    a.   IVP shows a mass in the upper pole of the left kidney. What are the possible causes of this?
    b.   Chest X-ray shows numerous round opacities scattered through both lungs. Does this alter your diagnostic impressions?
    c.   Will nephrectomy help this man?
    d.   Is there a place for cytotoxic drugs and/or radiotherapy?
    e.   How will you inform the patient of the problem?

W. F. Glastonbury, Adelaide

441   MR. R.D.   AGED 88   UNMARRIED, RETIRED CARPENTER

1.   How should his urinary problem be investigated?
    a.   Biochemical tests, bacteriology?
    b.   X-rays, bladder function tests?
    c.   Other investigations?

2.   What are the treatment options for benign prostate hypertrophy?
    a.   Surgical – indications?
    b.   Non-surgical – indications (if any)?

3. What other causes of anaemia, other than blood loss, should be considered?
   a. What investigations are indicated to consider feasible aetiological factors?
   b. Would you correct his anaemia by medical means prior to prostate surgery?

4. What assessment will be necessary prior to his return home?

C. T. Lamont, Ottawa

MR. F.C.M.   AGED 72   PENSIONER   442

1. How closely should the renal failure be monitored in the laboratory in this patient?
   a. Who benefits from such monitoring – doctor or patient?
   b. Should a patient who places great store in monitoring what he sees as a terminal illness be encouraged or discouraged?
   c. What are the costs of such monitoring? Who pays?
   d. How useful is the monitoring being employed in this case?
   e. Is it cost effective?
   f. Are other forms of renal function assessment indicated in this patient?
   g. Are they more or less cost effective than those being used?
   h. How can cost effectiveness be defined?

2. What criteria should one use when prescribing medication in a patient with renal failure?
   a. What are the pitfalls of prescribing when renal failure is present?
   b. How should dosage be adjusted?
   c. What is the place of serum assays?
   d. Does this patient need medication and if so are there not better drugs for the purpose?
   e. Is the giddiness related to the medication?
   f. What are the indications for prescribing quinine in the presence of renal failure?

3. What is the likely prognosis in this patient?
   a. What is meant by terminal illness?
   b. What is the natural history of chronic renal failure secondary to obstructive uropathy with delayed relief?
   c. Would you like to be a passenger in a car driven by this patient?
   d. What are the indications for renal transplantation?

D. Levet, Hobart

443 MISS K.E.   AGED 21   UNIVERSITY STUDENT

1. What are the common causes of vaginitis in women of child-bearing age?
   a. What is the type of discharge in each?
   b. Which are sexually transmitted?
   c. What office laboratory procedures are used to determine the diagnosis?

2. How do you treat vaginitis?
   a. What are the treatment options in gonorrhoea?
   b. How do you treat *Monilia* infection?
   c. How do you treat *Trichomonas vaginalis* infection?
   d. How do you treat *Haemophilus vaginalis* infection?
   e. When do you treat the male sex partner?
   f. How do you manage recurrent vaginal infections?

3. What are the predisposing factors for vaginitis?
   a. Do you always look for these or just with recurrent infections?
   b. Are most of the predisposing causes correctable?

4. How are older women with vaginitis different?
   a. Can atrophic vaginitis be successfully treated?
   b. Is it better to treat it locally or systemically?
   c. How quickly does oestrogen vaginal cream work?
   d. How long do you continue using oestrogen cream?
   e. Is there systemic absorption from the oestrogen vaginal cream?

5. How are children with vaginitis different?
   a. Why is it important to take a culture?
   b. How do you look for a foreign body?
   c. Is treatment systemic or local?
   d. What is the best psychological approach to these young patients?

R. L. Perkin, Toronto

444 MRS. X.Y.   AGED 29   HOUSEWIFE

1. What pattern of questioning would you use in such cases?
   a. What are the alleged associations with vaginal candidiasis?
   b. How many of them have a scientific basis?
   c. In fact her only symptom was a very offensive odour (and occasionally minimal discharge) most mornings after having had intercourse. What is your presumptive diagnosis?

2. What are the indications for laboratory (at the office or central) diagnosis of vaginal infection?
   a. Are there any indications for laboratory investigation of the partner or is initial empirical co-therapy justified in the majority of cases in which it is considered desirable?
   b. Why should an initial laboratory diagnosis be made, at least after the first episode, even if empirical therapy is applied before a result is obtained?
   c. Why do so many patients disclaim that the doctor examined her 'down there'?
   d. What can be done to increase the number of doctors who make an adequate inspection and examination of these patients?
   e. What are the laboratory findings on Gram stain for *Gardnerella vaginalis* (formerly *Haemophilis vaginalis*) and *Corynebacterium vaginale*?

3. What are the standard treatments for candidiasis of the pudendal area?
   a. Why are there so many 'effective' treatments and yet repeated 'recurrences'?
   b. Is there any justification for continuing with 2 or 3 week courses of intravaginal nystatin and natamycin when shorter courses of clotrimazole, econazole and miconazole appear equally effective?
   c. What are the indications for co-therapy of sexual partners?
   d. When should oral nystatin be considered? Why is it used so infrequently?
   e. What is the advantage of tinidazole over all other therapies for *Gardnerella vaginalis* and *Trichomonas* infections?

A. J. Radford, Adelaide

MRS. C.J.N. AGED 36   **445**

1. What are the most likely causes of this patient's symptoms?
   a. What are the two most likely pathogens?
   b. Does the previous history help to distinguish between them?
   c. Do the physical signs help to distinguish between them?
   d. How can a microscope help in the diagnosis at the time of consultation?

2. How could her marital state tie in with her symptoms?
   a. Could mental distress alone be the cause of her symptoms?
   b. Would the discovery of trichomonads or *Candida* lead you to suspect that she had been having an extra-marital sexual affair?

    c.   Would the discovery of trichomonads or *Candida* lead you to suspect that the husband had been having an extramarital sexual affair?

    d.   Could masturbation result in these clinical features?

3.   Does a previous experience of a similar episode help you in your management

    a.   If the diagnosis is uncertain and laboratory tests (taking two days) are ordered, what should the interim management consist of?

    b.   From a pharmacological point of view would it be better to mistakenly prescribe tinidazole tablets or mistakenly prescribe econazole suppositories?

    c.   From the point of view of not losing this patient to another doctor, would it be better to mistakenly prescribe tinidazole or econazole?

D. Levet, Hobart

146   MRS. L.B.   AGED 35

1.   What investigations are necessary to confirm the diagnosis of diabetes mellitus?

    a.   Is a full glucose tolerance test always necessary?

2.   What treatment is required?

    a.   Are ketones always an indication for treatment with insulin?

    b.   Discuss the indications for the use of oral hypoglycaemic agents.

3.   Would you refer this patient to hospital or treat her yourself?

    a.   Discuss the long-term care of a patient with diabetes mellitus. Is this best carried out in a hospital clinic or in general practice?

    b.   What advantage does home monitoring of blood sugar offer over urine testing? Which patients would most benefit from this?

A. G. Strube, Crawley, UK

147   MISS A.H.   AGED 20   SECRETARY

1.   What alternative diagnoses would you consider?

    a.   Of what organic illnesses may amenorrhoea be a concomitant?

    b.   At what point in recovery from anorexia nervosa does the menstrual cycle re-establish itself?

    c.   What, if anything, should be done about 'post-pill' amenorrhoea?

2. What steps would you take to distinguish between them?
    a. What are the diagnostic features of anorexia nervosa?
    b. If she 'gets her periods back' and wants advice on contraception, what advice would you give?
    c. How would you diagnose pregnancy at 8 weeks amenorrhoea?
    d. What difficulties may you face in reaching a correct diagnosis?

3. What is meant by the term 'denial' as used in psychology?
    a. With what models explaining anorexia nervosa are you familiar?
    b. Can anorexia nervosa be cured? What would 'cure' mean?
    c. What is meant by 'a unimodal distribution of a symptom'?

P. Freeling, London

MRS. VERA S.   AGED 27   CLEANER   448

1. What is she suffering from?
    a. What are the features of premenstrual tension?
    b. What variants of this condition occur?
    c. How common is this condition?

2. What would you do for her?
    a. What explanation would you give her?
    b. What treatment is usually effective?
    c. What alternate strategies do you use?
    d. How would you help the family to cope with Mrs. S.'s premenstrual tension?

3. In people who suffer severely from this condition, what is your opinion about their culpability if they exhibit criminal behaviour?
    a. What do you feel about the recent cases where women were not convicted of homicide which occurred during premenstrual tension?

W. E. Fabb, Melbourne

MRS. Y.B.   AGED 36   HOUSEWIFE   449

1. What conditions affect the uterus in a woman of child-bearing age?
    a. To what complications might fibroids give rise?
    b. What are the signs and symptoms of endometriosis?
    c. What factors are believed to predispose to the development of carcinoma of the cervix?

2. How would you investigate abnormal uterine bleeding in a 36 year old woman?
    a. How do you assess menstrual loss?

    b.   What do you understand by breakthrough bleeding?

    c.   What conditions other than carcinoma can be identified on cervical smear?

    d.   What is the significance of cervical carcinoma in situ?

3.   What are the indications for hysterectomy?
    a.   What factors influence the incidence of hysterectomy in a population?
    b.   What is the natural history of carcinoma of the body of the uterus?
    c.   How would you recognize a choriocarcinoma?
    d.   What explanation would you give to a patient about to undergo hysterectomy?

4.   What hormonal changes take place after hysterectomy?
    a.   What is the post-hysterectomy syndrome?
    b.   How do you treat the post-hysterectomy syndrome?
    c.   What other conditions may present with the same symptoms?

T. A. I. Bouchier Hayes, Camberley, UK

450 MRS. Y.L.   AGED 52   WIFE OF COMPANY DIRECTOR

1.   Is the menopause an ovarian deficiency disease?
    a.   Can a process which will affect every woman be viewed as pathological rather than physiological?
    b.   Which symptoms are specific to the menopause and which coincidentally experienced with it?
    c.   What other factors might be at work producing symptoms in women of this age?

2.   What are the disadvantages of treating flushes with hormone replacement therapy (HRT)?
    a.   Is HRT more effective than placebo?
    b.   Do flushes clear up spontaneously for long periods?
    c.   Will HRT delay the natural resolution of symptoms?
    d.   Does withdrawal of oestrogen provoke rebound flushing?

3.   Is it better to submit to, confront, or bargain with this patient?
    a.   Is her mind made up or will it be amenable to reasonable explanation?
    b.   Should one try to elicit further why she really wants HRT?
    c.   Would agreeing only to prescribe hormones for a specified period solve the problem or just delay a confrontation?
    d.   If she was a private patient would she be more likely to be prescribed long-term HRT?

A. J. Moulds, Basildon, UK

MRS. I.F. AGED 25 HOUSEWIFE **451**

1. What are the possibilities in the differential diagnosis?
   a. What is hirsuitism? Discuss the patho-physiology of hirsuitism.
   b. How can careful history taking and physical examination assist you in ascertaining the probable diagnosis?

2. How would you carry out your investigations?
   a. What is Stein-Leventhal syndrome?
   b. How may the diagnosis be confirmed?

3. What further aspect of management is of importance to the patient?
   a. The patient is distressed about her excessive hair. How would you manage this aspect?
   b. How would you manage her obesity?
   c. Should she wish to start her family, what would you advise?

F. E. H. Tan, Kuala Lumpur

MRS. Q. AGED 35 HOUSEWIFE **452**

1. Identify the problems presented by the patient.
   a. What is the natural history of carcinoma of the cervix?
   b. Do you agree with the management suggested by the gynae-cologist?
   c. Discuss the role of hormonal replacement therapy.

2. What are the possible reasons for the patient's refusal of operation?
   a. How would you educate the patient regarding the operation?
   b. What is the prognosis should she still refuse the operation?

3. How would you manage her?
   a. What valuable information may be obtained by going into her sexual and marital history?
   b. How would you rule out gonorrhoea in this patient?
   c. What method of contraception would you suggest?

4. How would you manage her husband?
   a. How do you educate her husband about her problem?
   b. How would you conduct conjoint therapy for the couple?

F. E. H. Tan, Kuala Lumpur

MR. S.M. AGED 22 MORMON MISSIONARY **453**

1. What are the likely causes of urethral discharge?
   a. Is it a feature of a urinary tract infection?

    b.   Should it be assumed to be due to a venereal disease until proved otherwise?

    c.   Can it be caused by prostatitis?

2.   Was prescribing Septrin a reasonable course of action?
    a.   What is its spectrum of activity?
    b.   Would it be the treatment of choice for either gonorrhoea or non-specific urethritis?
    c.   Would another antibiotic have been better?
    d.   Was any prescription necessary at that time?

3.   How often does social stereotyping interfere with the making of rational clinical judgements?
    a.   If he denied any sexual activity would you believe him?
    b.   If he wasn't a missionary and denied sexual activity would you believe him?
    c.   Where does the term 'missionary position' come from?

4.   How would you proceed to manage the case?
    a.   Should he be referred to a special clinic to exclude syphilis and gonorrhoea?
    b.   If so, how would you persuade him to go?

A. J. Moulds, Basildon, UK

454   ALLAN F.   AGED 26   LONG DISTANCE TRUCK DRIVER

1.   What would you advise him about telling his wife?
    a.   Do you feel he should attempt to give an alternative story?
    b.   Would truthfulness on his part lead to breakup of the marriage or could it have serious psychological consequences at this stage of pregnancy?

2.   What tests would you perform?
    a.   Describe the actual tests to be performed.
    b.   Would you take blood – if so for what tests?

3.   What advice regarding resumption of sexual activity would you give to Allan?
    a.   Would you tell him to refrain until all tests were negative?

4.   How would you initiate treatment as he is allergic to penicillin?
    a.   What drugs can be used as satisfactory alternatives?
    b.   What length of course would you use?

5.   How would you organize follow up and subsequent testing?
    a.   Should efforts be made to trace his contact?

b. When should swabs and blood tests be repeated?
c. What are his chances of recurrence if no re-infection occurs?

6. What are the dangers to the baby?
   a. How common is gonococcal infection of the newborn, and how does it show?
   b. How common is congenital syphilis and how does it present?

K. C. Nyman, Perth, Australia

MR. C.D.   AGED 32   CAR SALESMAN   455

1. How would you treat his gonorrhoea?
   a. What is your regime of antibiotic treatment?
   b. How would you follow-up the patient?
   c. How would you follow-up his contacts?

2. How would you investigate his wife?
   a. Is a culture a sensitive test for gonorrhoea in women?
   b. How would you contact and treat his wife?

3. What would you do about the marriage relationship?
   a. Do you think the marriage is really improving?
   b. How would you re-establish the relationship?

E. V. Dunn, Toronto

SAMUEL N.   AGED 47   BANK MANAGER   456

1. What is your clinical management of this patient?
   a. What additional questions could be important?
   b. What laboratory examinations would you order?
   c. What factors would you consider in selecting appropriate therapy?
   d. How does gonorrhoea commonly present in men and women?

2. What further action would you consider?
   a. How would you ensure that the young secretary is examined for venereal disease?
   b. How would you ensure that Dorothy N. is examined for venereal disease?
   c. How would you respond to Samuel's request for complete secrecy?
   d. What laws and regulations apply to the treatment of venereal disease?

3. Can you make any predictions as to the interpersonal family relationships which could have contributed to Samuel's one-time infidelity?
   a. What possible factors in Samuel?
   b. What possible factors in Dorothy?
   c. What possible factors in the children?
   d. How might you assist this family to cope with their problems?

4. What is the role of the family physician in preventing venereal disease in his practice population?
   a. Which population groups are at special risk?
   b. What is the relevance of contraceptive advice?
   c. How could he contribute to sex education in the local schools?
   d. What health education measures could be instituted in his practice?
   e. What educational resources are available in the community?

M. R. Polliack, Tel-Aviv, Israel

457 PHINEAS Z. AGED 22 SOLDIER

1. How might inguinal adenopathy, if present, influence your diagnosis?
   a. What is the possible aetiology?
   b. How complete an examination is necessary?

2. Should sexually transmitted disease be notifiable?
   a. Might it not be driven underground?
   b. Where it is notifiable by law, do you believe that a high proportion of cases are notified?
   c. Is gonorrhoea on the increase
      – in notifying countries?
      – in non-notifying countries?

3. How can we combat the problems of sexually transmitted disease?
   a. By correctly treating every case which presents?
   b. By correct treatment and contact tracing?
   c. By strictly controlled brothels?
   d. By banning prostitution?
   e. By education?
   f. By reverting to a strict paternalistic society?

R. T. Mossop, Harare, Zimbabwe

458 JOE M. AGED 23 UNEMPLOYED

1. What was the differential diagnosis?
   a. Is this likely to be gonorrhoea? Can acute purulent gonorrhoeal urethritis present without dysuria?

b. What else is possible?

c. How would you differentiate in the city, in the rural town?

d. Can you get a painless penile sore (and buboes) with gonorrhea?

e. Can you get associated urethritis in lymphogranuloma venereum?

2. What would be your line of questioning about his illness?

a. Is any diagnosis other than gonorrhoea likely if there has been sexual contact only within the last week?

b. Is it necessary to swab other areas? Which? Why?

c. If he had not presented with urethritis what symptoms might have led you to ask about it?

3. What line of questioning would you choose regarding contacts?

a. His 'primary' contact is pregnant and she did prove to have gonorrhoea – how would you manage her?

b. What would you ask her about her past history and this pregnancy before treatment?

c. One other contact was 'involved' with 'the whole football team', another a teacher's wife. What would your public health conscience encourage you to do in managing the whole problem?

4. What clinical follow-up is now regarded as essential for gonorrhoea cases?

a. Why?

b. What types of penicillin resistant gonorrhoea occur?

c. What are the most favoured injectable and oral treatments for such cases?

d. Would you have him return in one and six weeks for further tests? Which? If not, why not?

5. What are the treatment alternatives for acute gonorrhoea, other urethritides and lymphogranuloma venereum?

A. J. Radford, Adelaide

MR. WILLIAM R.   AGED 77   RETIRED CLERK   459

1. What are the most likely causes of this condition in this man?

a. What are the features of balanoposthitis due to *Candida albicans*?

b. What would you conclude if a swab of the discharge grew penicillin-resistant *Staphylococcus aureus*?

2. How would you deal with this problem?

a. If the condition was due to *Candida albicans*, what treatment would you use?

   b. If the situation was complicated by the presence of penicillin-resistant *Staphylococcus aureus*, under what circumstances would systemic therapy be warranted?

   c. In this circumstance, what local therapy would you use?

3. How could this situation be avoided in the future?
   a. What instructions would you give the patient about hygienic measures?
   b. Would you consider circumcision? Under what circumstances?

4. If the patient was 27, unmarried and sexually active, what causes would you consider and how would you manage them?
   a. What are the features of herpes simplex genitalis?
   b. What is the epidemiology of this condition in your country?
   c. How do you manage this condition?
   d. Is there any way of avoiding or minimizing recurrences of this condition?
   e. What is the prognosis for this condition?
   f. What are the fears and psychological sequelae in patients with this condition?
   g. What health education measures about this condition are being instituted in your country?

W. E. Fabb, Melbourne

160   MR. T.K.   AGED 28   WOODWORKER

1. What is the cause of the haemospermia?
   a. Is this a normal presentation for the condition involved here?
   b. What might be a more common presentation?
   c. What do you think the wife's concerns might be?

2. What is the simplest way of making a diagnosis in this case?
   a. Why did the doctor ask for X-rays?
   b. Why did he X-ray the heel?
   c. What other investigations might he have done?

3. How does the fact that this man is a Jehovah's Witness complicate the case?
   a. Does this make a difference to the approach in the way of therapy?
   b. X-rays of this man's pituitary fossa showed a mass the size of a small egg. What would the complications be if this were allowed to grow?
   c. What are the dangers involved in performing surgery?

J. K. Shearman, Hamilton, Canada

MRS. JANET K.   AGED 24   HOUSEWIFE

461

1. Would you speak to both parents in this situation? If so, what points would you make?
   a. Discuss the role of custom in promoting unnecessary circumcision.
   b. What is the current view held by paediatricians?
   c. Describe in lay terms the reasons the foreskin is there and the reasons for circumcision in the past and the present views held regarding the rare necessity for intervention.

2. What are the advantages and disadvantages of circumcision?
   a. What is the relationship of the operation to cancer of the cervix, venereal disease, cancer of the penis?
   b. What is the treatment of meatal ulcer in the circumcised baby?
   c. What advice should be given to the parents, regarding foreskin retraction and cleanliness?

3. If you decided to circumcise the baby, discuss what you would tell the parents.
   a. Anaesthetic or no anaesthetic?
   b. Hospital or office procedure?
   c. Feeding before or after, and how long will it take?
   d. When would you review following operation, and what would you tell mother about aftercare?

4. Discuss the doctor's role in breaking down parents' prejudices about health matters.
   a. Are there fields other than this where you can draw parallels?
   b. What would influence your decision to make exceptions in any case?
   c. Should you decline to perform procedures where your views and the parents' wishes do not coincide?

K. C. Nyman, Perth, Australia

GARRY J.   AGED 18 MONTHS

462

1. What factors govern accessibility and availability of doctors to patients in general family practice?
   a. What are the advantages and disadvantages of the various methods available to answer telephone calls?
   b. What factors might govern a response to a call such as that made by Garry's mother?

2. What diagnostic processes are used by clinicians?
   a. What specific advantages over the hospital-based doctor are enjoyed by the family doctor as regards clinical diagnosis?

b. What factors influence a family doctor's awareness of differential diagnoses to be applied to a given situation?
c. What might cause a maculopapular rash in Garry's case?
d. What justification is there for using invasive techniques to make a firm diagnosis in a situation such as Garry's?
e. What diagnostic tests, if any, might be employed?

3. If the doctor diagnoses an infective disease in Garry's case, what are the implications?
    a. What factors determine 'secondary attack rate'?
    b. Should the siblings (Lisa and Ian) be kept off school?

4. Might the issue of notification of infectious diseases arise?
    a. What functions does 'notification' serve?
    b. What diseases are 'notifiable'?
    c. What roles might family doctors have in developing a more efficient and effective information system concerning morbidity and health problems?

J. D. E. Knox, Dundee

163 M.E.   AGED 8   SCHOOLBOY

1. Why has this child been brought to you?
    a. Does the mother have no idea what the trouble is?
    b. Does the mother want confirmation of what she suspects the trouble is?
    c. Does the mother think that you can prescribe effective treatment?
    d. Does the mother need advice and/or certification regarding schooling?
    e. Does the mother/father see this as an opportunity to get back some of the premiums paid for medical insurance?
    f. Is it reasonable to enquire into the expectations of a patient (or in this case a parent)?

2. What are the most likely causes of this rash?
    a. Do second attacks of chickenpox often occur?
    b. Would recent contact with a case of shingles help in the diagnosis?
    c. Would a family history of 'hives' in an elder brother help in the diagnosis?
    d. Do mosquito bites ever present in the manner?
    e. What would your reaction be had you been called in by a trainee to confirm that this was a case of dermatitis herpetiformis?

3. Your record sheet has a space for 'diagnostic plans'. What would you put in there?

    a.   Do you feel comfortable leaving blank spaces in a medical record sheet?

    b.   Do you feel comfortable with clinical diagnoses without laboratory confirmation?

    c.   Are there any specific tests for chickenpox?

    d.   What are the advantages and disadvantages of a positive diagnosis as opposed to one made by exclusion?

4.   Your record sheet has space for 'treatment plans'. What would you put in there?

    a.   Do GPs feel compelled to provide 'treatment' for everything? If so where does the compulsion come from?

    b.   How much illness in general practice is unaffected by the treatment given?

    c.   What is the role of phenol applied to the skin?

    d.   Does calamine lotion contain phenol?

    e.   In prescribing an antihistamine in this case are you treating the mother, merely reducing the itch, actually reducing the rash, or giving a drug that will help your alternative diagnoses should your tentative one turn out to be wrong?

5.   Your record sheet has a space for 'patient education plans'. What would you put there?

    a.   What illnesses are notifiable in your area?

    b.   Have you a rule of thumb method for remembering incubation periods?

    c.   Have you a rule of thumb method for remembering when the rash appears in the various exanthemata?

    d.   What factors govern periods of isolation and exclusion from school in respect of infectious diseases?

    e.   What infectious diseases are known to be harmful to the unborn child?

D. Levet, Hobart

A.W.   AGED 15   FEMALE STUDENT   **464**

1.   What other information would you seek from any patient with a skin rash?

    a.   Can you forecast the course of the condition described?

    b.   How does distribution of a rash assist diagnosis?

    c.   Can you offer examples of distribution specificity?

2.   What are the commonest types of skin rashes you see now in general family practice?

    a.   How might you differentiate rubella rash from others?

b. When during pregnancy does this become important?
c. How would you assess its importance?
d. What are the features of pityriasis rosea?

W. D. Jackson, Launceston, Australia

465   MISS A.   AGED 16   SCHOLAR

1. What is the most likely diagnosis?
   a. Why is the history so important?
   b. What criteria make it unlikely to be tinea circinata?

2. What prognosis can you give the patient?
   a. Discuss any therapy that is useful.
   b. What is the average duration of this condition?

3. Is there need for notification to health authorities?
   a. Would you find it necessary to ask this person about sexual habits?
   b. What condition may be a possibility?

D. S. Muecke, Adelaide

466   MR. F.   AGED 40   TEACHER

1. Frank resentment is not a common component of doctor–patient relationships: why may it be 'buried'?
   a. What elements in patient behaviour might suggest its presence?
   b. What are characteristics of a 'good patient'?
   c. What options are open to doctors in dealing with dissatisfied patients?
   d. What options are open to patients dissatisfied with their doctors?

2. What is generally implied by 'fringe medicine'? What governs a family doctor's attitude to it?
   a. How might the doctor have responded had Mr. F. sought advice about consulting the faith healer?
   b. The faith healer consulted by the F. family uses a pendulum device. What 'unorthodox' methods are commonly sought by patients?

3. What is eczema?
   a. What forms have been described?
   b. Does a relationship exist between the activity of eczema and a patient's emotional state?

4. What treatment would help Mr. F. at this stage?
   a. If Mr. F. should require long-term topical steroid, how may potential adverse reactions be minimized?
   b. What factors govern a doctor's choice of topical steroid in eczema?

J. D. E. Knox, Dundee

KAREN M.   AGED 5   467

1. What is the treatment for Karen's itch?
   a. Are corticosteroids indicated?
   b. What long term effects do they have?
   c. How would you assist the family problem?
   d. Are tranquillizers indicated?

2. Would you expect a permanent cure?
   a. Is atopy a life-long affliction?
   b. Is any treatment effective as a long-term cure?

3. Are there any associated conditions?
   a. Would you expect her to develop asthma or hay-fever?
   b. Does eczema leave any long term damage?

4. How would you use the opportunity to discuss the real problem?
   a. Who is the patient?
   b. Would counselling help?
   c. How would you deal with the underlying problem?

R. M. Meyer, Johannesburg

AILEEN Z.   AGED 10   SCHOLAR   468

1. What is the diagnosis?
   a. What are the characteristic features of her condition?
   b. Does associated atopy in the patient and family assist in your diagnosis?

2. What is the treatment of this disease?
   a. Are corticosteroids of value in treatment either systemically or topically?
   b. Avoidance of precipitating factors?
   c. Are antibiotics of any value?
   d. How do you prevent a recurrence?

3. What is the management of this disease?

    a.   A clear understanding of the condition by both patient and parent?

    b.   Therapeutic triangle between patient, doctor and parent?

    c.   Is frequent counselling required?

B. M. Fehler, Johannesburg

469   MR. P.B.   AGED 24   PUBLIC SERVANT

1. How would you manage this man?
    a.   Can you use the same steroid for both areas?
    b.   What are the risks of long-term local steroids?
    c.   Should he have a course of parenteral steroids?
    d.   What other treatment is available?

2. Why has his eczema returned?
    a.   Can you accept his statement indicating no emotional problem at face value?
    b.   Is it wise to delve deeper?
    c.   Could he be sensitive to other ingested allergens, e.g. preservatives or dyes?
    d.   What significance can be placed on the IgE and RAST tests?

3. Should he be desensitized again despite lack of respiratory symptoms?
    a.   Did desensitization years ago really help his asthma?
    b.   Do grasses, weeds, dust and cat epithelia produce eczema?
    c.   Are there any dangers in desensitization?
    d.   Is desensitization effective in eczema?

P. F. Gill, Hobart

470   MR. C.A.   AGED 34   LABOURER

1. What are the essential problems in development of a problem list?
    a.   Is the groin rash likely to be an isolated problem?
    b.   What skin problems are more likely to occur in a patient who is obese?
    c.   What underlying medical problems may lead to this type of skin problem?
    d.   In what way may his wife's symptoms relate to this patient's medical problem?

2. What differential diagnostic possibilities exist in the male in the development of a groin rash?
    a.   What environmental factors influence the development of a 'jock itch' (tinea cruris)?

b. Can other skin diseases, including such papulosquamous diseases as psoriasis, affect the inguinal area and offer diagnostic difficulties?

c. What would positive physical findings be in a case of candidal intertrigo?

d. What physical findings and diagnostic aids would be helpful in diagnosing erythrasma (bacterial intertrigo)?

3. What factors in patient education would be important in this case?

a. Would it be helpful diagnostically and therapeutically to request that the patient's wife have a pelvic examination?

b. What evaluative procedures should be undertaken to rule out diabetes mellitus in this patient?

c. What factors at work would help lessen the likelihood of continuation or recurrence of this skin rash?

d. What factors are likely to be successful in gaining compliance regarding this patient's obesity?

L. H. Amundson, Sioux Falls, SD, USA

MR. J.B.   AGED 23   INFANT SCHOOL TEACHER

471

1. Where would you look to ensure the proper diagnosis?
   a. Any other pathognomonic features?

2. What would make you think it was not psychological?
   a. What distribution would you expect?

3. What investigations are necessary to prove the diagnosis?
   a. If a scraping was negative what would be your next move?

4. What is the appropriate treatment?
   a. What special advice would you give the patient?
   b. How would you describe to him the degree of contagiousness?

D. S. Muecke, Adelaide

BRETT A.   AGED 13   SCHOOLBOY

472

1. What is your immediate management?
   a. What specific measures for pain relief local and systemic?
   b. What questions might help to establish a possible cause?
   c. What significance has it that contact with water exacerbated the condition?

2. What is your working diagnosis?

    a.   Assuming a contact irritant or caustic, what likely substances might be encountered on a playing field?

    b.   What specific instructions would you give about care of the affected areas?

3.   What further steps would you take to establish the cause and plan further treatment?

    a.   The groundsman tells you that the pitch was recently dressed with superphosphate and freshly marked with 'lime'. Which is the culprit?

    b.   What is 'lime' as used for marking pitches?

    c.   Why was this particular 'lime' corrosive?

J. A. Stevens, Ulverstone, Australia

473   RITA W.   AGED 47   FARMER'S WIFE

1.   To what is she allergic?

    a.   What is the significance of the distribution?

    b.   What are the likely agents to affect this patient's hands?

    c.   She has not changed her detergent or handled any fresh irritant recently. Why has it just appeared?

    d.   On further questioning she says she has bought her latest batch of wool from a craft shop. Is this relevant?

2.   How would you confirm the diagnosis?

    a.   Is patch testing necessary?

    b.   Would you patch test now?

3.   What is the management?

    a.   Would you use local steroids? If so, what type, strength and base?

    b.   What advice about washing and care of the hands would you give?

J. A. Stevens, Ulverstone, Australia

474   JACOB H.   AGED 29   ACCOUNTANT

1.   What is your provisional diagnosis?

    a.   What specific questions might you ask?

    b.   How detailed should your examination be?

2.   What are the possible causes of this condition?

    a.   What initial investigations would you perform or arrange?

    b.   The ESR is 30 mm in one hour and chest X-ray shows hilar gland enlargement. What would you suspect as the underlying cause and how would you confirm it?

3. What would be your management?
    a.   Would you include prednisolone in your treatment and what would lead you to do so?
    b.   What advice would you give as to exercise, diet, and occupation?
    c.   How would you explain the illness, outline it's course and indicate the prognosis?
    d.   How would you follow up?

J. A. Stevens, Ulverstone, Australia

MRS. BARBARA F.   AGED 60   HOUSEWIFE   **475**

1. What treatment would be suitable for such an ulcer?
    a.   What do you think of the treatment by the two consultants?
    b.   In the event of circulatory insufficiency is radiotherapy safer than surgery?

2. The patient is thinking of litigation – what would your attitude be?
    a.   How do you feel about attending court as a witness?
    b.   Do you feel you owe loyalty to your colleagues under such circumstances?

R. M. Meyer, Johannesburg

MRS. B.Z.   AGED 52   HOUSEWIFE   **476**

1. What are the possible aetiological factors in this lady's presenting complaint of blue toes?
    a.   What systemic diseases should be considered?
    b.   How might smoking be incriminated in this lady's problems?
    c.   How does one discriminate between large vessel, small vessel, and embolic peripheral vascular disease?

2. What intrinisic problems might have an aetiological bearing on, or serve as aggravating factors in, this lady's medical disease?
    a.   What non-invasive and invasive procedures might be helpful in arriving at a diagnosis?
    b.   What aetiological factors could be ruled out by serum protein electrophoresis, antinuclear antibodies, LE preparations and latex fixation tests?
    c.   What are the differential diagnostic possibilities of medial versus lateral malleolar ulcers?

    d.   What diagnostic gains can be expected from plain films of the feet and abdomen in addition to Doppler ultrasonic blood flow studies?

3.   What therapeutic measures constitute good foot care irrespective of the diagnosis?
    a.   What approaches should be used to ensure appropriate nail care?
    b.   What precautionary measures will ensure the prevention of cold injury?
    c.   Will modifications be necessary in this lady's use of hot soaks and bathing, due to the nature of her illness?

L. H. Amundson, Sioux Falls, SD, USA

477   MRS. MARILYN B.   AGED 33   SINGLE PARENT

1.   How would you manage the physical aspects of this problem?
    a.   Under what circumstances do you aspirate a breast lump?
    b.   How do you do it?
    c.   How diagnostic are mammography and thermography?
    d.   If she requires an excisional biopsy, should the surgeon follow his routine of having a quick frozen section and immediate mastectomy if indicated?

2.   How would you manage the social aspects?
    a.   What options for care of the children are available in your community?
    b.   How are these options organized, who pays and how much notice must be given?
    c.   What convalescence arrangements would you make?
    d.   Is any income supplement possible in your community?

3.   What emotional supports can you offer this patient?
    a.   Can you help her to maintain contact with her children during hospitalization?
    b.   Does your local cancer organization have personnel who help patients deal with the loss of a breast and advise them on prostheses?

D. H. Johnson, Toronto

478   MRS. J.D.   AGED 35   HOUSEWIFE

1.   What is the likely diagnosis?
    a.   How do you determine possible malignancy on clinical grounds?
    b.   What does skin tethering indicate?

2. How could you prevent this situation?
   a. Do voluminous breasts pose a special problem?
   b. What radiological screening procedures are appropriate?
   c. What are the criteria to biopsy lumpy breasts?
   d. Do doctors tend to become careless with anxious patients who are regular attenders?

3. How would you manage this problem?
   a. Would you refer this patient for immediate surgery?
   b. What would you tell this patient?
   c. Would you refer the patient for radiological investigation?

4. How would you conduct a management interview?
   a. How could you explain the management without causing anxiety?
   b. Should you tell the patient the sad hard facts immediately?
   c. How would you rationalize the previous assessment to the patient?
   d. How would you rationalize the previous assessment to the husband?
   e. What predictions could you make about the natural history of this problem?
   f. Would you admit an error of judgement on the last visit?
   g. How would you cope with the possibility of litigation for medical neglect?

J. E. Murtagh, Melbourne

MRS. LINDA A.   AGED 39   SALESLADY   479

1. What is your presumptive diagnosis?
   a. Compare the clinical significance of breast lumps, at various ages, in both sexes?
   b. Which women are at special risk for developing breast cancer?
   c. What steps would you take to confirm your diagnosis?
   d. On what criteria would you base your prognostic prediction for Linda?

2. How would you answer Linda's question?
   a. What factors in the doctor–patient relationship could influence your response?
   b. What would you tell her?
   c. How should the problem be explained to her husband?
   d. What would you tell her daughters?
   e. What is 'informed consent' prior to operation?

3. Discuss your management of Linda after the performance of radical mastectomy.

    a.   What problems could you anticipate for Linda and her family?
    b.   What is 'body image'?
    c.   What groups or organizations in the community could assist Linda to cope with her problems?
    d.   What problems could you anticipate from the post-operative use of cytotoxic drugs or radiotherapy?

4.   Could the diagnosis have been established earlier?
    a.   What are possible reasons for delay in her diagnosis?
    b.   How effective is mass screening for breast cancer?
    c.   How effective is self-examination for early detection?
    d.   What health education measures could be used in the practice?
    e.   What are the roles of the practice nurse and health visitor in the early detection of breast cancer?

Z. Cramer, Tel-Aviv, Israel

480   RACHEL S.   AGED 57

1.   How serious a problem is carcinoma of the breast?
    a.   What is the prognosis for the individual?
    b.   What is the incidence of carcinoma of the breast?
    c.   How does it compare in incidence and prognosis to other malignant disease?
    d.   Is any effective screening available?

2.   What treatment is available for carcinoma of the breast?
    a.   What side effects do the various forms of treatment have?
    b.   How effective are they?

3.   How might the doctor react to Rachel's reluctance to undergo treatment?
    a.   What factors would influence his management?
    b.   How far should he explain in detail the outlook?
    c.   Is Rachel's attitude reasonable?

J. C. Hasler, Oxford

481   MISS G.Y.   AGED 22   UNIVERSITY STUDENT

1.   How do you decide if a neck lump is significant?
    a.   What are the clinical characteristics of a lymphoma?
    b.   What are the clinical characteristics of secondary carcinoma?
    c.   Do you investigate such a patient right away, or is a period of observation indicated?
    d.   What about a therapeutic trial of antibiotics?

2. How would you proceed to investigate this patient?
   a. If secondary carcinoma is suspected, what steps would you take in searching for the primary?
   b. At what point do you biopsy the neck lump?

3. What determines the prognosis in a patient with lymphoma?
   a. What is meant by staging of Hodgkin's disease or other lymphomas?
   b. What influence does the cell type have on prognosis?
   c. Does response to initial treatment give clues to prognosis?
   d. What do you tell the patient and the family?

R. L. Perkin, Toronto

MR. J.B.W.   AGED 84   RETIRED SAILOR   **482**

1. How serious is this problem?
   a. What is the incidence of parotid tumour?
   b. If this is a secondary metastatic deposit, where might the primary neoplasia be found?
   c. What changes may need to be contemplated in his home situation with increasing ill health?

2. What treatment do you recommend?
   a. How much further investigation should be considered?
   b. What risks are involved in excision of the lump?
   c. What undesirable sequelae may be expected to occur if radiotherapy is performed?

G. M. Dick, Hobart

MR. B.P.   AGED 49   UPHOLSTERER   **483**

1. What do you think is the nature of the lesion in this man's axilla?
   a. What would your approach be in dealing with this?
   b. What investigations might you perform?
   c. Would you admit the patient to hospital or investigate as an outpatient?

2. How do you think this man's past contact with the medical profession might affect his attitude to his present illness?
   a. Who do you think might give him the best support during this illness?
   b. How important is it for him to have a physician he can trust?

3. How would you treat the pain this man is suffering from?
   a. The biopsy shows this process to be Hodgkin's disease. What kind of prognosis can we give this man?

    b.   What factors will affect the prognosis we give?
    c.   What modes of therapy do we have available?
    d.   What are the advantages and disadvantages of each?
    e.   How will this affect his livelihood?
    f.   Will strong narcotics be dangerous for him?

J. K. Shearman, Hamilton, Canada

484   MISS SHEILA B.   AGED 23   TYPIST

1.   What is the nature of her condition?
    a.   What is the pathology of this form of wry neck?
    b.   What are the common precipitating factors?

2.   What would you do about it?
    a.   What is the place of manipulation?
    b.   Would you X-ray the neck before manipulating it?
    c.   What physiotherapy might help?
    d.   What advice would you give the patient after treatment?
    e.   What advice would you give to prevent a recurrence?

W. E. Fabb, Melbourne

485   MS. H.Z.   AGED 35   AIRLINE HOSTESS

1.   Is this likely to be a pathological or functional problem?
    a.   Is 'fibrositis' a reality in general practice?
    b.   What conditions aggravate muscle spasm?
    c.   What relationship has this condition to the URTI?

2.   What is the natural history of this condition?
    a.   How long does this condition take to resolve?
    b.   Is this period shortened by therapy?
    c.   Would you write fibrositis on a medical certificate?

3.   What advice would you give the patient?
    a.   Does local heat help in the management of this condition and
        what types would you favour?
    b.   Does drug therapy have any place in the management of this
        condition?
    c.   What simple measures may the patient undertake to help?

T. D. Manthorpe, Port Lincoln, Australia

486   MRS. E.C.   AGED 59   HOUSEWIFE

1.   To what extent can legal proceedings complicate the management of
    an accident-related medical problem?

a. How do lawyers and insurance companies arrive at appropriate settlement?
b. If both the doctor and the lawyer have the patient's/client's best interests at heart why is it that their interventions have been futile if not destructive?

2. How does a prolonged disability affect the patient's self-image, relationships with family and friends, and finances?
   a. What would be the best approach regarding rehabilitation in this case?
   b. What can be done to resolve the legal matter as soon as possible?
   c. What therapeutic modalities could be used?
   d. Is there an indication for counselling – psychotherapy?

E. Domovitch, Toronto

MR. B.B.   AGED 23   STOREMAN   487

1. What is the most likely diagnosis here?
   a. List the possible differential diagnoses at this stage.
   b. What other information could be sought from his workmates?

2. What would you expect to find on examination?
   a. Detail your neurological examination and the probable findings.
   b. What other systems should be examined?

3. What immediate investigations could you arrange?
   a. What other investigations are required?

4. What is the immediate management?
   a. What would you do for pain relief?
   b. Should hospital or home management be undertaken? What instructions would you give?
   c. What certificates would be required?

5. After the immediate episode, what then?
   a. When should mobilization commence?
   b. Is physiotherapy of any advantage?
   c. What arrangements should be made about return to work?
   d. Is recurrence or permanent disability likely?
   e. What preventive measures would you take?
   f. What opportunities does this illness provide for health promotion?

D. U. Shepherd, Melbourne

488   MR. NATHAN S.   AGED 42   BUTCHER

1. Where are the possible sites of Mr. S.'s back pathology?
   a. What is the significance of the narrowed intervertebral space?
   b. What pathology could there be in other intervertebral joints?
   c. What soft tissue changes could be present in his back?
   d. Do any bone diseases have to be excluded?

2. What investigations are appropriate in chronic lumbar backache?
   a. What help might discography be?
   b. How can myelography help?
   c. What biochemical investigations could be indicated?

3. How can recurrent backache and sciatica be treated?
   a. When are cold and/or heat therapy used?
   b. When is rest and when is mobilization indicated?
   c. What back exercises are of value?
   d. What forms of manipulation are helpful?
   e. Should anti-inflammatory drugs be prescribed?
   f. When should a corset or brace be prescribed?
   g. What is the place of surgery?

4. When is functional overlay or malingering diagnosed?
   a. How often are psychosomatic factors involved in chronic backache?
   b. In the absence of physical signs how can the genuineness of back pain be assessed?

D. G. Chambers, Clare, Australia

489   MR. J.D.   AGED 48

1. What is the nature and pathogenesis of the relatively common 'lumbago' seen in general practice?
   a. In what ways may the clinical findings in 'lumbago' differ from those in a classical prolapse of, say, L5–S1 disc?
   b. What is the natural history of acute lumbago?

2. In Mr. D.'s case psychological and social elements are intertwined with the 'medical' condition. List as many (stated and implied) as you can.
   a. What steps might Mrs. D. have already taken in relation to
      – the marriage?
      – tenancy of the house?
   b. In general, what significance may be attached to the phenomenon 'Did not attend'?

J. D. E. Knox, Dundee·

MRS. V.S.   AGED 48   HOUSEWIFE   **490**

1. What is the mechanism of this type of low back pain?
   a. Is it a part of lumbar disc disease?
   b. Is it usually precipitated by a more significant injury than in the case of Mrs. V.S.?
   c. What will the X-rays show?

2. What is the natural history of such an episode of low back pain?
   a. How long does the pain usually last?
   b. Does the patient usually develop nerve root irritation with leg pain?
   c. Does the patient usually experience sensory or motor symptoms in the lower extremities?

3. How would you treat the patient?
   a. How much bed rest will be required?
   b. Will manipulation help?
   c. Will acupuncture help?
   d. Do you prescribe analgesics or muscle relaxants or both?
   e. Do muscle relaxants really work?
   f. What is the role of exercise in treatment?
   g. Can future attacks be prevented?

R. L. Perkin, Toronto

MR. R.   AGED 40   TRADESMAN   **491**

1. Does Mediterranean back exist?
   a. Is the prolonged compensation back injury more prevalent in migrants?
   b. Is it a manifestation of an underlying depression, phobia or anxiety?
   c. Should the doctor seek the help of an interpreter to elicit symptoms related to emotional problems?
   d. Does it respond to compensation?

2. Should the doctor have departed from his usual practice of treating back injuries with rest and analgesics and immediately embarked on a course of injections and manipulation which would appear to be closer to the treatment regime offered in the country of origin of this workman?
   a. Is the practice of 'ethnic medicine', outlined above, ethical?
   b. Is it cost effective?
   c. Should new arrivals be educated to expect and accept the medical standards and customs of their new country?

    d.   With a national and a community funded health service is it justifiable to provide expensive and non-proven remedies on the basis of ethnicity?

3.   How would you treat this injury?
    a.   Do X-rays help in the diagnosis?
    b.   What is the value of physiotherapy?
    c.   Do alternative medicine practitioners have any role in treatment, e.g. chiropractors?
    d.   What part does poor posture have in the causation?

P. F. Gill, Hobart

492   MR. P.M.   AGED 38   SHIP'S CAPTAIN

1.   Is it possible to pick which cases of backache will do well?
    a.   What anatomical structures give rise to backache?
    b.   What is the natural history of disc lesions?
    c.   What features suggest nerve root involvement?

2.   How much does one's knowledge of the patient's personality influence management?
    a.   If this man had been a man with a poor work record would his management have been different; if so, why?
    c.   Should the general practitioner try to influence the orthopaedic specialist?

3.   Do unusual pain features rule out organic disease?
    a.   How would one distinguish the organic from the 'functional'?
    b.   What are the merits of the various investigations for backache?
    c.   Is headache a feature of lumbar disc disease?

A. L. A. Reid, Newcastle, Australia

493   MR. A.B.   AGED 38   LABOURER

1.   Why has this patient returned to the physician?
    a.   What is and what should be your reaction to his improvement?
    b.   What is the place of chiropractic in the management of musculoskeletal problems?
    c.   Can an effective doctor–patient relationship continue to exist here?

2.   How can motivation be accurately assessed in problems with compensation, insurance, and medicolegal complications?
    a.   To what extent do physicians prejudge such cases?

b. What is the 'secondary gain' which is attributed to this patient because of his disability?
c. How is our ability to provide optimal care hindered in cases in which we must make a medical report to a third party?
d. Is the first priority in these cases always the optimization of health for the patient?

E. Domovitch, Toronto

MR. D.F.   AGED 65   SEMI-RETIRED   494

1. What are the essential problems in his problem list?
   a. What are the differential diagnostic entities to be entertained in this case?
   b. What general category of diseases should be entertained with the presence of these skin findings?
   c. What are the ramifications of a normocytic, normochromic anaemia in a 65 year old male with backache?

2. If in the clinical management of this patient, an intravenous pyelogram is considered, what factors should be kept in mind?
   a. In what conditions is there a higher than normal chance of developing anuria after an intravenous pyelogram?
   b. What measures may be instituted before the X-ray study to lessen the likelihood of anuria?
   c. Certain radio-opaque dyes are more likely to induce anuria after intravenous injection in a patient with this diagnosis. Which is one of the safest dyes for the contrast study?

3. What are the main diseases to be considered in the differential diagnosis in a patient with this degree of back pain?
   a. What tests can reliably rule out gout, rheumatoid arthritis, and ankylosing spondylitis as a cause of this problem?
   b. What salient laboratory tests should be ordered if one entertains the diagnosis of multiple myeloma as a cause of this problem?
   c. What are the likely primary sites if this is a case of metastatic cancer of the spine?

L. H. Amundson, Sioux Falls, SD, USA

MR. J.T.   AGED 50   495

1. Why might the BP have become difficult to control?

2. How can a doctor establish whether or not the patient is compliant?
   a. What are the causes of poor compliance?

  b. What steps can be taken to improve compliance?
  c. Are any investigations necessary?

 3. Are there any underlying emotional factors?
  a. To what extent are lifestyle changes possible?
  b. Can a doctor influence a patient's motivation and insight?
  c. Is psychotherapy indicated in a patient in whom motivation and insight are lacking?

 4. What should be done about the coin lesion?
  a. What further tests would help make the diagnosis?
  b. What are the indications for surgery?
  c. What are the risks and benefits of surgery in this case?

E. Domovitch, Toronto

496 MR. M.S.   AGED 68   RETIRED STEELWORKER

 1. What disease do you think the family physician is looking for?
  a. If the X-ray is negative, is the bone scan likely to be helpful?
  b. What do you think the doctor noted in the rectum?
  c. What blood test(s) would you order?
  d. If these tests are not helpful, what else might assist in making the diagnosis?

 2. If the diagnosis is made, is there any treatment?
  a. What surgical treatment is used?
  b. Is there any other form of treatment?
  c. What is the prognosis?
  d. Should he alter his gardening activities?

 3. What discussions might take place between the physician and the patient and his wife?
  a. What is the effect of orchidectomy on potency?
  b. Is sexuality an issue in a 68 year old man and his spouse?
  c. Should this be discussed with either or both of them?

C. A. Moore, Hamilton, Canada

497 MRS. R.S.   AGED 24   HOUSEWIFE

 1. What are the possible causes of backache?
  a. Why is backache a symptom of pelvic infection?
  b. How can backache result from a psychosomatic cause?

 2. How could you diagnose this case?
  a. What tests would you perform?

b. What is the relevance of the husband's present behaviour and past history?

3. How would a VD clinic manage this case?

4. What would be your management approach?
   a. Would physiotherapy play any part in the treatment?
   b. How would you counsel in this case?
   c. Who should be treated?

E. J. H. North, Melbourne

MR. S.P.Y.   AGED 24

498

1. What is your assessment of this situation?
   a. What pathological processes underly his pain?
   b. What is the connection between symptoms and radiological signs?
   c. What part has his work played in the causation?
   d. What responsibility does his employer have for his problem?
   e. In these days of unemployment is he at risk of losing his job?
   f. How much trouble is his back going to cause in the future?
   g. Why does he need a swivel chair and has he been using it properly?
   h. What role does a GP have in industrial medicine?

2. What are your treatment plans for this man?
   a. Does he need time off work and if so for how long in the first instance?
   b. Should your certificate give an estimate of likely time off in total or should it merely cover the period until you see him next?
   c. Does he need bed rest?
   d. What is meant by bed rest?
   e. Does he need physiotherapy?
   f. Does the physiotherapist come to him or does he go to the physiotherapist?
   g. Does he need medication? If so, what medication?
   h. Does he need hospitalization?
   i. Does he need home visits?
   j. Does he need a district nurse or home help?

3. What additional patient education plans are indicated.at this stage?
   a. If the patient had read the X-ray report, is there a need to explain and interpret?
   b. Do plastic models of the lumbar spine have a role in patient education?
   c. Is there a need to anticipate a patient expectation for a second opinion?

    d.   Where can a GP direct a patient to get an explanation of his rights and obligations under the appropriate legislation – e.g. Worker's Compensation, Social Security?

    e.   Is sexual intercourse compatible with advice to spend the next week in bed?

D. Levet, Hobart

499 MR. A.S.   AGED 18   LABOURER

1. What were the likely diagnoses at the initial presentation?
    a.   What investigations may be appropriate at this stage if you suspect a prolapsed intervertebral disc?
    b.   What treatment would you advise and why?
    c.   What are the risks of treatment for this condition?
    d.   What are the implications for subsequent employment?

2. How do you cope with a situation in which you or one of your colleagues may have missed an important diagnosis?
    a.   Is honesty the best policy?
    b.   Should the threat of litigation affect your clinical practice?
    c.   What precautions should you take if confronted by a medico-legal problem?

3. What pathological process might account for the findings at the later consultation?
    a.   What investigations might be appropriate at this stage?
    b.   What is the most likely cause of inferior vena caval obstruction in a young man?
    c.   What treatment is available?

E. C. Gambrill, Crawley, UK

500 ROBERT P.   AGED 4

1. What is 'irritable hip'?
    a.   Do you think this diagnosis is justified in the first instance?
    b.   What pathological process is taking place?
    c.   Who does the making of an immediate initial diagnosis benefit most, the patient or the doctor?
    d.   What are the dangers of making an immediate diagnosis?

2. Why did Robert limp?
    a.   What other symptoms would have been important?
    b.   Under what circumstances would you have referred him to a consultant?

3. Is rest an important part of the treatment?
   a. What purpose did the four day period of rest serve?
   b. Is it important to make a correct diagnosis when the patient is first seen?

4. What are the dangers of making a diagnosis of irritable hip?
   a. What are the alternative diagnoses?
   b. How does tuberculosis of the hip present?
   c. How should it be managed?
   d. Is early diagnosis important?

5. What would you have done about Robert?
   a. What investigations could have been done to make the diagnosis clearer?
   b. How do you decide whether to carry out further tests?

G. Strube, Crawley, UK

MR. FRANCIS M.   AGED 50   INVALID PENSIONER   **501**

1. Both general practitioner and orthopaedic surgeon suspected osteomyelitis. What steps were taken as a result of this provisional diagnosis?
   a. What blood tests should be performed to identify the cause of Mr. M's symptoms and signs?
   b. What other investigations are indicated?
   c. In the absence of any radiological signs to explain the symptoms and signs what alternatives are left to the surgeon?

2. After exhaustive tests the orthopaedic surgeon is unable to explain Mr. M's symptoms and signs and has referred him back to his GP. Meanwhile, Mr. M. has lost 26 lb in weight, his pains continue in his left leg and his fever and sweats persist. What possibilities must the GP now consider?
   a. A full blood count reveals a Hb of 10.7 g, a WCC of 8000/cmm with 11% band forms, a moderate lymphopenia and marked rouleaux formation. Occasional myelocytes and metamyelocytes are seen and the ESR is 117 mm in 1 hour.
      – What pathological process or processes should now be suspected?
      – What investigations are indicated in the light of these suspicions?
      – How are these investigations best arranged?

3. In view of the fact that Mr. and Mrs. M. are very dependent upon each other and that she is confined to a wheelchair, what special considerations should govern the GP's management of the situation?

a. If Mr. M.'s treatment involves oral prednisone what responsibilities now rest with the GP?

b. If reduction of the steroids results in a resurgence in Mr. M.'s symptoms, what signs should be looked for and what investigations should be carried out?

W. L. Ogborne, Sydney

502 JOHN Q. AGED 15 SCHOOLBOY

1. What is the likely diagnosis and what diagnoses must be excluded?
   a. What forms of osteochondritis (osteochondrosis) can you recall? At what age does each tend to occur?
   b. Is Osgood-Schlatter's disease (osteochondrosis of the tibial tuberosity) usually limited to that bone?
   c. What may be clinical pointers to the diagnosis of acute osteomyelitis? Are there any clinical pointers to the diagnosis of sarcoma of a bone? Are there any clinical pointers to the diagnosis of septic arthritis?

2. What are likely to be John's major worries when he presents?
   a. What do you know about adolescents and their concepts of identity?
   b. What defence mechanisms do adolescents commonly use to deal with problems concerning independence?
   c. What treatment advice would you give John if he proves to have osteochrondrosis of the tibial tuberosity?

3. Do you have any views concerning teenagers who are brought to you for treatment?
   a. Are you comfortable speaking to both parent and child in the same consultation?
   b. What are the advantages and disadvantages of trying to see an adolescent brought by parents separately from them?

P. Freeling, London

503 MR. W.K. AGED 82 RETIRED SCHOOLMASTER

1. What common joint diseases are likely to be causes of his symptoms?
   a. What tests would you carry out to confirm the diagnosis?
   b. Is oral therapy likely to be helpful?
   c. What groups of drugs can be tried, and in what sequence?

2. Is a surgical opinion required now?
   a. What operation is likely to help an osteoarthritic hip?
   b. How soon can the patient expect mobility after surgery?

   c.   What long-term hazards are there to surgery?
   d.   Are the patient's home conditions important?

J. Grabinar, Bromley, UK

MRS. E.B.   AGED 71   **504**

1. What was the diagnosis given by her own doctor?
   a.   How could this have been confirmed?
   b.   What treatments are available?
   c.   What are the dangers of long-term Butazolidin (phenyl-butazone)?

2. What is the true diagnosis?
   a.   How can this be confirmed?
   b.   What other conditions can cause secondary hyperparathyroidism?
   c.   What treatment is available?

3. How could this condition have been prevented?
   a.   Discuss the problems of long-term surveillance in general practice.
   b.   What other conditions require long-term surveillance?

A. G. Strube, Crawley, UK

MR. DONALD V.   AGED 48   **505**

1. What problems for Mr. Donald V., apart from his obvious medical illness, should have been considered by his physicians during his hospital care?
   a.   What is the effect of separating a seriously ill man from the security of his family, spouse and community?
   b.   What factors determine the successful outcome of hospitalization apart from the medical management?
   c.   What are the psychological stresses of an undiagnosed illness?

2. What are the unusual features of this illness?
   a.   How often does this illness occur in males?
   b.   How often is the antinuclear antibody titer negative in cases of lupus erythematosus?
   c.   What are the chances that all lab work up, apart from the skin biopsy and an elevated sedimentation rate, would have been unremarkable?

3. Considering Mr. Donald V.'s inexperience with serious illness or hospitals, what further questions, apart from a medical history, should have been asked by his physicians?
   a. What are the most likely diseases that Mr. D.V. would have guessed he was suffering from?
   b. How much patient education is required for an illness such as this?
   c. Other than his doctors, what persons are likely to share information with the patient regarding the seriousness of the disease and its prognosis?

4. What effects could the illness have had on Mr. D.V.'s psychological coping skills?
   a. What are the central nervous system manifestations of systemic lupus?
   b. What effects could the fever and debilitation of the illness have had?
   c. Are there any important side effects of the drug used to treat Mr. Donald V.'s illness?

C. Driscoll, Iowa City

506   **MRS. B.**   **AGED 75**   **WIDOW**

1. What are the most common causes of nocturnal leg cramps in a 75 year old lady?
   a. If the arterial circulation in the legs is normal, are any further investigations indicated?
   b. Does restless legs syndrome exist and if so how is it defined?
   c. What role do benzodiazepines play in the management of leg cramps at any age?

2. What are the most common causes of an elevated serum potassium in an otherwise physically and biochemically healthy individual?
   a. In a healthy person what level of serum potassium is tolerable?
   b. What is the probability of a laboratory error accounting for a serum potassium of 6.2 mmol/l on the first occasion and 6.4 mmol/l on the second report?
   c. Discuss the reasons why the investigation of the problem should or should not be conducted in a general practitioner's office rather than by an endocrinologist.

3. If the elevated serum potassium was persistent, what steps could be taken to prevent potentially serious consequences?
   a. How high a level of serum potassium is acceptable in a 75 year old?

b. What would be the simplest treatment of this problem that would not interfere with the lifestyle of this lady?
c. What are the consequences of labelling an otherwise completely healthy woman with an illness?

W. W. Rosser, Ottawa

MR. BRUNO G.   AGED 54   SHOP ASSISTANT   **507**

1. What organs can be damaged by cigarette smoking?
   a. What are the lung changes produced by smoking?
   b. How might his coronary thrombosis be related to his smoking?
   c. What relation is there between intermittent claudication and smoking?
   d. What percentage of lung cancers occur in cigarette smokers?

2. What is the significance of Mr. G.'s symptoms and signs?
   a. How common are specific lung symptoms and signs in lung cancer?
   b. When does clubbing of the fingers occur?
   c. What relation do peripheral neuritis, bone pains and non-pitting oedema of the extemities have to lung cancer?
   d. What investigations does he require?

3. How can the morbidity from cigarette smoking be reduced?
   a. How can health education on this subject be promoted?
   b. What forms of help can be offered to smokers who wish to stop?
   c. What is the success rate of the various smoking cure methods?
   d. What is the place of hypnotherapy and group therapy?
   e. What is the role of the family doctor in reducing smoking morbidity?

D. G. Chambers, Clare, Australia

MRS. A.J.   AGED 43   HOUSEWIFE   **508**

1. What is the most likely diagnosis?
   a. What movements of the joint would prove the diagnosis and why?

2. Would any investigations help you?
   a. Does a negative X-ray for calcification help you?
   b. Did you suspect a possible secondary carcinoma – If not, why not?

3. How would you manage this problem?

    a.   Is there a need for physiotherapy?
    b.   Could acupuncture be of benefit?
    c.   If not, why not?

D. S. Muecke, Adelaide

509   SYLVIA BLACK   AGED 26   APPLE PACKER

1. What is the diagnosis?
   a. Describe the symptoms and signs of tenosynovitis.
   b. What is your 'whole person' diagnosis?

2. How would you treat her forearm?
   a. What is the main first line treatment?
   b. What other treatment is appropriate?
   c. What further treatment may be indicated if initial response is poor?

3. What are the other aspects of managing this patient?
   a. How can she avoid losing her job?
   b. Would you involve her husband or her parents?
   c. Who else in the community might you involve?
   d. Is she eligible for worker's compensation payments?
   e. What preventive advice would you give?

R. P. Strasser, Melbourne

510   MRS. P.R.   AGED 51   HOUSEWIFE

1. What process is at work?
   a. How is it caused?
   b. Why does movement aggravate it?
   c. What other things can aggravate it?

2. How can it be treated?
   a. What complications could follow injection?
   b. Is operation ever indicated?
   c. What operation?
   d. Are there any other methods of treatment?
   e. Can manipulation help?

3. What is the prognosis?
   a. How long do patients have it before seeking help?
   b. What is the recurrence rate?
   c. What is the prognosis if left alone?

E. J. H. North, Melbourne

MOLLY A.   AGED 63

511

1. What is your provisional diagnosis?
   a. What other conditions should you exclude?
   b. How?

2. What treatment would you prescribe?
   a. Would you use corticosteroids?
   b. If so, by what route? In what form? How much? For how long? With what precautions?

3. How would you monitor the course of the disease?
   a. There is an initial dramatic improvement on prednisolone with a fall in the ESR to normal levels on 10 mg daily by mouth but attempts to reduce this dose are met with a recrudescence both symptomatic and objective. How long do you persevere?
   b. Even on 10 mg prednisolone daily the ESR is tending to climb after some six weeks. Should you hang on? Put up the dose? Think again?
   c. What complication is likely to result if not adequately controlled?

J. A. Stevens, Ulverstone, Australia

MR. B.Z.   AGED 26   DENTIST

512

1. What is the differential diagnosis?
   a. Enumerate the essential differences between rheumatoid and osteoarthritis.
   b. What are the features of Reiter's syndrome?
   c. Which joints are usually affected by psoriatic arthropathy?
   d. What are your criteria for diagnosing gout?

2. What further aspects of his history might be important?
   a. What is the significance of fleeting pains?
   b. Of which conditions may carpal tunnel syndrome be a feature?
   c. What infectious illnesses might affect the joints?
   d. What are the non-articular complications of rheumatoid disease?

3. What investigations would help in making your diagnosis?
   a. What percentage of rheumatoid arthritics have a positive RA latex test?
   b. What conditions would you suspect if the ESR were over 100?
   c. What blood tests would help to substantiate a diagnosis of SLE?
   d. What tests should be requested on the aspirate from a joint effusion?

4. What particular problems will be posed for this patient?
   a. What agencies might help with the support of chronic arthritics?
   b. What allowances may be claimed by the physically disabled?
   c. What does 'arthritis' mean to the patient?
   d. What is the role of 'alternative medicine' in the management of chronic disease?

T. A. I. Bouchier Hayes, Camberley, UK

513 JULIE FREDRICKSON   AGED 28   TYPIST

1. What are the possible diagnoses?
   a. How does rheumatoid arthritis present?
   b. Could this be osteoarthritis?
   c. What are the seronegative arthritides?

2. What investigations are indicated?
   a. What would you expect to find on X-ray?
   b. Does a negative rheumatoid factor rule out rheumatoid arthritis?
   c. Would any other blood tests be helpful in making the diagnosis?
   d. How much do all these tests cost?

3. How would you manage this problem?
   a. What medication(s) would you use?
   b. Are there any side effects to be concerned about?
   c. Will any particular diet prevent progression of rheumatoid arthritis?
   d. Does regular exercise help?
   e. What about a copper bracelet?

R. P. Strasser, Melbourne

514 MR. G.C.   AGED 49   MANUFACTURER

1. What factors may influence the activity of rheumatoid disease?
   a. How may activity be assessed?
   b. What is the significance of the positive RA factor?

2. Discuss the treatment of rheumatoid arthritis.
   a. What are the advantages of the new anti-inflammatory agents compared with aspirin?
   b. What are the toxic effects of gold therapy and how can these be avoided?
   c. Is there a place for immuno-suppressive therapy?

A. G. Strube, Crawley, UK

MISS E.W.   AGED 52   UNEMPLOYED CLERK

515

1. What are the major causes of severe disability in middle-aged people?
   a. How many patients with rheumatoid arthritis are permanently crippled by the disease?
   b. What steps can the doctor take to minimize disability?
   c. What aids to daily living are available for patients handicapped by a chronic disease?

2. What major problems are likely to arise for this family in the future?
   a. How would you assess the ability of a patient to cope in his/her social situation?
   b. What alternative accommodation might be available for this lady when she is left alone?
   c. What resources are available in your community to help with this type of problem? When would be the correct time for referral?

3. What do you understand by the terms 'reactive' and 'endogenous' depression?
   a. What implications does this classification have for choosing appropriate management?
   b. What criteria would you use in assessing the need for specialist referral or hospital admission in a case of depression?
   c. In what, if any, circumstances might you consider compulsory admission to hospital to be in the best interests of the patient?

E. C. Gambrill, Crawley, UK

MR. P.   AGED 68   SELF-EMPLOYED ENGINEER

516

1. What are the major management problems here?
   a. Should he be on antibiotics?
   b. What about steroids?
   c. What about his bone marrow depression?

2. How should his arthritis be treated?
   a. Should he have a non-steroidal anti-inflammatory agent?
   b. Which ones may produce bone marrow depression?
   c. What about gold?

3. What is the natural history of rheumatoid arthritis?
   a. Is late onset unusual?
   b. Are our diagnostic tests sensitive enough to pick up early rheumatoid illness?

    c.   Do some elderly folk develop the typical destructive type joint lesions without complaining of symptoms?

P. F. Gill, Hobart

517 S.C.   AGED 6 MONTHS

1. What aetiology should the doctor be thinking about in this case?
    a.   Should he confront the mother?
    b.   Should he voice his suspicions to her?
    c.   How likely is it that the child could have sustained this injury unknown to anyone?
    d.   Do you have any other suggestions?
    e.   How common is this?

2. Are there any features which might lead the family physician towards the causation of the fracture?
    a.   What are the features of families in which child abuse occurs?
    b.   Is there a relationship to parental age, family history and alcohol?

3. If the doctor's concerns are confirmed, what course of action should he take?
    a.   Is he compelled to report his suspicions to any agency or authority?
    b.   Should he hospitalize the child because of the injury?
    c.   Should he hospitalize the child for any other purpose?
    d.   Are there community agencies or self-help groups to whom this family might be referred?

C. A. Moore, Hamilton, Canada

518 BILL D.   AGED 12   SCHOOLBOY

1. What actions would you take immediately?
    a.   What are the features of concussion?
    b.   Could the clinical features be consistent with an extradural haemorrhage?
    c.   What is the most likely diagnosis in this case?

2. What actions would you take?
    a.   What observations would you make?
    b.   What investigations would you carry out?
    c.   What would be the indications for hospital admission?
    d.   Under what circumstances would you send Bill home?

3. What follow up would you order if it is decided to send Bill home?
   a. What general instructions would you give the parents?
   b. For what warning signs would you ask them to look?
   c. When would you arrange to review the patient?
   d. What preventive advice would you offer?

W. E. Fabb, Melbourne

MR. DAVID D.   AGED 28   SCHOOLTEACHER   **519**

1. What diagnostic hypotheses would you entertain?
   a. What particular injury must be excluded in this case?
   b. Over what period do the features of extradural haemorrhage usually appear?
   c. What are the most reliable signs of an enlarging extradural haemorrhage?
   d. What importance do you ascribe to pupil signs in such cases?
   e. What is the most likely diagnosis in this man?

2. What would you do for this patient?
   a. What are the indications for skull X-ray in cases of head injury?
   b. How often does the skull X-ray alter management?
   c. What observations are needed in this case?

3. What follow up would you order?
   a. If the skull X-ray is normal and the patient is clinically normal after four hours of observation, what would you do if this man was to stay alone overnight in a hotel room?
   b. Would you take different action if he was to return home to his wife and two children?
   c. When would you see him again and what review would you carry out?
   d. What opportunities does this situation present for preventive care?

W. E. Fabb, Melbourne

MR. GEORGE K.   AGED 48   UNEMPLOYED   **520**

1. What actions would you take immediately?
   a. What is the usual way of controlling scalp bleeding?
   b. What techniques can be used if these measures fail?

2. What actions would you take next?
   a. What investigations would you carry out?
   b. What observations would you make?
   c. If after four hours the patient is still apparently intoxicated, what would you do?

3. What condition(s) would you be watching for?
   a. If this patient does have an intracranial haemorrhage, which is more likely – a subdural or an extradural haemorrhage?
   b. Why are alcoholics more prone to subdural haematomas than normal people?
   c. Over what time period is the patient at risk of subdural haematoma?

4. What follow-up care would you order when the patient is ready for discharge to his home?
   a. What instructions would you give the patient?
   b. What arrangements would you make for the patient to be observed?
   c. What dietary advice would you give?
   d. What analgesics, if any, would you prescribe?
   e. What opportunity does this situation present for health promotion and preventive care?

W. E. Fabb, Melbourne

521 MASTER P.H.   AGED 8   SCHOOLBOY

1. What are the implications of this injury?
   a. What complications could occur?
   b. How would you detect them?
   c. What are the implications of signs of cord trauma?

2. What will you do immediately?
   a. What is the most important precaution?
   b. How can you stabilize an injured cervical spine?

3. What will you do next? (You are a long way, 120 miles, from the nearest orthopaedic surgeon.)
   a. What transportation is most suitable?
   b. What precautions would you take during transportation?
   c. Should a doctor or nurse travel with him?

Follow-up note. This boy's head was sandbagged. He was transported with care to Edmonton. The orthopaedic surgeon confirmed your diagnosis and took him to theatre to position traction. During the operation the boy stopped breathing, but they were able to revive him and he subsequently made an uneventful recovery.

J. K. Shearman, Hamilton, Canada

MRS. CARLA de P.   AGED 36   HOUSEWIFE   **522**

1. What conditions would you suspect?
   a. What damage may occur in extension – flexion (whiplash) injuries?
   b. Why are odontoid views advisable in such injuries?

2. What would you do for her?
   a. What sequence of steps would you carry out in assessing her injury?
   b. If no fracture is revealed, what treatment would you give her?
   c. What instructions would you give her as she leaves?
   d. What follow-up arrangements would you make?
   e. What long-term sequelae may occur in such injuries?
   f. What steps would you take to prevent these sequelae?

W. E. Fabb, Melbourne

G.H.   AGED 9   SCHOOLBOY   **523**

1. How does a doctor gain a 'sixth sense' about clinical matters? In such a case as this, it was a valuable positive influence.
   a. Should a doctor place any reliance on intuition to persuade him toward non-interference?
   b. Should all traumatic injuries be X-rayed?
   c. Would the doctor have been unwise to delay X-ray, given 2 to 3 weeks symptomatology?

2. What is the morbid condition involved?
   a. What is the most likely clinical course of osteosarcoma in this position?
   b. Is surgical amputation advisable or practicable?

3. Clearly the technical treatment of this patient will be outside the province of the family doctor, but how does he go about supporting the rest of the family?
   a. What support agencies are available?
   b. What can the family doctor do personally?

P. L. Gibson, Auckland

MR. KERRY McC.   AGED 39   SCHOOLTEACHER   **524**

1. What is the probable diagnosis?
   a. What are the clinical features of supraspinatus tendonitis?
   b. What is the natural history of this condition?

    c.   What is the relationship of this condition to frozen shoulder?

    d.   What variants in presentation are seen?

2.   What would you do for this man?
    a.   What investigations are appropriate?
    b.   What is the place of steroid injections into the subacromial space?
    c.   What is the value of anti-inflammatory drugs?
    d.   How much analgesia do such patients need?
    e.   If an X-ray of Mr. McC.'s shoulder showed marked calcification of the supraspinatus tendon, what would you do?

3.   What preventive measures would you advise?
    a.   How can this man minimize recurrence?
    b.   How would you explain his condition to him?
    c.   What advice would you give about what to do at the onset of a recurrence?
    d.   What prognosis would you give Mr. McC.?

W. E. Fabb, Melbourne

525   MR. B.F.   AGED 42   BUSINESSMAN

1.   How do you make your diagnosis?
    a.   What diagnostic investigations are necessary?
    b.   Is gout one of your differential diagnoses?

2.   What is the treatment plan?
    a.   Physical treatment of splints and rest – are these necessary?
    b.   Are anti-inflammatory and anti-uricosuric agents of benefit to the patient?
    c.   Can local steroid infiltration cure the condition?

3.   Future management problems?
    a.   How common is this condition?
    b.   What is the recurrence rate?
    c.   Do you advise the patient to discontinue all sport?

B. M. Fehler, Johannesburg

526   PETER N.   AGED 3½

1.   What are likely causes?
    a.   What might the X-ray show?
    b.   Describe the process of the lesion?
    c.   What are the age limits for this condition?
    d.   Why is this so?

2. How would you treat it?
   a. Is it likely to recur?
   b. How can it be prevented?
   c. What is the frequency of this condition?

E. J. H. North, Melbourne

MRS. H.　　AGED 55　　　　　　　　　　**527**

1. What is the most likely diagnosis?
   a. Describe the classical signs of a Colles' fracture
   b. Describe the anatomical deformities.
   c. Describe the accepted treatment.
   d. What are the anticipated disabilities resulting from incorrect or inadequate reduction of this fracture?

2. Was the general practitioner justified in making the initial decision on his own behalf?
   a. What factors should be considered when making a clinical judgement?
   b. What is the meaning of responsibility in reference to medical care?
   c. How does this incident exemplify the concept of treating the problem and not the disease?
   d. Was the type of conservative treatment instituted the correct one?

3. What is the basis to support or otherwise a claim for liability under Worker's Compensation legislation for an injury sustained while taking the employer's dog for a walk?
   a. What is the general practitioner's function in relating injury to cause in such cases?
   b. Should Mrs. H.'s pre-existing disability influence her rights under such legislation?
   c. Is it preferable for all compensatable injuries to be treated at special accident clinics?
   d. What is the relationship between the general practitioner and expert medical assessors?

D. A. Game, Adelaide

MR. DONALD G.　　AGED 24　　CLERK　　　　**528**

1. What possible injuries may result from this trauma?
   a. How important is a fracture of the proximal phalanx?
   b. What is the mechanism of injury in Bennett's fracture?

2. How would you establish the diagnosis?
   a. What clinical signs would you seek?
   b. What X-ray views are needed?

3. How would you manage each of the possible diagnoses?
   a. How would you manage a fracture of the proximal or terminal phalanx?
   b. What is your management of Bennett's fracture?
   c. What rehabilitative measures would you arrange?

W. E. Fabb, Melbourne

529 **MISS DEBORAH C.   AGED 16   SCHOOLGIRL**

1. What specific enquiries would you make?
   a. How will knowledge of the mechanism of injury help in diagnosis?
   b. How relevant is the sequence of events following injury?
   c. What significance do you place on the occurrence of rapid swelling of the knee joint following injury?

2. What conditions can result from knee injuries sustained at sport?
   a. What are the most common knee injuries in body contact sports?
   b. How often is tibial condyle fracture an accompanying injury?

3. What examination would you carry out?
   a. What are the diagnostic signs of ruptured lateral ligament, ruptured medial ligament, ruptured cruciates and meniscus injury?
   b. If you are unable to examine the knee because of severe pain, what would you do?

4. What are the indications for X-ray in knee injuries?
   a. What views would you order routinely?
   b. What value is there in a 'skyline' patellar view?

5. How would you manage this situation?
   a. If under anaesthesia, the knee was found to be stable, if no fracture was detected on X-ray, but blood was aspirated from the knee joint, what would you do?
   b. What rehabilitative measures would you arrange?
   c. What opportunity does this situation present for preventive care?

W. E. Fabb, Melbourne

MRS. R.   AGED 36   HOUSEWIFE

530

1. Is it justifiable to continue episodic treatment when surgery will probably remove the need for treatment?
    a. What are the patient's rights?
    b. What are the risks with medical treatment?
    c. What are the risks of surgical treatment?
    d. What is the prognosis of both?

2. Why has this patient avoided surgery?
    a. Is it because she failed to achieve rapport with the consultant?
    b. Should the doctor suggest a second consultant?
    c. How far should the doctor explore the patient's reluctance for surgery?
    d. Should the doctor insist on surgery as a better option?

P. F. Gill, Hobart

J.F.   AGED 17   STUDENT

531

1. What conditions have to be considered?
    a. How would you explain to the patient the anterior tibial (shin splint) syndrome?
    b. What are the complications of the anterior tibial syndrome?
    c. What is a stress fracture?
    d. Of what group of disorders is Osgood-Schlatter's disease an example?

2. What investigations would you do?
    a. How long does it take for a stress fracture to show up on X-ray?
    b. What are the characteristic X-ray changes of chondromalacia patellae?
    c. What part does joint aspiration play in the management of a traumatic effusion?

3. What advice would you give this patient?
    a. Outline a training programme for an athletic 17 year old male preparing for a five mile run with boots and pack.
    b. How would you modify the programme for a female?
    c. What are the characteristics of a good running shoe?
    d. How can blisters be avoided?

4. What is the role of the general practitioner in the management of minor sporting injuries?
    a. Explain ICE.
    b. For which sports are special medical examinations required?
    c. What is the immediate treatment of heat exhaustion?

T. A. I. Bouchier Hayes, Camberley, UK

532 MR. DOMINIC F. AGED 32 ACCOUNTANT

1. What is the likely cause of this man's injury
   a. What are the features of a ruptured plantaris muscle?
   b. Could this man have torn his gastrocnemius muscle?
   c. Is he likely to have a ruptured achilles tendon?

2. What would you do for him?
   a. What immediate treatment would you give?
   b. Would physiotherapy help; what would you order?

W. E. Fabb, Melbourne

533 MR. PETER M. AGED 18 CIGARETTE SALESMAN

1. What specific enquiries would you make?
   a. How relevant is it to determine the mechanism of injury?
   b. To what extent is the sequence of events following injury of diagnostic importance?

2. What examination would you carry out?
   a. What diagnostic features would you seek?
   b. How do you test for ankle instability?

3. What conditions can result from ankle injuries at sport?
   a. How would you recognize a complete rupture of the lateral ligament of the ankle?
   b. How would you recognize a malleolar fracture?
   c. How would you be certain of the diagnosis of sprained ankle?

4. What are the indications for X-ray in ankle injuries?
   a. What special views are needed sometimes to exclude fractures about the ankle?
   b. How do you ascertain when the tibio-fibular ligament is ruptured?
   c. What are the X-ray signs of ruptured lateral ligament of the ankle joint?

5. How would you manage this situation?
   a. What are the basic principles of management of a sprained ankle?
   b. When is surgery indicated in ankle injuries?
   c. What rehabilitative measures do you use in ankle injuries?
   d. What opportunity does this injury provide for preventive care?

W. E. Fabb, Melbourne

MISS A.M.   AGED 17   SHOP ASSISTANT

1. What are the possible diagnoses?
   a. Is an X-ray indicated?
   b. What would lead you to suspect a fracture?
   c. What features would lead you to suspect rupture of the lateral ligament?

2. Describe your management.
   a. Do anti-inflammatory agents help?
   b. What limits do you place on exercise?
   c. Is proprioception or balance affected by such an injury?
   d. What place has strapping in ankle sprain?
   e. Would a cold compress help?

R. W. Roberts, Ravensthorpe, Australia

MR. DEREK J.   AGED 29   SPORTS GOODS SALESMAN

1. What is the likely cause of this man's injury?
   a. What are the features of ruptured achilles tendon?
   b. Could anything else produce this clinical picture?

2. What would you do for him?
   a. What is the definitive treatment for ruptured achilles tendon?
   b. What rehabilitative measures would you arrange?
   c. What would you say if Mr. J. asks you when he is likely to be able to resume running?
   d. What opportunity does this situation provide for preventive care?

W. E. Fabb, Melbourne

MISS R.B.   AGED 14   SCHOOLGIRL

1. Why are these conditions seen more commonly in the adolescent?
   a. Ingrowing toe nails and plantar warts are often seen in the active, sporting types. Why does this occur?
   b. How could these conditions be prevented or minimized?
   c. What process is at work with acne and painful heavy periods in this 14 year old lass?

2. How would you go about treating this girl?
   a. Is there a priority? What?
   b. How would you treat plantar warts?
   c. How would you treat plain warts?
   d. What advice would you give for acne?

e. How would you treat the menstrual disorder?
f. How would you go about giving hormone treatment?
g. What concerns would the lass have, and the mother have?

E. J. H. North, Melbourne

537   MRS. S.W.   AGED 38   LIBRARIAN

1. What is the natural history of a fractured proximal phalanx of a minor toe?
   a. Should the fracture have healed after 24 days?
   b. Can pain persist after a fracture has united?
   c. Was the treatment and advice given by your partner appropriate?
   d. Has healing been delayed by inappropriate management?
   e. Has healing been delayed by non-compliance with his advice?

2. What are the indications for re X-ray?
   a. Do fractures of minor toe phalanges normally require follow up X-ray?
   b. Is this case any different?
   c. Will an X-ray alter the management of this situation?
   d. Does the fact that the injury comes under Worker's Compensation legislation affect the case for re X-ray?
   e. Is it reasonable to offer a re X-ray if clinically you feel it is not warranted?
   f. How much expertise should a GP have in interpreting progress of healing fractures?

3. Assuming the re X-ray report reads 'fracture line remains evident' what will your further management be?
   a. Will a metatarsal bar fitted to the shoe be of any benefit?
   b. How should the patient arrange for this to be done?
   c. Is she fit for work?
   d. Is there potential for prescribing a sedentary job as a temporary measure?
   e. Is there a need for further follow up?
   f. If so, when?
   g. Would this include radiological follow up?
   h. What if the fracture hadn't united by then?
   i. Should you speak to your partner?

D. Levet, Hobart

538   MISS HELEN C.   AGED 18   TYPIST

1. What structures might have been damaged?
   a. What structures are most vulnerable to transverse wrist lacerations?

b. In such injuries, are structures remote from the wound likely to be damaged?

2. How would you assess the damage?
   a. How do you assess tendon damage at the wrist?
   b. How do you assess nerve damage at the wrist?
   c. How do you exclude a foreign body in the wound?

3. What would you do immediately?
   a. How would you stop arterial haemorrhage at the wrist?
   b. How soon should a surgeon see the patient – immediately or in the morning?
   c. What rehabilitative measures would you expect to be instituted?
   d. What is the prognosis when nerves and tendons are divided at the wrist?
   e. What preventive action should be instituted at her workplace?

W. E. Fabb, Melbourne

MR. HARRY L.   AGED 42   SHEETMETAL WORKER   539

1. How would you assess this injury?
   a. What aspects of the physical examination are essential in the assessment of hand injuries?
   b. How do you assess the viability of crushed tissues?

2. What would you do immediately?
   a. What emergency care would you give for the crushed hand?
   b. What do you say when he asks, 'How bad is it, doctor; how long will I be off work?'

3. What might be done for this man by the hand surgeon?
   a. What are the basic principles of the management of a crushed hand?
   b. What rehabilitative measures should be undertaken, and when?

4. What factors other than the physical injury will be important in managing this man?
   a. What psychological and family problems would you be attempting to avoid?
   b. What economic and financial problems might occur?
   c. What opportunity does this accident provide for preventive action?

W. E. Fabb, Melbourne

540 WAYNE K.   AGED 3

1. How would you assess this situation?
   a. How do you assess the depth of a burn?
   b. What is the difference between this burn and burns caused by flame or boiling water?
   c. What would be the likely reaction of Wayne's mother?

2. What would your management be?
   a. What special problems do burns of the hand present?
   b. What is your immediate management?
   c. How would you cope with Mrs. K.'s feelings?
   d. What advice and assistance would you seek?
   e. What would be appropriate management for this burn?
   f. What rehabilitative measures would be needed?
   g. If this child's parents were musicians, what prognosis would you give when asked by his mother whether he will ever be able to play the piano in the future?
   h. What opportunity does this situation present for preventive care?

W. E. Fabb, Melbourne

541 MR. F.M.   AGED 50   PHARMACIST

1. How should you approach the patient with multiple somatic complaints?
   a. What are the main differential diagnostic possibilities of each of these somatic complaints?
   b. What is the importance of a general, screening type of initial workup for this kind of problem?
   c. What is the importance of age and sex in the decision regarding the scope of a workup in this setting?
   d. What are the advantages in recommending a general, preventive/prospective evaluation and workup when this has not been done for a period of time, regardless of the narrow scope of the current problem?
   e. What are the main factors to be considered in the treatment of endogenous depression?

2. What classifications of drugs are available for use in the therapy of depression?
   a. How can one assess improvement in the depression during therapy?
   b. What factors should be considered in the frequency of revisits and the anticipated duration of drug use?

3. How can the family physician ensure a continuation of the primary
    care role before, during, and after diagnosis and therapy?
    a. What are the importance and benefits of this continuing role to
        the patient?
    b. Is it important to consider patient preferences and choices in
        management and treatment plans?
    c. What is the optimal way to arrange for consultation and/or
        referral when indicated?

L. H. Amundson, Sioux Falls, SD, USA

MRS. D.H.   AGED 37   HOUSEWIFE   542

1. What is the likely diagnosis?
    a. Could there be a physical cause for the fatigue and insomnia?
    b. Is a physical examination indicated, and if so, what in particular
        will be sought?

2. Why does the recent death of her dog appear to have precipitated
    this problem?
    a. What is your concept of a 'family'? Can it include a pet?

3. Should the sexual problem be followed up? How?

4. Who else should be involved in this problem with her permission?
    a. Should she bring her husband on a future visit?
    b. Should she obtain another pet?

D. U. Shepherd, Melbourne

MR. CLEMENT K.   AGED 82   RETIRED FARMER   543

1. What was the chain of events leading to the consultation?
    a. Why do depressed patients often present requesting examin-
        ation?
    b. Could his presenting symptoms have been mainly physical?
    c. What is the risk of a busy family doctor treating only the
        physical complaints?

2. What sexual problems can arise in old age?
    a. What is the changing pattern of sexual activity as couples age?
    b. How does the decline in libido differ between the sexes?
    c. Why are old people more reluctant to mention sexual problems?
    d. What effect does degenerative disease have on sexual relations?

3. How should this man and his wife be treated?
    a. Does an aged man need to ejaculate to enjoy sexual intercourse?

b. Must he be able to sustain an erection to satisfy his wife?
c. Could the wife's jealousy be aggravated by senile dementia?
d. Could anti-depressants have a place in the treatment of this man?
e. What precautions are necessary in the use of anti-depressants in the elderly?

D. G. Chambers, Clare, Australia

544   MRS. E.N.   AGED 78

1. What are the causes of atrial fibrillation in an elderly person?
   a. What are the symptoms of hyperthyroidism in the elderly?
   b. What is the forme fruste of hyperthyroidism?
   c. What are the risks of tricyclic anti-depressants in the elderly?
   d. Are any special precautions needed in prescribing for patients with thyroid disease?

2. What is the connection between a life crisis such as bereavement, and physical disease?
   a. What diseases are especially likely to occur after a life crisis?
   b. Does concern and sympathy for emotional distress make it more difficult for the doctor to recognize a second diagnosis?

G. Strube, Crawley, UK

545   MRS. JOAN W.   AGED 70   HOUSEWIFE

1. What primary hypothesis might the locum make?
   a. Too much digoxin?
   b. Too much propranolol?
   c. Hypothyroidism?
   d. Involutional melancholia?
   e. Reactive depression?

2. What action might he take, regarding her drugs and the further elucidation of her problems?
   a. Add an anti-depressant?
   b. Arrange for thyroid function tests?
   c. Take her off all the drugs and arrange for thyroid function tests, and if necessary institute replacement therapy?
   d. Add thyroid replacement to her present list of drugs?

3. How often may slowly developing changes in a patient escape the notice of a family doctor?
   a. What dangers are engendered by familiarity?
   b. How often should frequent attenders have detailed reviews?

R. T. Mossop, Harare, Zimbabwe

MR. H. McG.　　AGED 68　　BREWERY WORKER

546

1. What aspects of history taking are highlighted?
   a. What differentiates relevant historical facts from 'red herrings'? How do you select historical truth from untruth? When is it appropriate to seek historical facts from another person?

2. What features would you expect to find to clinch your diagnosis?
   a. Which of the special tests listed would assist in proving your clinical diagnosis:
      – X-ray chest
      – ECG
      – Thyroid function tests
      – Renal function tests
      – Serum lipids
      – X-ray skull
   b. Describe features of chosen tests which would be appropriate to a diagnosis of myxoedema.

3. Does treatment pose problems?
   a. What therapeutic regime would you commence?
   b. How would you monitor response?
   c. Are there risks attending such treatment?
   d. What measure of recovery can you expect?

W. D. Jackson, Launceston, Australia

MRS. E.M.　　AGED 50

547

1. Why did her own doctor miss the diagnosis of hypothyroidism?
   a. Would there have been clues to the diagnosis if he had investigated her more fully at an earlier stage?
   b. What are the signs of hypothyroidism and what confirmatory tests would you apply?
   c. What type of anaemia is present in hypothyroidism?
   d. Are there other ways in which hypothyroidism may present?

2. How would you treat Mrs. E.M.?
   a. What is the dose of thyroxine in this condition?
   b. What complications can arise during treatment?

A. G. Strube, Crawley, UK

MRS. D.J.　　AGED 47　　HOUSEWIFE

548

1. How would you define 'mental illness'?
   a. What 'mental illness' may account for this lady's behaviour?

    b.   What physical disorders might account for her condition?
    c.   What is your ethical position in respect of the solicitor's request?

2. On what grounds should society admit a person to hospital against their will?
    a.   What is the legal situation locally in respect of compulsory admission to a mental hospital?
    b.   Which professionals need to be involved?
    c.   How do you contact them? What are their individual roles?

3. How might you manage this particular problem?
    a.   What specific questions would you ask in order to establish a diagnosis?
    b.   What investigations might you order?
    c.   What treatment is available for a nutritional megaloblastic anaemia?
    d.   What treatment is available for hypothyroidism? What are the hazards?

E. C. Gambrill, Crawley, UK

549 SCOTT D.   AGED 13   SCHOOLBOY

1. Is his condition mental, physical or both?
    a.   How far should you go in seeking and eliminating physical illness?
    b.   A blood examination shows a normal Hb and 'occasional atypical lymphocytes of the type found in viral disease'. The glandular fever screening test is negative. Is this relevant?
    c.   At what point should you discuss possible stress factors?

2. What would you see as the most pressing emotional elements?
    a.   Should you explore or ventilate his attitude to grandfather's illness and death?
    b.   How would you deal with his worries about his weight?
    c.   How would you allay his mother's anxieties and explain his symptoms?

3. Would you approach his teachers and coaches?
    a.   Would you make contact directly or via his mother?
    b.   Do you see the family doctor as having any place in planning athletic programmes for children or advising on classroom teaching on fitness and prevention?

J. A. Stevens, Ulverstone, Australia

MISS F.T.   AGED 19   STUDENT

550

1. What other parts of the body would you specifically examine?
   a. Is it important to examine other gland areas?
   b. Is it important to examine for enlargement of liver and spleen?

2. To determine if this is a physical illness, or an emotional problem or both, what questions would you ask?
   a. In relation to physical problems – previous attacks of tonsillitis, appetite and diet, menstruation?
   b. In relation to an emotional component – previous separation from home, social activity, friends, study habits, drugs?

3. What special investigations would you perform?

4. What other important questions should be asked?
   a. Immune status – diphtheria immunization?
   b. Contact with other infections – viral sore throat, tuberculosis, mononucleosis?

5. If the diagnosis is confirmed as infectious mononucleosis, what advice would you give?

D. U. Shepherd, Melbourne

ANDREW M.   AGED 15   SCHOOLBOY

551

1. What is 'glandular fever'?
   a. Can it be diagnosed solely on clinical grounds?
   b. How infectious is it?
   c. Does it spread through a family?
   d. Is it really more prevalent during examination periods or does it only appear to be so?

2. Should the doctor have performed any further investigations before making the provisional but confident diagnosis of glandular fever in Andrew?
   a. Can glandular fever be present in the absence of a confirmative haematological abnormality?
   b. How soon after the onset of glandular fever does the mono spot test become positive?

3. Should Andrew be allowed to sit for the examinations?
   a. What are the complications?
   b. What is the treatment?
   c. What is the prognosis?

P. F. Gill, Hobart

552 **MRS. VENERSTIA D.** **AGED 30** **PEASANT HOUSEWIFE**

1. What is the life cycle of the hookworm?
    a. In what environmental conditions do they flourish?
    b. By what route do they enter the body?
    c. What is the mechanism causing anaemia?
    d. What habits are necessary for the transmission of the disease?

2. Do you agree with Venerstia that the clinician had done a good job?
    a. Was he wrong to make a provisional diagnosis and act on this without laboratory confirmation?
    b. Was he right to allow her to continue to believe that he possessed magic capable of overcoming the effects of her bewitchment?
    c. What chances has he of seeing Venerstia and her family back again with the same problem?

3. How may attempts to promote health be hindered by a firm belief in witchcraft (or even a belief that all illness arises from the will of God)?
    a. Can one convert a belief in a supernatural aetiology to an understanding of explainable cause and effect?
    b. Which belief leads to easier motivation to personal action towards better health?
    c. In what ways can community health be improved without requiring active co-operation of the individuals concerned?
    d. What health promotive measures require active and enthusiastic co-operation?

R. T. Mossop, Harare, Zimbabwe

553 **MRS. C.A.** **AGED 75** **PENSIONER**

1. What is her problem?
    a. Does this blood picture represent a serious condition?
    b. Can this condition be labelled iron deficiency anaemia?
    c. If not, why not?

2. Are any other laboratory investigations necessary?
    a. Do you think any serum assays are essential for correct diagnosis? If so, which ones?
    b. If she showed normal serum results, is she suffering from an iron deficiency anaemia?
    c. If the serum results are normal, is she an 'old age' anaemia?

3. How would you manage this problem?
    a. If the serum assays performed are found to be reduced, how would you treat her?

b. If the serum assays are found to be normal, does she need **any** treatment?

T. D. Manthorpe, Port Lincoln, Australia

MRS. V.G.   AGED 32   DOMESTIC   **554**

1. What diagnoses would you consider at this time?
   a. What diagnostic steps could help differentiate leukaemia, lymphoma, tuberculosis, sarcoidosis and endocarditis at early stages?

2. What tests would you order at this point?
   a. What findings on chest X-ray might you expect in tuberculosis, sarcoidosis, lymphoma?

3. What would you tell the patient about her problem?
   a. Is it significant that she waited until the end of the examination to mention the lump in her neck?
   b. What does this behaviour tell you about her reason for consulting you now and how would you address yourself to this problem?

K. F. Weyrauch, Charleston, SC, USA

MR. W.P.   AGED 24   BANK TELLER   **555**

1. What are the implications of the diagnosis of acute myeloblastic leukaemia?
   a. How would you break the news to the patient?
   b. Is this disease universally fatal in a 24 year old?
   c. What treatments are used?
   d. How does the prognosis compare with acute lymphoblastic leukaemia in a child and in an adult?
   e. Does bone marrow transplant have a place in therapy? If so, when?
   f. What additional information would you wish before considering a bone marrow transplant?
   g. What is the incidence of this disease?
   h. Are there any suggested aetiological agents?

2. What are the apparent dynamics in this case?
   a. Why does the patient refuse to eat?
   b. Why does he skip appointments?
   c. Can the physician do anything to assist managing this very difficult case?
   d. Are there organizations which might help him?
   e. Is patient compliance with medications usual or unusual?

3. What are the issues related to the pregnancy?
   a. Should termination be considered?
   b. Is the foetus at risk from the chemotherapy?
   c. How can foetal development be monitored?
   d. Should sperm be collected from this patient for banking?

C. A. Moore, Hamilton, Canada

556   **MRS. M.R.**   **AGED 70**   **WIDOW**

1. What is the relationship between smoking and bronchitis?
   a. Are there strategies which family physicians can employ to assist patients to stop smoking?
   b. Do family physicians have a responsibility to encourage healthy lifestyles?
   c. Are such proposals effective?

2. Why has the patient waited so long to consult her physician?
   a. Was she afraid?
   b. Was she sufficiently informed to be aware of the danger signs of cancer?
   c. Do you think guilt about her continuing to smoke may have delayed her visit?
   d. What might the physician do to prevent patients' guilt delaying the seeking of needed care?
   e. What potential barriers exist in the health care system, preventing patients from seeking out their physician early, for indefinite symptoms?

3. What is the significance of a patient presenting with fatigue?
   a. Is it a common presentation?
   b. How can you sort out if it is organic or non-organic?
   c. What clues might help you sort out the types of fatigue?

4. Is it unusual to have this lesion in a patient of 70 years of age?
   a. What is the incidence?
   b. What is the prognosis?
   c. Could it have been prevented?
   d. Who is at particular risk?
   e. What screening programs are used at the present time?
   f. Are the recommendations similar for all age groups?
   g. How would you discuss your findings with the patient?

C. A. Moore, Hamilton, Canada

MR. I.J.   AGED 45   ENTERTAINER

1. How would one manage the physical illnesses?
   a. How does the doctor go about the initial treatment of the diabetic condition in such a patient?
   b. What treatment regime is most suitable for the hypertension?
   c. What instructions does he give his office about the management of the patient at subsequent visits?

2. What other elements are there in the 'total diagnosis' of this patient?
   a. How does the doctor motivate the patient to
      - reduce or cease smoking?
      - check his diabetic state regularly?
      - continue pharmacological treatment for hypertension?

3. What are the likely effects of his illness on himself and his life, his family and his employers?
   a. What is the patient's prognosis
      - if he cooperates optimally in the treatment regime?
      - if he complies only spasmodicaly and never loses enough weight?
      - if he ignores the proffered medical advice?
   b. How does the doctor go about motivating this patient for weight reduction? His livelihood of some years' standing depends on his obesity.

4. What are the likely psychological and social effects of his illness?
   a. What support agencies are available if this man loses his livelihood as a result of necessary medical management?

P. L. Gibson, Auckland

MR. B.   AGED 55   CIVIL SERVANT

1. What further investigations would be indicated in arriving at a differential diagnosis?
   a. What special psychological history would be of assistance?
   b. Would a chest X-ray be of assistance?
   c. Are there any specific blood or skin tests that would be helpful?

2. Should this man be admitted to hospital for further investigations?
   a. What investigations are necessary that could not be done on an out-patient basis?
   b. Would removing this man from his environment be of benefit in diagnosing the problem?

3. What role does organic illness play in the development of depression?

   a.   What is the impact of chronic illness of unknown aetiology on family dynamics?

   b.   What role do physical problems play in the development of depression in an individual?

W. W. Rosser, Ottawa

559   MISS K.   AGED 21   AU PAIR GIRL

1. What are the most likely causes of hypokalaemia in an otherwise healthy 21 year old female?
   a.   How dangerous is hypokalaemia in a 21 year old female?
   b.   At what level of potassium would you be worried about increased risks of cardiac arrest?
   c.   Would giving supplementary potassium be of any assistance to this woman?

2. What simple investigations would help you to decide whether this was a psychologically or organically based problem?
   a.   What is the most common organic cause of this problem?
   b.   What is the most common psychological cause of this problem?
   c.   How would you differentiate between these problems?

3. How would you manage this problem if it were psychologically based?
   a.   Would you confront the patient with the problem?
   b.   What type of counselling would be most helpful?
   c.   What would you suggest to the patient as a solution for the problem?
   d.   How urgent would this solution be, based on the level of her serum potassium?

W. W. Rosser, Ottawa

560   PAUL S.   AGED 6   SCHOOLBOY

1. What other conditions may present in a similar fashion to measles?
   a.   How do you manage a febrile child when there are no localizing signs or symptoms?
   b.   What rashes may be confused with that of measles? What are the distinguishing features?
   c.   What is the evidence for and against the use of prophylactic antibiotics in uncomplicated measles?
   d.   What are the common complications of measles?

2. What factors may influence the degree of anxiety which parents feel about a sick child?

a. What are the effects of a serious illness in a child on parents and siblings?

b. What can the doctor do to help the family cope in this situation?

3. What conditions may account for the deterioration in Paul's condition?

a. What is the incidence and prognosis of post-measles encephalitis?

b. How would you exclude diabetes in this child?

c. How could the measles have triggered off diabetes? Is the association purely coincidental?

d. What further management is indicated?

E. C. Gambrill, Crawley, UK

MR. B. AGED 59 BRICKLAYER, MRS. B. HOUSEWIFE 561

1. What are the possible diagnoses of Mr. B.'s condition?

a. Which is the most likely?

b. How could you confirm this?

c. Is this an unusual presentation of diabetes?

d. Should the diagnosis have been made at the first contact?

2. What are the possible diagnoses of Mrs. B.'s condition?

a. What is the most likely?

b. How could you confirm this?

c. Is this an unusual presentation for thyrotoxicosis?

d. Should the diagnosis have been made at the first contact?

3. Could the general practitioner have anticipated Mrs. B.'s condition?

a. What are the early indications of thyrotoxicosis?

b. Would earlier elucidation have affected the final outcome?

4. What is the management of this family?

a. How should Mr. B.'s diabetes be managed?

b. How should Mrs. B.'s thyrotoxicosis be managed?

c. If the conditions are related in any way, does this influence management?

d. What are the possible final outcomes of both their conditions?

5. Was the general practitioner justified in accepting his own diagnosis and instituting treatment for these disease processes?

a. How far does the responsibility of the general practitioner go?

b. Was reference to a specialist mandatory?

c. Would referral to a specialist have been desirable?

d. What are the determining factors in referring a patient to a specialist?

D. A. Game, Adelaide

562 MRS. R.H. AGED 23 HOUSEWIFE

1. What is the most likely cause of Mrs. H.'s symptoms?
   a. Is it likely that there is a psychiatric disease?
   b. What type(s) of neoplastic disease might this be?
   c. What type(s) of infectious or inflammatory disease could this be?
   d. In what age group is Graves' disease most common?
   e. In what sex is Graves' disease most common?

2. What advice would you offer this lady regarding treatment?
   a. What are the indications for surgery in an individual with Graves' disease?
   b. What are some of the advantages and disadvantages of treatment with radioactive iodine?
   c. What are some of the indications for the use of propylthiouracil in the treatment of hyperthyroidism?
   d. What are some of the indications and contraindications for the use of propranolol in the treatment of hyperthyroidism?

3. If Mrs. H. suggested that she was about 6 weeks pregnant and you were able to confirm this, how might your recommendations for investigation or treatment be modified?
   a. Is the use of radioactive iodine for investigation or treatment contraindicated in pregnancy?
   b. If surgery was required, at what stage in pregnancy should it be performed?
   c. Are the guidelines (dose, suppression of symptoms etc.) for the use of propylthiouracil different in the pregnant versus the non-pregnant individual with hyperthyroidism?
   d. Is propranolol ever of use in the treatment of hyperthyroidism in pregnancy?

G. G. Beazley, Winnipeg

563 JOHN P. AGED 48 LABOURER

1. What are the most likely causes of muscular weakness and weight loss in a man of this age?
   a. How can you distinguish between hyperthyroidism and an anxiety state?
   b. Is there any link between hyperthyroidism and stress?
   c. What investigations are useful?
   d. What exactly do the results quoted mean?

2. What other methods are used in treating hyperthyroidism?
   a. Under what circumstances would you refer the patient to a consultant?
   b. If he had not developed an allergy to carbimazole, would you have continued this instead of giving I^{131}?
   c. What are the advantages of surgery over other forms of treatment?

3. What was the rash and arthralgia due to?
   a. How common a reaction to carbimazole is this?
   b. What other risks does treatment with this drug carry?

4. What is the value of routine follow up in thyroid disease?
   a. What should it consist of?
   b. Who should carry it out?
   c. How common is hypothyroidism after I^{131}?
   d. How long after treatment does it most commonly occur?

5. How would you have managed this patient?

G. Strube, Crawley, UK

MR. MARK L.   AGED 56   WARDSMAN   564

1. What other symptoms would you enquire about? What is the value of checking:
   a. What his appetite is like?
   b. What his diet consists of?
   c. Is there any abdominal or rectal pain?
   d. Is there any change in bowel habit?
   e. Is there any family history of similar conditions?
   f. Has there been any stress in his life recently?

2. What would your physical examination include? What is the value of checking:
   a. What his overall physical condition is like?
   b. If there are any signs of anaemia or cachexia?
   c. What his abdominal examination shows?
   d. If a rectal examination and protoscopy has been done?
   e. The haemoglobin?

3. What would you say to the patient before any other investigations are carried out?
   a. How would you explore with the patient what his fears about his condition are?
   b. What would you say about possible diagnoses e.g. haemor-rhoids, diverticulitis or cancer?

    c.   What would you tell him about what the different investigations will involve? e.g. sigmoidoscopy, barium enema with air contrast, colonoscopy.

M. D. Mahoney, Brisbane

565   MR. M.N.   AGED 63   INSURANCE AGENT

1.   What investigation would you conduct?
    a.   Does the sequence make any difference?
    b.   Can you save money by ordering a few tests first?

2.   While you are investigating him how would you explain to him what you are doing?
    a.   What are you investigating?
    b.   Is it serious?

3.   What might be the therapy?
    a.   Would you prescribe iron?

4.   What would you do if he refuses investigation?
    a.   Would you refuse to look after him?
    b.   Would he accept referral to a colleague?

E. V. Dunn, Toronto

566   MRS. G.S.   AGED 76

1.   What do you think is wrong with Mrs. G.S.?
    a.   How important is her symptom of dysphagia?
    b.   How reliable is a barium swallow and meal in excluding malignant disease?
    c.   Can carcinoma of the bronchus occur in non-smokers?
    d.   Can carcinoma of the bronchus present with oesophageal symptoms?
    e.   What is the prognosis of carcinoma of the bronchus presenting with infiltration of the oesophagus?

2.   What would you do next?
    a.   Is there any other test which might be useful?
    b.   What might a consultant do if the patient were to be referred?

3.   What are the risks of delay in investigating this problem?
    a.   What treatment might she be offered?
    b.   If the prognosis is poor, why bother to investigate, refer and treat?

c. What problems might you anticipate during her terminal illness?
d. How would you manage them?

G. Strube, Crawley, UK

MR. W.   AGED 67

567

1. What investigations would seem to be appropriate?
   a. How is one influenced by a raised ESR?
   b. What significance can one attach to a raised IgA?
   c. How does blood chemistry alter with normal ageing?

2. Could all this have been caused by 'getting old'?
   a. What hallmarks distinguish dementia from treatable confusion?
   b. What are the causes of confusion in the elderly?
   c. How does the general practitioner feel when refused a hospital bed?

3. What are the diagnostic possibilities in this case?
   a. Does his increased deafness give any clues?
   b. His heart murmur is considerably louder than it was.
   c. The disease was probably not diagnosable at presentation.
   d. If he had given a history of recent dental extraction the ultimate diagnosis would have been obvious.

4. The general practitioner is frequently concerned with undifferentiated illness. How does he manage this?
   a. What special strains does this impose upon general practitioner and patient?
   b. Time **can** be a useful diagnostic tool.
   c. What are the special difficulties of referral of undifferentiated illness?

A. L. A. Reid, Newcastle, Australia

MISS L.   AGED 66

568

1. What illnesses does this patient probably have?
   a. Are there tests which could definitely exclude some disease(s)?
   b. Which of the complaints may be iatrogenic?
   c. What disease might be caused by this drug regimen?

2. What difficulties might one encounter in reducing therapy?
   a. 'Some patients enjoy ill health'. Does going to the doctor satisfy emotional needs?
   b. What practical steps would be most appropriate to reduce therapy?

3. What do we know about the patient's doctor?
    a. How would one feel recounting this patient's treatment to a colleague?
    b. Do systems of payment influence doctors' behaviour?
    c. What strategies can a doctor adopt to prevent a patient from becoming dependent?

A. L. A. Reid, Newcastle, Australia

569 MRS. D.   AGED 55

1. List this patient's problems?
    a. Does she have iatrogenic disease?
    b. Is iatrogenic disease complicating organic illness?
    c. Is she taking drugs which are incompatible?
    d. What are the dangers of thyroid hormone usage in the presence of coronary artery disease?

2. List the doctor's problems?
    a. How long does it take for thyroid functions tests to return to a baseline following cessation of therapy?
    b. Was the doctor justified in stopping treatment?
    c. Should the doctor simply have acceded to the patient's request for repeat therapy?

3. What responsibility does a hospital outpatient department have in such cases?
    a. Who should review polypharmacy?
    b. Is repeat prescription writing without seeing the patient justifiable?
    c. Should there be regular review of diagnoses made years ago?

P. F. Gill, Hobart

570 MRS. ANNIE W.   AGE 86

1. Are you worried about continuing these drugs and these doses?
    a. What are the major changes in pharmacokinetics with ageing?
    b. Which of these drugs is heavily dependent on renal excretion?
    c. Which of these drugs have a very prolonged half life in the elderly, unrelated to renal clearance?
    d. What changes would you suggest in her medications and doses?

2. What adverse drug reactions might occur in this patient?
    a. What are the symptoms of excess dosage for each of these drugs?
    b. Are there any drug interactions or effects here, which might be offset by adding a supplementary drug?

3. Do the risks of treating hypertension in the elderly outweigh the benefits?
   a. How many elderly patients have you treated for falls due to light-headed spells? How many of these were on hypotensive agents?

D. H. Johnson, Toronto

MRS. MARGARET S.   AGED 78   **571**

1. What further history do you want from the patient or her husband?
   a. What symptoms of disease would you inquire about?
   b. What happens to such symptoms in the elderly?
   c. Could this be an adverse drug reaction?
   d. Would you remember to take a drug history from the husband?

2. What is your plan of investigation?
   a. What is your screening for endogenous disease?
   b. What is your screening for exogenous causes? (This patient was receiving a calcium supplement for osteoporosis from another MD. Serum calcium was elevated. Mental state cleared when calcium was stopped.)

3. What community help can be offered to help maintain this person in optimum health at home?
   a. Would a move to a safe institutional setting help her state of mind?
   b. Are there any programmes you might offer to help her reality orientation?

D. H. Johnson, Toronto

ERNEST W.   AGED 78   **572**

1. Can you make a provisional diagnosis?
   a. What pathological processes could be occurring?
   b. Could his symptoms have anything to do with his medication?
   c. What are the indications for digoxin?

2. Are there any tests which could be useful?
   a. What is the significance of a raised blood urea in this situation?
   b. Are thyroid function tests useful in old people without clinical evidence of disturbed thyroid function?

3. What would you do next?
   a. Would a period of observation be helpful?
   b. What would you expect to happen during the next few days?
   c. Would you change his medication?

G. Strube, Crawley, UK

573 MRS. A.D.   AGED 83

1. What is the significance of the serum potassium?
   a. Who should receive a potassium supplement?
   b. What form should it be in?
   c. Are there any risks in taking potassium?
   d. Can extra potassium be provided in the diet? How?

2. What are the symptoms of potassium depletion?
   a. Is a serum potassium a useful test?
   b. On whom should it be carried out, and when?
   c. What are its limitations?

3. What are the dangers of potassium depletion?
   a. Who is at special risk from it?
   b. How can it be guarded against?

4. How can a doctor guard against missing a new diagnosis in an old patient with multiple pathology whom he sees frequently?
   a. What special features should alert him?
   b. What is the role of digitalis in this situation?

G. Strube, Crawley, UK

574 MR. J.F.   AGED 80

1. Are there any other investigations worth pursuing?
   a. What attendant pathology is common in haemolytic anaemia due to cold agglutination?
   b. If bone marrow biopsy is normal, what other investigations might reveal pathology?
   c. If a lymphoma or other proliferative disorder is discovered, would treatment significantly prolong life?

2. How long will symptomatic treatment give relief?
   a. How frequently may transfusions be necessary?
   b. Was there any rationale for ceasing methyldopa?
   c. What ordinary precautions should the patient take?
   d. What special precautions must be observed when transfusing?

G. M. Dick, Hobart

575 MR. A.B.   AGED 79   PENSIONER

1. Who defines an emergency? Should it be the patient, the receptionist, the relatives or the doctor?

a. How should a group practice deal with emergencies?
b. Should one consulting room be specially reserved for emergencies?
c. How can emergencies be fitted into the normal consulting times without causing routine patients undue delay?

2. Who is responsible in a group medical practice for each patient's care?
   a. How should the medical records be organized to ensure that each patient's chronic problems are highlighted?
   b. What sort of problems should be stressed?
   c. What is the best system for ensuring that the treatment for one problem does not interfere with that of another condition?
   d. How should differences in therapeutic approach by different doctors in the same group practice be resolved?

3. In this case, how much care should be provided by the primary care doctor?
   a. What immediate diagnostic and therapeutic steps should be taken?
   b. How could this problem be solved non-surgically?
   c. What long-term treatment would be useful for this man's gastro-intestinal tract?
   d. What advice should be given to his wife?

B. H. Connor, Armidale, Australia

JAN WILLIAMSON   AGED 21   PRIMARY TEACHER   576

1. Will you treat Jan's hypertension?
   a. The cardiologist describes her problem as 'labile hypertension' – 'What is that?'
   b. What are the risks of not treating mild hypertension?
   c. What drug treatment would you consider?

2. Will you continue her on the pill?
   a. Is there any association between the pill and hypertension?
   b. What risks are involved in continuing the pill?
   c. What risks are involved in not continuing the pill?

3. What non-drug treatment is appropriate?
   a. What non-drug contraception is appropriate at this time?
   b. What about a less hectic lifestyle?
   c. What is her fiancee's place in all of this?
   d. What opportunity is there for health promotion?

R. P. Strasser, Melbourne

577 GILLIAN A.   AGED 24   SCHOOLTEACHER

1. What is the significance of a blood pressure of 160/100 in a 24 year old female taking oral contraceptives?
   a. What are the critical elements of history that must be covered by the doctor in assessing this patient?
   b. What elements of physical examination are mandatory in the doctor's assessment of this patient's blood pressure?
   c. What investigations, if any, should be performed?

2. What factors would influence the doctor's decision to advise Gillian for or against continuing to take her oral contraceptive?
   a. What are the risks to this patient if she continues to take her oral contraceptive?
   b. What other factors in the history must the doctor consider in order to assess this patient's risk if she continues her oral contraception?
   c. What information should the doctor seek in his or her physical examination in order to assess other factors which may compound the risk to this patient should she continue to take her oral contraceptive?

3. What alternatives are available to Gillian if a decision is taken to stop her oral contraceptive?
   a. What factors in the history should be considered when assessing alternative contraception?
   b. What information should be sought in the physical examination in order to assess the most suitable alternative method of contraception?

W. L. Ogborne, Sydney

578 MISS C.T.   AGED 33

1. To what extent should an attempt be made to persuade her to alter the use of her medication?
   a. Would psychotherapy be of value?
   b. What facilities are available to you in the management of drug and alcohol related problems?

2. Is the medical profession in any way culpable for this patient's addiction?
   a. What guidelines in the use of benzodiazepines and similar drugs would prevent this situation from recurring?

3. If the doctor feels that he cannot in all good conscience fulfil her request, how should he manage the case?

a. Is there any approach which leaves a possibility for a successful outcome?
b. How is 'success' defined?

E. Domovitch, Toronto

MR. O.P.   AGED 27   UNEMPLOYED
579

1. Should the doctor carry out a full clinical examination?
   a. What are a doctor's professional and legal obligations toward casual patients?
   b. If the doctor suspects the symptoms are due to withdrawal of the medication, what information would support this view?

2. Should he make out the prescription or refuse to do so?
   a. If the doctor thought the patient was suicidal, but the patient refuses referral to hospital, what action should he take?

3. Should he try to communicate with the prison doctor concerned to see if the patient's story is correct?
   a. If the prison doctor is not available, and the doctor deems it proper to refuse the request for a prescription, how responsible is he for subsequent eventualities? How does he plan his approach to such contingencies as attempted suicide or assault on a third party?
   b. If he does manage to locate the prison doctor, and it is confirmed that the patient was in fact taking Valium (diazepam), does he proceed at once to prescription? What arrangements does he make about seeing the patient again?
   c. What is the incidence of iatrogenic illness resulting from the abuse of psychotropics and how can it be reduced?

P. L. Gibson, Auckland

MR. K.   AGED 66   PAINTER
580

1. What are the disease processes, if any, in this man?
   a. What is the basis for the diagnosis/es?
   b. How can the general practitioner be sure he is correct?
   c. What are the possible underlying causes?
   d. Was Mr. K. over-investigated or under-investigated?

2. How should this case be managed?
   a. Did the medical attention contribute to his condition?
   b. Does he require any medications, if so, what?
   c. Could other agencies assist?

3. Were sickness certificates and later the Invalid Pension justified?
    a. Could this have been avoided?
    b. What is meant by dependent patients?
    c. Should functional illness or disability be grounds for invalidity benefits?

D. A. Game, Adelaide

581 MR. G.   AGED 45   WORKSHOP MANAGER

1. What is or are the disease process/es exemplified here?
    a. What was the justification of the intern for diagnosing angina pectoris and prescribing trinitrin tablets?
    b. How common is the hyperventilation syndrome?
    c. What symptoms can it cause?
    d. What were the grounds for the general practitioner making this diagnosis?
    e. What treatment should he have prescribed?

2. How does the general practitioner cope with the ongoing 'medical' problems created by others?
    a. What is 'cardiac neurosis'?
    b. How is it perpetuated?
    c. What are the roles of adequate initial assessment and repeated further assessment?
    d. How should the general practitioner manage Mr. G.'s problem?

3. Are there any grounds for compensation for Mr. G. under the provisions of Worker's Compensation legislation?
    a. What advice should the general practitioner have given Mr. G. when he specifically sought such advice?
    b. What are the possible motives behind Mr. G. seeking such compensation?
    c. If subsequently the general practitioner is requested for a medical report by the appropriate authorities what should be the outline and basis of this report?

D. A. Game, Adelaide

582 MRS. A.W.   AGED 74

1. What complications of diabetes threaten life?
    a. Do we have a duty to oppose every threat to life in all circumstances?
    b. What did we hope to achieve for this patient with her latter management?

2. Does sympathectomy or bypass surgery have much place in treating vascular complications?
   a. Should we have striven to keep her at home?
   b. What would you perceive as the determinants of home care?
   c. Could such terminal catastrophes as listed have been avoided?

W. D. Jackson, Launceston, Australia

MASTER M.C.C.   AGED 6

583

1. What are the problems?
   a. What are the complications of long term use of steroids?
   b. How should steroids be withdrawn?
   c. Does the problem lie with the mother, the unregistered 'doctor', or is it a social problem?

2. What is the role of the GP as a health educator?
   a. Educating the individual patient?
   b. Educating the community?
   c. Bringing about health reform in the control of undesirable practitioners?

Footnote: Herbalists do not require registration in Hong Kong. Keeping and selling Part 1 poisons, e.g. antibiotics and steroids, is illegal, but they are easily obtainable without prescription.

N. C. L. Yuen, Hong Kong

Index

The index is a vital part of this book. It gives access to cases categorized in ways other than by chapter headings. In addition to indexing symptoms and illnesses, the processes of care used by the family physician and the concepts of family medicine are indexed, enabling the reader to extract cases which illustrate, for example, whole-person care, preventive care, health promotion, health education, the bereavement process, family dysfunction, and so on. It should be noted however, that the majority of cases illustrate such concepts as whole-person care and preventive care; the index lists only those cases in which such concepts are a major feature.

Where a disease entity is listed, it does not mean that this disease was necessarily 'the diagnosis' in the particular case. Disease entities have been indexed wherever they form part of the differential diagnosis, as well as the definitive diagnosis. Likewise, where a symptom is indexed, it is not necessarily the most prominent or significant symptom in that case. Sometimes a disease or symptom is indexed to a case because it is relevant to the questions and sub-questions rather than to the case history.

The index concludes with a listing of cases in age groups. Each case has been listed according to the age indicated in the heading of the case. Where more than one person is involved, the lesser age has been chosen. This part of the index will enable readers studying a particular age group to identify a series of suitable cases.

For the convenience of the reader, cases have been indexed by CASE NUMBERS, not page numbers. This will enable the reader quickly to refer to the case history and major questions in the first part of the book and the corresponding questions and sub-questions in the second part of the book. The case numbers are to be found in large bold type on the free edge of each page.

It is believed that careful use of the index will augment the value of this book for teachers and learners in general family practice. We hope it will provide further insight into the nature of the discipline.

Index

Age Group Index